Marine Biopharmaceuticals: Scope and Prospects

Authored by

Santhanam Ramesh
Karuna College of Pharmacy
Kerala University of Health Sciences, Palakkad
Kerala, India

Ramasamy Santhanam
Fisheries College and Research Institute
Tamil Nadu Veterinary and Animal Sciences University
Thoothukudi, India

&

Veintramuthu Sankar
P.S.G. College of Pharmacy
Coimbatore, Tamil Nadu
India

Marine Biopharmaceuticals: Scope and Prospects

Authors: Santhanam Ramesh, Ramasamy Santhanam & Veintramuthu Sankar

ISBN (Online): 978-981-5196-47-4

ISBN (Print): 978-981-5196-48-1

ISBN (Paperback): 978-981-5196-49-8

© 2024, Bentham Books imprint.

Published by Bentham Science Publishers Pte. Ltd. Singapore. All Rights Reserved.

First published in 2024.

need for a court order if at any point you breach any terms of this License Agreement. In no event will any delay or failure by Bentham Science Publishers in enforcing your compliance with this License Agreement constitute a waiver of any of its rights.

3. You acknowledge that you have read this License Agreement, and agree to be bound by its terms and conditions. To the extent that any other terms and conditions presented on any website of Bentham Science Publishers conflict with, or are inconsistent with, the terms and conditions set out in this License Agreement, you acknowledge that the terms and conditions set out in this License Agreement shall prevail.

Bentham Science Publishers Pte. Ltd.
80 Robinson Road #02-00
Singapore 068898
Singapore
Email: subscriptions@benthamscience.net

BENTHAM SCIENCE

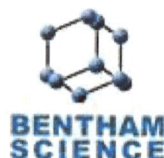

CONTENTS

FOREWORD

I am delighted to write this foreword, not only because Prof. Ramasamy Santhanam, one of the authors, has been my teacher and colleague for more than 30 years, but also because I believe deeply in the educative value of the contents of this book for all the stakeholders in Fisheries and pharmaceutical Education.

Nature is considered to be an ancient pharmacy serving as the solitary source of therapeutics for thousands of years. Almost all of the current natural product-derived therapeutics have their terrestrial origins. The marine environment has also become a promising source of bioactive molecules and drugs of therapeutic use. Recent research findings have shown that marine organisms possess a higher incidence of significant bioactivity compared with terrestrial organisms. In a National Cancer Institute preclinical cytotoxicity screening, 1% of the examined marine samples exhibited anti-cancer potential versus 0.1% of the tested terrestrial samples. The number of new marine bioactive compounds reported each year is also increasing considerably, and more than 1000 new such compounds have been reported each year. However, the path to drug discovery from marine organisms faces several challenges. Lack of advancements in sampling techniques, taxonomic identification of therapeutically important marine species, compound structure determination strategies, etc. represent crucial steps in marine drug discovery.

The present volume titled "Marine Biopharmaceuticals: Scope and Prospects" the first of its kind is written by both the experts of pharmaceutical and fisheries disciplines and it deals with the pharmaceutically important marine organisms; and their bioactive compounds, chemical classes and modes of action. It also deals with the techniques in the development of marine biota-derived drugs; and the constraints and remedial measures. The chapter on the introduction of an inter-disciplinary PG degree program on the hitherto unknown but productivity course viz. Marine Bio-Pharmacy will help drug companies acquire trained personnel in the development of new marine drugs.

I congratulate the authors for their timely publication for the benefit of the Fisheries and Pharmaceutical sector.

Dr. G. Sugumar
Vice-Chancellor, Tamil Nadu Dr. J. Jayalalithaa Fisheries University
Tamil Nadu
India

PREFACE

Our marine ecosystems including the seas and oceans cover about 70% of the earth's surface and contain over 80% of the world's biodiversity. Unfortunately, only 5% of these ecosystems have so far been explored and only 9% (about 200,000) of the total species have been adequately researched. The marine biodiversity is an exceptional reservoir of natural products (bioactive compounds or secondary metabolites) owing to their different structural features from those of terrestrial natural products. During the last 50 years, about 15,000 bioactive compounds with potential applications as medical drugs have been isolated from these species. However, only less than 1% of these compounds have so far been examined for their pharmacological activities. The study of marine organisms for their bioactive potential has therefore increased in recent years. As there is a great demand for the discovery of new medicines, researchers are nowadays increasingly looking towards these marine ecosystems

for the isolation and development of novel compounds, treatments, and solutions to combat human disease.

Though some books are presently available on marine natural products, a comprehensive book on marine biopharmaceuticals and their scope and prospects is still needed. Further, a book dealing with the most promising pharmaceutical compounds derived from the major groups of marine organisms with an aim of utilizing them in the development of new drugs is the need of the hour. Keeping these in consideration, this publication is being brought out for the first time by bringing together the experts in Pharmaceutical Sciences, Marine Biology, and Marine Biochemistry disciplines. Aspects relating to Marine Bioprospecting; Promising Pharmaceutical Compounds of Marine Biota with their Therapeutic Applications; Marine Biopharmaceuticals in the Pipeline; and Scope and Career Prospects of Marine Bio-Pharmacy (= Marine Biopharmaceutical Sciences) and Pharmaceutical Marine Biology courses are dealt with .It is strongly hoped that this title would largely help the researchers and students of disciplines like Marine Bio-Pharmacy, Marine Biology, Marine Microbiology, Marine Biochemistry and Marine Biotechnology; as a standard Reference for all Libraries of Colleges and Universities; and as a guide for the drug companies involved in the development of new drugs from marine biopharmaceuticals.

Santhanam Ramesh
Karuna College of Pharmacy
Kerala University of Health Sciences, Palakkad
Kerala, India

Ramasamy Santhanam
Fisheries College and Research Institute
Tamil Nadu Veterinary and Animal Sciences University
Thoothukudi, India

&

Veintramuthu Sankar
P.S.G. College of Pharmacy
Coimbatore, Tamil Nadu
India

CHAPTER 1

Introduction

Abstract: This chapter deals with the role of seas and oceans in human life; marine biodiversity; marine drugs and their origin; groups of marine biota as sources of drugs; importance and advantages of the production of marine drugs; pharmaceutical marine biodiversity in the development of marine drugs; existing problems in the development of new marine drugs; and remedial measures for the adequate supply of bioactive compounds for the production of cost-effective new drugs for various diseases.

Keywords: Marine biodiversity, Marine organisms as drug sources, Origin of marine drugs, Pharmaceutical marine biodiversity, Problems in marine drug development.

INTRODUCTION

Although 71% of the earth's surface is covered in water, 97% of this is found in our seas and oceans. But, only 5% of our oceans have so far been explored. Further, the first marine organisms appeared about 3500 million years ago and even after 250 years of active marine research, only 9% of the species present have been adequately researched and the remaining 91% of the species present in the seas and oceans still lack a detailed description. The marine environment is the richest biosphere on earth and its living conditions differ significantly from those on the earth. The temperature range of this environment is huge as it varies from $-1.5°C$ in ice sea to $350°C$ in deep hydrothermal systems; pressure from 1 to over 1,000 atmospheres; light from complete darkness to extensive photic zones; and nutritional conditions from nutrient-rich to nutrient-sparse.

Role of Seas and Oceans in Human Life

The seas and oceans play an important role in the human life. As per available reports, about one billion people depend on seafood as their primary source of animal protein. These water bodies are known to produce over half of the oxygen we breathe besides storing 50 times more carbon than the atmosphere. The coastal habitats adjoining the seas such as coral reefs and mangrove swamps provide protection from tsunamis and storms, while the ocean currents regulate largely our climate and weather systems. The seas and oceans also provide humans with several unique recreational activities which include fishing, boating, and whale watching. These water bodies are also known to help largely in transportation and 76% of all US trade is done involving some form of marine transportation. Recent research on marine organisms has shown that these organisms are the reservoirs of several drug-producing natural products especially for the treatment of cancer, arthritis, Alzheimer's disease, and heart disease [1].

Marine Biodiversity

Only a fraction of the types of organisms that live in the sea are known today. As per the World Register of Marine Species, there are 240,000 known species (2016, http://www.marinespecies.org/) of which the highest number of species (about 33000) was found in the seas around Australia and Japan. Of the 36 animal phyla so far reported, about half are exclusive to the sea and among the marine animals, 60% belongs to the invertebrates [2].

Origin of Marine Drugs

Throughout history, nature and medicine have shown a strong relation, as highlighted by the wide use of therapeutic biomolecules in traditional medicines for thousands of years. During the ancient Greece and early Byzantium periods, the therapeutic applications of marine invertebrate organisms were deeply rooted in Mediterranean populations. Amazingly these invertebrates were used therapeutically in the forms of beverages, pulverized products, juices, broth, unguent, or eaten as fresh or dry flesh. The use of marine herbs and their formulas belongs to a thousand-year tradition. The Chinese Marine Materia Medica, a kind of encyclopedia is considered to be the best compendium about blue-green algae (cyanobacteria), seaweeds and marine animals. This encyclopedia is also considered the starting point in the development of new marketed drugs. This long tradition amply testifies that the interest in marine natural products developed in the ancient world, though the current research has been emphasizing the beneficial effects of these natural products and their molecules [3].

Marine Organisms as Sources of Drugs

Nowadays, most drugs in use come from nature. For example, while aspirin was first discovered from the willow tree, penicillin was isolated from the common bread mold. Further, the majority of drugs derived from natural sources have their origin from land-dwelling organisms. However, as there is a great demand for the discovery of new medicines, researchers are nowadays increasingly looking towards the ocean. Systematic and continuous searches for new drugs have shown that marine invertebrate organisms are capable of producing several anticancer, antibiotic, and anti-inflammatory substances than any group of terrestrial organisms. Such promising invertebrates include sponges (Porifera), corals and jellies (Cnidaria), flatworms (Platyhelminthes), polychaetes (Annelida), moss animals (Bryozoa), lamp shells (Brachiopoda), crustaceans (Arthropoda), mollusks (Mollusca), sea stars and other echinoderms, (Echinodermata), acorn worms and relatives (Hemichordata), tunicates, (Urochordata) and elasmobranchs and teleost fishes (Chordata). Across these animals, the marine sponges (Porifera) account for almost half of new natural products since 1990. An interesting feature of the habitats of these drug-producing organisms (except the cone snail) is more or less sessile (non-moving) invertebrates. The possible reasons for this phenomenon are: these sessile invertebrates use these chemicals to repel predators because they cannot escape from their habitat easily; and since many of these sessile species are filter feeders, they may use these powerful chemicals to repel parasites or as antibiotics against disease-causing organisms. [2, 4].

Need for the Production of Marine Drugs

Of late, diseases, such as Alzheimer's and Arthritis have been reported to create greater threats to the quality of human life. Heart disease, on the other hand, has become a major threat, while cures for cancer and AIDS continue to be challenging. Unfortunately, many of the drugs formulated over the past several decades have now become less useful due to the development of drug resistance. Some forms of cancer have evolved multiple drug resistance which has made all drug treatments ineffective. In this context, the organisms of the seas and oceans could be a new source of biodiversity and novel drugs. Unlike the terrestrial environment, ethnomedicinal information to guide marine research is very much limited. It is interesting to know that about one-half of all cancer drug discovery focuses now on marine organisms. It was only after the 1950s, scientists began to explore the seas and oceans for useful therapeutics and this was largely due to the advent of scuba diving and new sampling technologies. Marine drug discovery, however, began in the late 1970s, and programs were formulated in the 1980s in the USA, Japan, and Australia. These programs have led to the development of novel new drug leads. Significant progress in the clinical development of marine-derived drugs has been achieved during the last 20 years and during this period, six out of nine currently used drugs of marine origin have been approved [5].

Pharmaceutical Marine Biodiversity and Drug Development

The high diversity of marine species and associated high competition for survival make their compounds unique in chemical structures and biological activities compared to terrestrial natural products. The marine life yielding bioactive compounds includes mainly microorganisms such as microalgae, cyanobacteria,

bacteria, fungi, and other protists; seaweeds (green, brown, and red algae); sponges, cnidarians, bryozoans, molluscs, tunicates and echinoderms; and mangrove plants and other intertidal plants. The number of marine bioactive compounds isolated has increased considerably over the last two decades. As of December 2020, about 36,000 bioactive compounds have been isolated from about 3,400 species. The compounds marketed as drugs or are under drug development are, however, relatively few. It is also worth mentioning here that intensive research has always been focused on the cytotoxic and anticancer activities of these compounds and this is largely due to the fact that the main source of funds for Marine Natural Product Drug Discovery Research in the US was the National Institutes of Health (NIH) / National Cancer Institute (NCI) [5]. It is also reported that only 9,000 marine biopharmaceutical compounds have so far been screened for potential therapeutic value and of these, only 16 have been marketed (11 of them for cancer indications). According to the marine pharmacology/pharmaceutical pipeline website, as of August 2021, there were 30 marine biopharmaceutical compounds in the clinical pipeline, 5 in phase III, 9 in phase II and 16 in phase I [6].

Problems in the Development of New Marine Drugs

a. Bottleneck in the permanent availability of sufficient amounts of organisms.
b. Difficulties in harvesting the organism.
c. Difficulties in the identification of marine species.
d. Limited quantities of bioactive compounds from original source organisms.
e. Complex chemical structures of bioactive compounds.
f. Difficulties in isolation and purification procedures.
g. Difficulties in synthesizing bioactive compounds.
h. Enormous time it takes to reach the market (*i.e.* about 12 years to develop one approved drug from about 5,000-10,000 bioactive compounds) and the cost of drug production.

Remedial Measures for the Supply of Bioactive Compounds

a. In order to ensure a sustainable supply of drug candidates, marine biotechnology processes *viz.* aquaculture/mariculture/ fermenter cultivation, genetic engineering, enzymatic synthesis, chemical synthesis or semi-synthesis need to be encouraged.
b. Sufficient investment by pharmaceutical companies.
c. Enhancing the research in pharmaceutical companies with staff with adequate expertise.

Present Status of Marine Drug Discovery

a. The concept of Marine Bio-pharmacy, Marine Pharmacology, or Marine Pharmacognosy is either new to India or in an infant stage.
b. Although the pharmaceutically important marine species diversity is enormous in India, no intensive research has been done on this aspect due to the absence of an interdisciplinary approach.
c. Although few research papers are presently available on the bioactivities of marine organisms from their extracts, no new bioactive compounds have been isolated from the marine organisms in our country.
d. The existing course *viz.* 'Fish Pharmacology' in the different institutes of India deals with only 'Drugs for fish diseases in Aquaculture systems' and not on the pharmaceutical potential of fish.

Scope for Active Research on the Development of Marine Drugs

The exploration of the marine environment is increasing in developed countries and this is largely due to the adoption of new techniques for sample collection, and improved spectrometric techniques and separation methods.

a. Starting of an inter-disciplinary course *viz.* Marine Bio-Pharmacy \
b. Collaborative research between academic marine scientists with biomedical researchers in the pharmaceutical industries.

CONCLUSION

The recent advances made in the development, approval, and therapeutic use of marine drugs amply reveal the enormous potential of the bioactive compounds derived from marine organisms. However, there are many challenges ahead to further exploit the potential of marine organisms for therapeutic purposes. In this regard, the following aspects need to be given more emphasis [2].

Taxonomy: As the correct taxonomic identification of the bioactive compound-producing marine organism is essential for further processes, this aspect needs to be given top priority.

Supply/cultivation: In order to ensure sustainable supply of marine organisms towards the development of drugs, advancement in sampling techniques needs to be discovered. Such techniques can allow access to marine samples not only near shore but also in the deep sea. Further, special fermentation technologies are to be devised to cultivate organisms living in marine environments under extreme conditions like high pressure.

Market access: As for terrestrial drugs, the requirements to get access to the market are more or less the same for marine-derived drugs. Presently a long time (8-15 year period) is required for the approval of drugs and a significant amount of money (about US$900 million) is involved from the discovery of drugs to market. Further, there is a very high risk in the procedures in the development of new drugs and many drug candidates have failed during the development processes because of toxicity, lack of sustainable availability, *etc.*

Collaborative venture: Intensive interdisciplinary collaboration between biologists, pharmacists, chemists, biotechnologists, medical doctors, *etc.*, and between universities, hospitals, and companies is the need of the hour in order to make marine pharmaceutical development a great success.

CHAPTER 2

Marine Bioprospecting

Abstract: This chapter deals with the types of marine ecosystems and their pharmaceutical biodiversity; the present status of marine bioactive compounds and their chemical classes; therapeutic activities of marine bioactive compounds; level of contribution of bioactive compounds by different groups of marine organisms; green processing methods of marine drug development; and measures to tackle supply problems of bioactive compounds.

Keywords: Contribution of bioactive compounds by marine biota, Green processing methods, Marine ecosystems, Meeting supply problems, Status of bioactive compounds, Therapeutic activities of bioactive compounds.

INTRODUCTION

Bioprospecting or biodiversity prospecting is defined as the "process of collecting or surveying of a large set of flora (or fauna) for the purpose of biological evaluation and isolation of lead compounds" [7]. Marine bioprospecting is a process involving the collection of microorganisms like bacteria and fungi and microalgae and larger organisms (marine plants, invertebrates, and fishes) from the sea; categorization into species through valid taxonomical identification; and analysis in research and development. The result of such bioprospecting may be a purified molecule that is produced biologically or synthetically or the entire organism. From a business perspective, the purpose of marine bioprospecting is to find components, and compounds that may be included as components in products or processes. In other words, marine bioprospecting is not an industry but it may procure different compounds that may be used in many different industries. Due to its importance, marine bioprospecting is now lying at the forefront of industrial production as it is also considered as doing something new in order to create future wealth. Companies possessing high profile in the field of marine bioprospecting in recent decades include Diverse and New England Biolabs. In regards to the development of new biopharmaceuticals, the marine bioprospecting (also known as Marine biodiversity prospecting) can be described as a targeted and systematic search for bioactive compounds (secondary metabolites/natural products/ ectocrines) from marine organisms. This unique venture in fact started in geographic territories with long coast-line with warm temperatures. Prominent countries where large-scale samplings were done for pharmaceutically important invertebrates (and probably also other groups of marine organisms) include Asia followed by Oceania, America, Africa, and Europe [2]. Further, the bioprospecting approach is not new, as more than 10,000 pharmaceutically important compounds have already been reported from marine sources, although very few of them have been put on the market.

Marine Ecosystems and their Pharmaceutical Biodiversity

The marine ecosystem is the largest ecosystem of our blue planet. Its biotic and abiotic components play an important role in maintaining proper balance in this ecosystem. Compared to other ecosystems of the planet, the marine ecosystem supports great biodiversity. The different types of marine ecosystems are open deep sea, salt water wetland, coral reefs, estuaries, mangroves, sandy beach, kelp forests, polar marine and rocky marine ecosystems [8]. The salient features of the different types of marine ecosystems are given below.

Open Marine Ecosystem

This is the upper layer of the ocean with adequate light penetration and the sun rays reach quite easily in this ecosystem. This open marine ecosystem which extends up to 150 m from the ocean surface provides habitat to a variety of sea creatures such as plankton, algae, whales, jellyfish, *etc.*

Deep-Sea Ecosystem

The deep-sea marine ecosystem inhabits various animal species up to its 1000 m depth. As there is poor light penetration at the seafloor of this ecosystem, its inhabiting species possess several adaptations. The important animals of this ecosystem include squids, fishes, elephant seals, sperm whales, crabs, worms, some sharks, *etc.*

Sandy Beach Ecosystem

Compared to other marine ecosystems, the biodiversity is quite poor in this ecosystem. However, the species of this sandy beach ecosystem such as mollusks, crustaceans, and polychaetes are very much adapted to a constantly variable environment.

Rocky Marine Ecosystem

The rock shores, rock cliffs, boulders, tide pools, *etc.* are the different constituents of this rocky marine ecosystem. The biodiversity of this ecosystem includes lichens, birds, and invertebrates such as lobsters, urchins, barnacles, sea stars, sea squirts, *etc.*

Coral Reef Ecosystem

It is a special type of marine ecosystem and is mostly found in tropical waters forming the most productive ecosystem of the earth. This ecosystem has been reported to provide food and shelter to about ¼ of marine species. Further, this ecosystem attracts exotic color fishes like sponges, snails, and seahorses; and occasionally large animals like sharks, dolphins, *etc.*

Kelp Forest Ecosystem

Kelp forests are underwater areas with a high density of kelp, (large brown algae) which has been reported to cover a large part of the world's coastlines. This ecosystem supports various animal species such as seabirds, shorebirds, invertebrates (like crabs, sea stars, snails, *etc.*), fishes, and mammals (like sea lions, seals, whales, sea otters, *etc.*).

Estuarine Ecosystem

The region around the river mouth where it connects with the sea is usually termed an estuarine ecosystem. The characteristic feature of this ecosystem is its salinity which largely depends on the influence of tides and it varies between 0 and 35 ppt. This ecosystem does not normally support a variety of species and it plays an important role as nurseries for various kinds of fishes, shrimps, *etc.*

Saltwater Wetland Ecosystem

The coastal regions of oceans and seas are commonly known as the saltwater wetland ecosystem which is classified into two types *viz.* saltwater swamps and salt marshes. While the saltwater swamps are dominated by trees, salt marshes are often covered with grasses. The most common animals of this ecosystem are shellfish, fishes, amphibians, reptiles, migratory birds, *etc.*

Mangrove Ecosystem

It is a special type of saltwater swamp found in some tropical and sub-tropical coastal regions. These mangrove swamps are home to special types of plants such as *Avicennia* and *Rhizophora*. This mangrove ecosystem provides shelter to various species such as shrimps, jellyfish, birds, sponges, crabs, fish, crocodiles, *etc.*

Polar Marine Ecosystem

As the climate of these ecosystems is extremely cold, its species have adapted to the adverse climatic conditions of this region. The most common species found in this ecosystem include planktons, algae, birds (like penguins,) polar bears, seals, walruses, *etc.*

Although all these marine ecosystems possess therapeutically important species, the continental shelves – the shallow waters (0-200m) of the seas have been reported to possess the majority of marine life due to the abundant penetration of sunlight and nutrient upwellings. Such favorable conditions create an ideal environment for the rich production of microalgae (phytoplankton), seaweeds (macroalgae and seagrass which in turn support vast food chains from microzooplankton to the blue whale, the largest animal of the Earth. However, our marine environment is under great threat due to several factors including overfishing, habitat destruction, pollution, climate change, and ocean acidification. This calls for strict measures to protect marine biodiversity and some of the recommendations to protect marine biodiversity are: safeguarding marine ecosystems and their species diversity through effective protection and management; tackling the major threats to marine ecosystems and their species diversity through improved policy and practice; and addressing the different stakeholders viz the people and organizations to protect their local marine environments through awareness programs [1].

Marine Bioactive Compounds

The bioactive compounds (natural products, secondary metabolites, pharmaceutical compounds, therapeutic compounds, biomedical compounds, or ectocrines) are derived from marine organisms and are quite diverse in their chemical structure. The different chemical classes of these metabolites are steroids, terpenoids, alkaloids, polyketides, phenolic metabolites, some carbohydrates, lipids, and peptides. Further, these secondary metabolites can also be classified on the basis of their biological functions as antibiotics, pheromones, hormones, toxins, *etc.* The soil microorganisms and higher terrestrial (land) plants were only considered for a long time to be the major biological sources of these natural products. However, when scuba diving in the deep sea became popular, the study of marine organisms significantly increased and this has led to the development of marine natural products. It is also known that the total number of studied marine natural products may exceed 120,000-150,000 though about 20,000 natural substances have so far been segregated. It is also worth mentioning here that marine organisms contain very rarely already-known compounds. Therefore, the biochemistry of the marine secondary metabolism differs substantially from that of terrestrial organisms [9].

Therapeutic Activities of Marine Bioactive Compounds

The therapeutic activities of bioactive compounds isolated from different groups of marine organisms [5] are given below.

1. Anti-infective

    i. Antiviral (anti-retroviral, anti-herpetic) (Anti-CoV, Anti-HBV, Anti-HCV, Anti-HIV, Anti-HSV, Anti- HAdV, Anti- influenza A (H3N2), Anti-Influenza (Flu) A virus, Anti- HMPV, *etc.*)
    ii. Antimalarial (antiplasmodial).
    iii. Antiprotozoal (antileishmanial and antitrypanosomal).
    iv. Antitubercular (antimycobacterial).
    v. Antibacterial.
    vi. Antifungal.

2. Anti-tumor (anticancer, antineoplastic, cytotoxic, cytostatic, antiproliferative, anticarcinogenic, antimitotic, antileukemic, antimetastatic).

3. Anti-diabetic, antidiuretic, diuretic and uretic.

4. Anthelmintic (anti-helminthic).

5. Angiostatic.

6. AChE (Acetylcholinesterase) inhibitory.

7. Analgesic and antipyretic.

8. Anti-Alzheimer (anti-dementia).

9. Anti-asthmatic.

10. Anti-hepatitis (hepatoprotective),.

11. Anti-hyperglycemic.

12. Anti-hypertensive.

13. Anti-inflammatory.

14. Antinociceptive.

15. Anti-oxidant.

16. Anti-osteoporotic.

17. Antitussive and expectorant.

18. Anti-ulcerogenic.

19. Anti-urolithiatic.

20. Cardiovascular effects (cardiotropic, anti-cardiovascular).

   i. Anti-hyperlipidemic
  ii. Anti-hypercholesterolemic.
 iii. Anti-atherosclerotic.
 iv. Anti-hypertensive.
  v. Angiotensin-converting enzyme (ACE) inhibitory.
 vi. Antithrombotic (anticoagulant, anticlotting, antiplatelet, platelet aggregation, hematopoietic, granulopoietic).

21. Central Nervous System (CNS) disorders [anti-epileptic (anticonvulsant), anxiolytic - anti-anxiety, tranquilizer and sedative, and anti-parkinsonian].

22. Cholinergic (neuromuscular).

23. Endocrine.

24. Haemolytic.

25. Haemostatic effect (coagulation, clotting, platelet activation).

26. Hypolipidemic (hypocholesterolemic, antihyperlipidemic).

27. Immunomodulatory (immunoregulatory).

28. Myoactivity (myotropic).

29. Neuromodulatory.

30. Neurodegenerative disorders (neuroprotective, brain diseases).

31. Neuropsychiatric disorder (hallucinogenic, psychotropic).

32. Protease inhibitor (anti-viral).

33. Wound healing.

34. Anti-obesity.

The therapeutic activities of biomolecules derived from the different constituents of marine life are shown below (Fig. **1**).

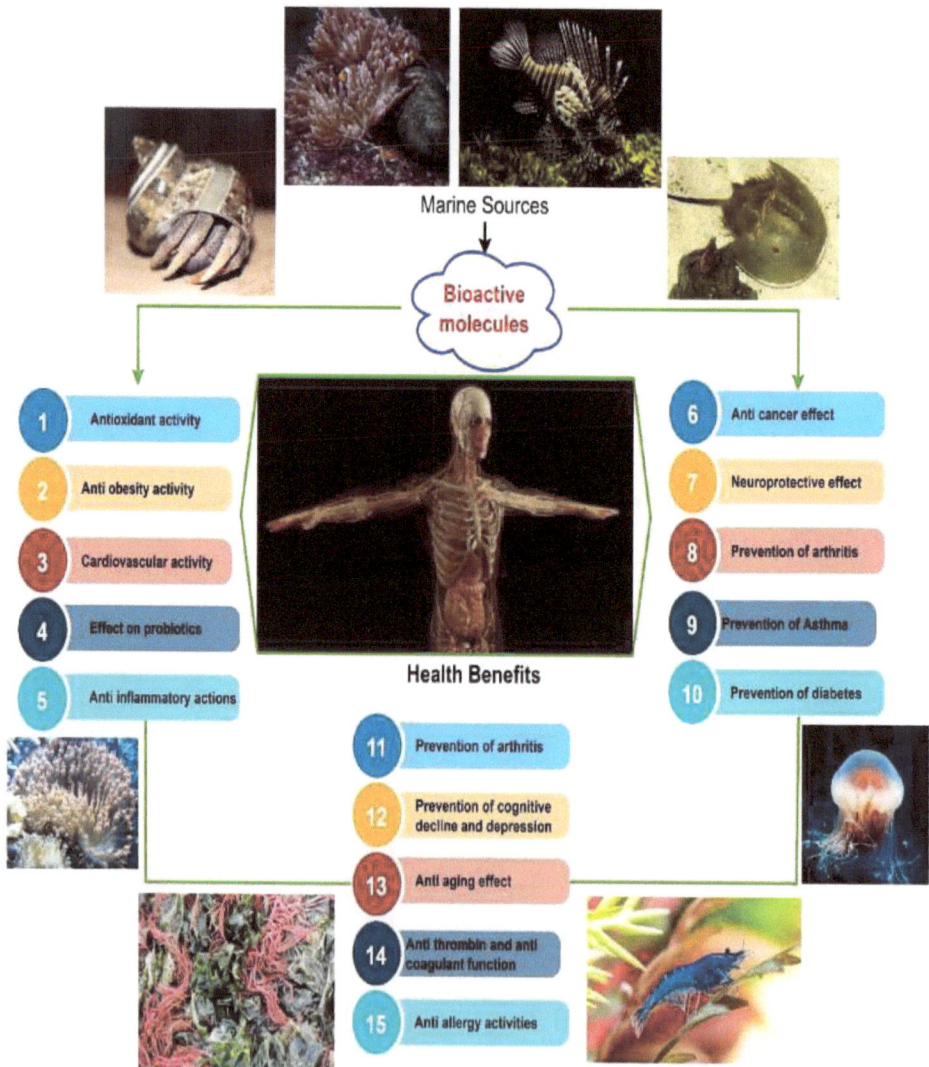

Fig. (1). Therapeutic activities of biomolecules derived from the marine life. Image credit: Ghosh *et al*. (CC as per message received).

Bioactive Compounds of Marine Organisms

Among the different groups of marine life, invertebrates such as sponges, cnidarians, bryozoans, mollusks, echinoderms, and tunicates have been found to be the most important sources for the isolation of pharmaceutically important bioactive compounds. The percentage contribution of bioactive compounds by the different groups of marine organisms is shown below (Table **1**).

Table 1. Percentage contribution of bioactive compounds of marine organisms [5].

Group of Marine Organisms	Percentage
Sponges	37
Cnidarians	21
Microbes	18
Macroalgae (= Seaweeds)	9
Echinoderms	6
Tunicates	6
Mollusks	2
Bryozoans	1

Chemical Classes of Marine Bioactive Compounds

Based on their chemical structures, the isolated marine bioactive compounds belong to chemical groups such as carbohydrates, proteins, alkaloids, peptides, lipopeptides, polyketides, terpenes, steroidal or triterpene saponins, aliphatic compounds, amino acids, *etc.* Among these chemical groups, alkaloids have been reported to contribute the maximum level (69%) followed by terpenes (17%), polyketides (13%) and glycosphingolipids (1%). Further, while the number of new terpenoids from the marine invertebrates is increasing, the discovery of new alkaloids and aliphatic molecules has shown a decreasing trend [2,10]. The percentage values of bioactive secondary metabolites of major marine invertebrates are shown below (Table **2**).

Table 2. Percentage values of bioactive secondary metabolites of major marine invertebrates [11].

Category	Sponges	Cnidarians	Mollusks	Tunicates
Alkaloids.	29	5	-	50
Terpenes	35	67	24	-
Lipids	22	-	-	-
Steroids	-	21	8	-

(Table 2) cont.....

Category	Sponges	Cnidarians	Mollusks	Tunicates
Peptides	-	-	31	13
Polyketides	14*	-	15	37
Polyphenols	-	-	22	-
Others	-	6	-	-

* Includes peptides also.

Potential Bioactive Compounds of Different Constituents of Marine Life

The potential bioactive compounds obtained from different constituents of marine life as reported by Ghosh *et al.* [12] are given below (Fig. **2**).

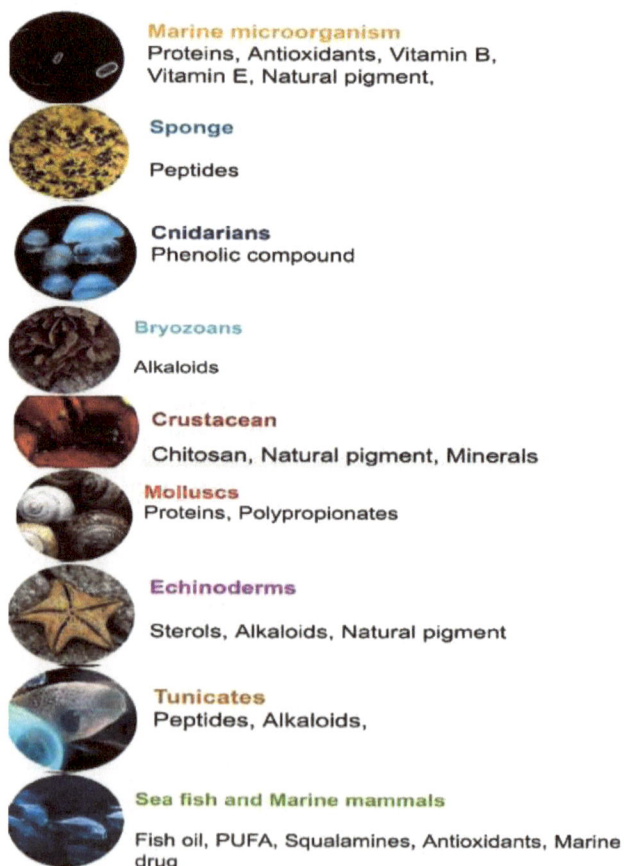

Fig. (2). Potential bioactive compounds obtained from different constituents of marine life. Image (modified) credit: Ghosh *et al.* (CC as per message received).

Bioactivity-based Contribution of Marine Bioactive Compounds

Among the bioactive compounds, more than half of the compounds discovered from 1985 to 2012 possess antitumor/anticancer, cytotoxic, and cytostatic activities. This is believed to be due to the medicinal need for new anticancer drugs; the conduct of intensive research on these need-based bioactivities; the availability of easily applicable *in vitro* test systems; and the support of more funding agencies. For instance, the main source of funds for Marine Natural Product Drug Discovery Research in the US was the National Institutes of Health (NIH) / National Cancer Institute (NCI) [2, 5]. The bioactivity-based percentage distribution of marine bioactive compounds is shown below (Table 3).

Table 3. Bioactivity-based percentage distribution of marine bioactive compounds [5].

Bioactivity	Percentage Distribution
Antitumor/Anticancer/Cytotoxic	64
Antibacterial	14
Antimalarial	6
Antifungal	3
Anti-inflammatory	3
Anti-HIV	3
CNS Disorders	3
Antioxidant	2
Antiviral	1
Antidiabetic	1

Romano *et al.* [11] reported on the percentage of bioactivities of major marine invertebrates such as sponges, cnidarians, mollusks, echinoderms and tunicates. Among the different bioactivities, cytotoxic/antiproliferative activity dominated in all these groups with percentage values of 50, 42, 36, 38 and 58, respectively. The individual bioactivities of the different groups of these marine invertebrates are given below (Fig. 3).

Status of Isolated Marine Bioactive Compounds

The number of marine bioactive compounds isolated has increased considerably over the last two decades. As of December 2020, about 36,000 bioactive compounds have been isolated from about 3,400 species. The status of marine bioactive compounds isolated from marine organisms from 1965 to 2020 is shown below (Table 4).

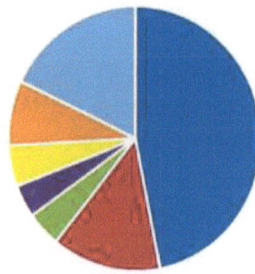

- Cytotoxic against cancer cells
- Antimicrobial
- Anti-fungal
- Antimalarial
- Anti-inflammatory
- Enzyme inhibitor
- Others

Marine Sponges

Bioactivity

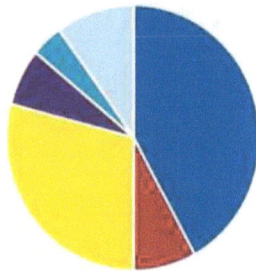

- Cytotoxic against cancer cells
- Antimicrobial
- Anti-inflammatory
- Antifouling
- Antiviral
- Others

Marine Cnidarians

Bioactivity

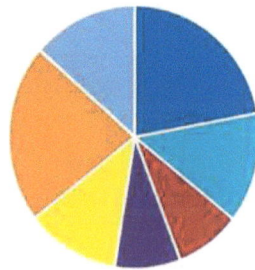

- Cytotoxic against cancer cells
- Anti-proliferative
- Antimicrobial/antibacterial
- Antioxidant
- Anti-inflammatory
- Neuroactive
- Others

Marine Molluscs

Bioactivity

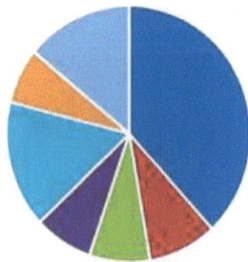

- Cytotoxic against cancer cells/anti-proliferative
- Antimicrobial
- Inhibition of colony formation
- Haemolytic
- Anticoagulant
- Neuritogenic
- Others

Echinoderms

(Fig. 3) contd.....

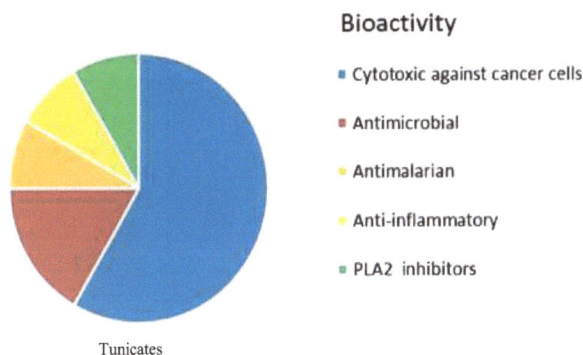

Bioactivity

- ■ Cytotoxic against cancer cells
- ■ Antimicrobial
- ■ Antimalarian
- ■ Anti-inflammatory
- ■ PLA2 inhibitors

Tunicates

Fig. (3). Bioactivities of marine sponges, cnidarians, mollusks, echinoderms and tunicates. Images credit: Giovanna Romano *et al.* (CC- Reproduced with his kind permission).

Table 4. Status of marine bioactive compounds isolated during the period 1965-2020 [5].

Period	No. of Compounds
1965-1975	Nil
1976-1985	3,000
1986-1995	10,000
1996-2005	18,000
2006-2016	29,000
2017-2020	36,000

MARINE BIOACTIVE COMPOUNDS AS DIAGNOSTICS AND EXPERIMENTAL TOOLS

Several bioactive compounds derived from marine organisms have been reported to serve as diagnostics and experimental tools [2] as detailed below.

Enzymes

The enzyme Taq polymerase isolated from the bacterium Thermus aquaticus living in hot springs; and the enzyme Pfu from the marine thermophile *Pyrococcus furiosus,* are used in Polymerase chain reaction (PCR).

Green Fluorescent Protein (GFP) and Phycoerythrin

The GFP isolated from the jellyfish *Aequorea victoria* is used as a biological marker for labelling cellular structures *in vitro* and *in vivo*. Phycoerythrin, a red protein-pigment complex isolated from the marine red algae is also used for the same purpose. The proteins are believed to act as light-driven electron transfer.

Okadaic Acid

This polyketide Okadaic acid (Fig. **4**) produced by the dinoflagellates *viz.* *Dinophysis* sp., and *Prorocentrum* sp is a useful tool to study mechanisms of diseases which are associated with protein phosphorylation, *e.g.* Alzheimer's disease.

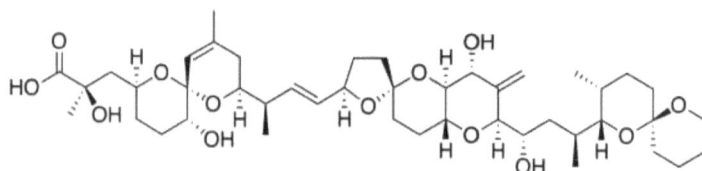

Fig. (4). Okadaic acid.

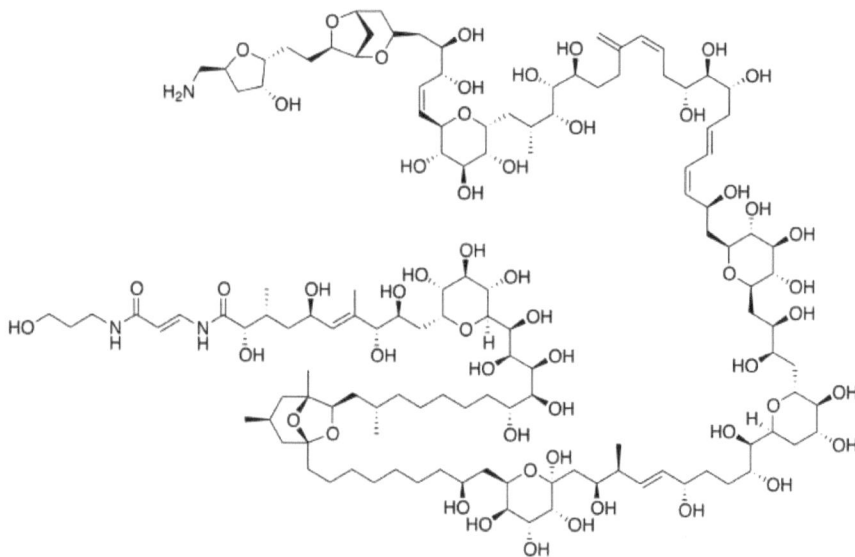

Fig. (5). Palytoxin.

Palytoxin

A very large polyketide, palytoxin (Fig. **5**) is produced by marine microbes associated with the marine sponge *Palythoa* sp. It can be used for the analysis of the structure and mechanisms of Na+/K+ pumps.

Limulus-Amoebocyte-Lysate (LAL)

It is an aqueous extract of blood cells (amoebocytes) from the Atlantic horseshoe crab *Limulus polyphemus* and is utilized in the LAL test for the sensitive detection of pyrogenic lipopolysaccharides (LPS) from gram-negative bacteria.

Keyhole Limpet Hemocyanin (KLH)

IKLH (Fig. **6**) is a large, oxygen-carrying metalloprotein found in the hemolymph of the giant keyhole limpet *Megathura crenulata*, a marine bivalve mollusk. It is used as a vaccine component for the treatment of bladder carcinoma).

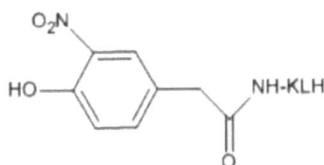

Fig. (6). KLH.

Tetrodotoxin

The chinazoline alkaloid, tetrodotoxin (Fig. **7**) is well-known as a secondary toxin in puffer fishes ("Fugu"). It is actually produced by marine bacteria and is transferred to these fishes through the food chain. This alkaloid has been reported to target very specific $Na+$ ion channels and therefore, it can be used for the investigation of physiological processes mediated by such ion channels.

MARINE BIOPHARMACEUTICALS

The term "biopharmaceutical" (used as both noun and adjective) was coined in the 1980s and it refers to (land plant and animal-based) pharmaceuticals produced in biotechnological processes using methods relating to molecular biology. Thus, this type of product was distinguished from the broad category of "biologics", which are pharmaceuticals produced using conventional biological methods. Further, biopharmaceuticals are produced in living cells, whereas synthetic drugs are the products of chemical processes. Since its introduction in 1982, the land-based biopharmaceuticals are very commonly used in all branches of medicine, and thus they have become one of the most effective clinical treatment modalities for a wide range of diseases, including cancers and other metabolic disorders [13].

Advantages of Biopharmaceuticals

Biopharmaceuticals have several advantages. They target only specific molecules with rare side effects which are invariably associated with conventional small-molecule, synthetic drugs. Further, compared to conventional drugs, biopharmaceuticals display high specificity and activity. Furthermore, the application of biopharmaceuticals has been reported to facilitate the treatment of patients who respond poorly to traditional synthetic drugs. It is also known that, unlike synthetic drugs, biopharmaceuticals are potentially immunogenic. Unlike synthetic drugs, the active pharmaceutical ingredients in biopharmaceuticals include nucleic acids and recombinant proteins.

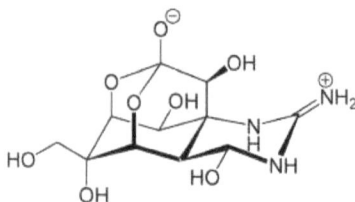

Fig. (7). Tetrodotoxin.

Generics *vs* Biosimilars

Generics are defined as drugs that are equivalents of the reference drugs possessing the same active pharmaceutical ingredient. However, the term "generic" is not used in reference to biopharmaceuticals. Biosimilars are biological medical products containing the active pharmaceutical ingredient which is found in the previously registered reference biological medicinal products. While the European Union (EU) uses the term "Biosimilars", FDA (US) uses the term "Follow-on biologics " for Biosimilars. Their introduction in the European Union and, recently, the United States markets has been reported to reduce the costs of biopharmaceutical treatment.

Bio-betters

Bio-betters are another group of biopharmaceuticals. Bio-betters are nothing but biopharmaceuticals that are structurally and/or functionally altered to achieve an improved or different clinical performance, compared to approved reference products. Bio-betters are different from the existing products and are therefore considered new drugs, in a standard approval procedure. Bio-betters also represent the next stage in the development of biopharmaceuticals in which proteins were purposefully altered equivalents of existing drugs. Both biosimilars and bio-betters are considered natural alternatives for the reference biopharmaceuticals and therefore they are likely to compete for the same market.

DEVELOPMENT OF MARINE BIOPHARMACEUTICALS (DEVELOPMENT OF MARINE DRUGS)

The development of a new drug begins from the study of the disease processes and pathways, at a cellular or molecular level, to identify targets for new treatments. The search for molecules and compounds that act on such targets will then begin. When a marine organism is considered to have therapeutic values, it is first administered in its entirety to cells or small laboratory/ experimental animals. Meanwhile, screening is made; the sample is separated into fractions (clusters of molecules that are separated by chromatography techniques), and subsequently biological tests are begun. If these tests display that some of the bioactive compounds reduce the growth of tumour cells, for example, a selection is then made, and fragmentation continues until an almost pure compound is derived. Mass spectrometry analysis is then done to measure the molecular weight and, through other analyses, such as infrared or nuclear magnetic resonance (NMR) spectroscopy, the structure of the selected bioactive compound can then be understood [6].

The process of marine drug development consists of several stages. First of all it starts with the supply which involves collection and identification of the marine organisms, an important stage which can be successfully completed only with the help of a marine scientist or marine biologist who is well-trained in Taxonomy. If this stage is not properly completed especially the identification of collected pharmaceutically important organisms, then the entire process may go waste. The collection of organisms from unexplored regions and depths is also possible nowadays due to trained SCUBA divers. Less availability of important species may be compensated by culturing them, following the standard aquaculture methods. The organisms so collected and identified are then well purified and dried for further analysis. Strictly speaking, the following steps are more or less the same as for terrestrial organisms. The other stages involve extraction; and isolation and structure elucidation of compounds with potential bioactivities. Subsequently, these compounds are subject to broad pharmacological investigations of biopharmaceutical (=drug) candidates for pharmacodynamics, and pharmacokinetics. Among the selected compounds, best suitable biopharmaceutical candidates are taken to clinical trials and subsequent registration according to valid legislation [2]. The general procedures for the marine biota-derived biopharmaceutical (drug) discovery are given below (Fig. 8).

Green Processing Methods to Extract Biomolecules from Marine Life

Due to the enormous diversity of marine life as well as the variances in the characteristics of its biomolecules, the extraction procedures are becoming crucial so as to derive a greater yield and greater target substances quality. In this regard, green extraction techniques are considered potential methods for recovering biomolecules from pharmaceutically important marine life [12]. The emerging, modern technologies which are more advantageous over the traditional methods for the extraction of bioactive compounds of the different constituents of marine life and their discards are given below.

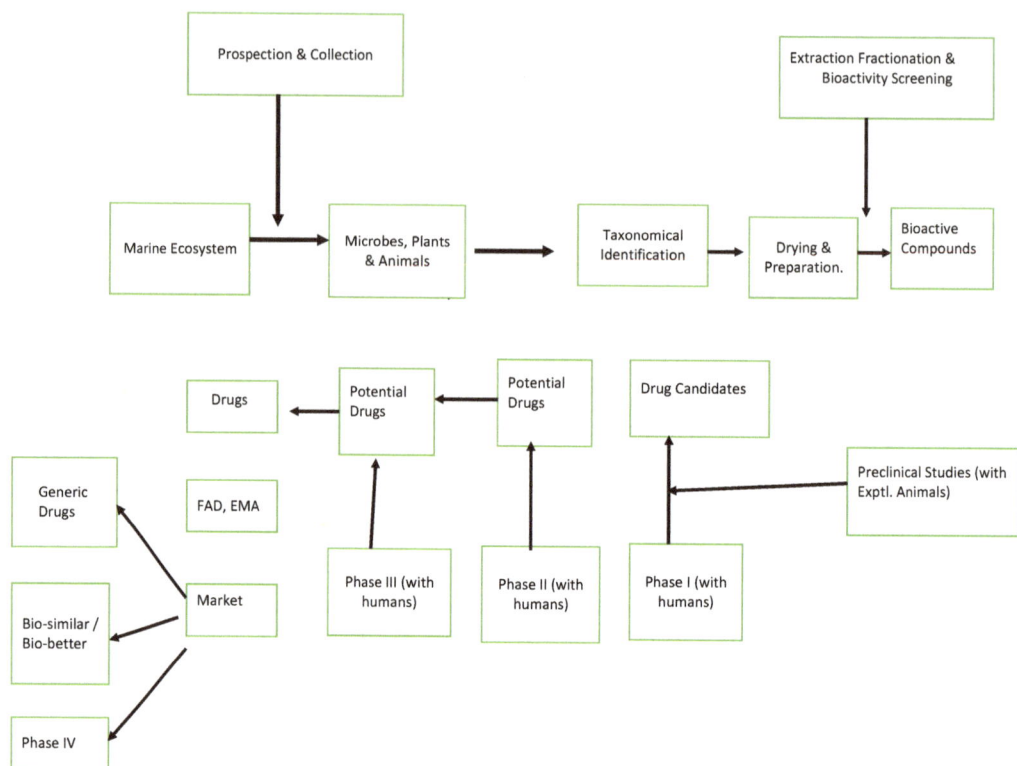

Fig. (8). Procedures for the marine biota-derived biopharmaceutical (drug) discovery.

Traditional Methods

Maceration, percolation, and Soxhlet extraction are the commonly available traditional methods for the extraction of compounds from organisms in general. Depending on the polarity of the molecules to be extracted, the most commonly employed solvents include acetone, water, methanol, ethyl ethanoate and ethanol in various combinations. Combining a solvent with acids like citric acid, tartaric acid, or hydrochloric acid has been reported to enhance the extraction efficiency of specific substances. Among the traditional extraction methods, the Soxhlet extraction method is commonly used as it is known to yield better results.

Modern Methods

Fermentative Extraction

Fermentation is considered to be a useful method for demineralization, deproteination, and proteolysis compared to ensilaging. This method is ideal for crustacean (shrimp) wastes as fermenting of these wastes yields a higher extraction yield than other chemical extraction methods. For example, during bacterial fermentation, the proteins and minerals of crustacean shells are successfully eliminated, thereby increasing the extraction efficiency of carotenoids besides safeguarding the quality. In such fermentations which often take a long period, maintaining a constant temperature is very much essential to achieve better results.

Enzymatic Extraction

Enzymatic extraction is believed to be a potential method as it has been reported to save energy and time by eliminating chemical contamination which is often caused by leftover solvents. It is therefore considered to be an ecologically acceptable method especially for the extraction of value-added compounds associated with nutraceutical applications. As enzymes are influenced by temperature, acidity, and other environmental factors, they can be used at different stages of the process in the creation of a wide range of products and by-products. In the processing of crustacean wastes, enzymatic digestion is utilized as the final step after fermentation and/or other digestion processes.

Supercritical Fluid Extraction

This method involves increasing temperature and pressure above their critical points while maintaining liquid characteristics. Carbon dioxide is the commonly used solvent for this method due to its non-toxicity, safety, and low cost. However, this method can only be employed to extract non-polar or low-polarity molecules though it can also extract polar chemicals.

Pressurized Liquid Extraction

The selectivity and solubility of the different substances in the supercritical fluid are normally influenced by the extraction conditions, particularly pressure and temperature. This extraction method uses small volumes of non-toxic solvents, high pressures (10–15 MPa), a temperature range of 50-200 °C and short processing periods. In this method, bioactive molecules are preserved and no breakdown seems to happen because CO_2 has a low critical temperature and pressure. Fatty acids, phytosterols, phenolics, carotenoids, and triglycerides are commonly seen in the extracts associated with this method.

Subcritical Water Extraction

As this method uses a small amount of the right solvent and is operated for a short time (5–10 min) at high temperatures (50–200°C) and pressures (50–300 psi), this method is believed to be the most promising technology for extracting bioactive molecules from marine organisms. Further, SWE is an environmentally friendly extraction method since it uses water instead of an organic solvent as a solvent. In this extraction method, the solvents are normally kept in a liquid state below their boiling point with the help of applied temperature and pressure. As the working temperature rises, the surface tension and viscosity of the solvent decrease, resulting in the improvement of solubility and mass transfer rate.

Supercritical CO_2 Extraction

As a non-flammable and non-toxic gas, the carbon dioxide is also used in this method. In this method, CO_2 makes the extraction process easier besides making the fluid behave both like a liquid and a gas. As this Supercritical CO_2 Extraction can be employed with several pressure-temperature combinations, this method is commonly employed for a wide range of end products. Further, this method allows for the use of low pressure (7.386 MPa) and low temperature. For example, a combination of low temperatures and pressure ensures the retention of thermolabile phytochemicals.

Pressurized Hot Water Extraction

It is also known as superheated water extraction (SHWE), subcritical water extraction, or pressurized low polarity water (PLPW) extraction owing to the use of water as a solvent in this method of extraction. It is a more environmentally friendly extraction method because it uses water instead of organic solvents. In this method, water is used at temperatures higher than its atmospheric boiling point while keeping it as a liquid by applying pressure. Under these conditions, the physical and chemical properties of water are known to change dramatically. Further, as the water temperature rises, the viscosity and surface tension decrease. This increases the diffusivity thereby improving the extraction method in terms of speed and efficiency. Furthermore, temperature affects the solubility of water, thus favoring the solubility of various types of compounds. Although PHWE is a promising technology, further research in the marine field is the need of the hour.

Pulse Electric Field-Assisted Method

This method is more acceptable due to its less energy consumption and other environmental and cost-effective benefits. Combined with other methods like osmotic shock and mechanical press, this developing technology is believed to be efficient in the extraction process. Further, the combination of PEF and solid/liquid extraction has been reported to produce less waste compared to the other existing methods. In the treatments associated with this extraction method, 1–20 kJ/kg specific energy and 0.7–3 kV/cm electric field intensity are commonly used.

Microwave-Assisted Method

Microwave radiation which is a non-ionizing radiation is a synergistic combination of two techniques namely energy and mass transfer that both work in the same direction. During the microwave processing, the moisture in the cells of the tissues evaporates as the temperature rises, resulting in high pressure in the cells. Further, due to the breaking of cell walls, porosity improves. The mass transfer is aided by raising the matrix porosity apart from increasing the temperature and pressure. Sample size, moisture of the sample, solvent type, extraction cycles, microwave power output, processing period, sample viscosity, frequency, pressure, *etc.* are known to affect the efficiency of the MAE process. By this method, polyphenols and polysaccharides can be extracted in open (at atmospheric pressure) or closed (at higher pressure) vessels.

Ultrasound-Assisted Method

In this method, ultrasonic waves (mechanical waves) in the range of 20–1000 kHz are commonly used to improve the extraction efficiency. When these ultrasonic waves propagate through the solvent, they create negative pressure; and when sound wave pressure of higher intensities propagates through the solvent, microscopically sized small holes or bubbles develop. When these bubbles are filled with gas or water vapor, the bubbles grow and shrink until they collide resulting in cavitation. Parameters such as frequency, power, and temperature are known to optimize this method of extraction. In this method, after the sample has been immersed in the ultrasonic bath, the ultrasonic probe is inserted into it. This method has been reported to be less expensive than other extraction methods, and it can be conveniently used with a variety of solvents. Further, the UAE operates at low temperatures which facilitates the preservation of thermolabile compounds.

High Hydrostatic Pressure

It is a non-thermal high hydrostatic pressure method and is more suitable for improving phytochemical extraction. HHP-assisted enzymatic treatment is known to improve the extraction of certain components like proteins, polysaccharides, and polyphenols. According to available research findings, treatment with HHP and hemicellulose may increase the antioxidant activity of isolated fractions by about 3 times. This method of extraction is invariably used to reduce microbial populations and inactivate enzymes in marine samples. For example, under high pressure (100–1000 MPa) and at a temperature of 5–35°C, cell permeability increases which in turn raises the pressure to the crucial threshold level, thereby improving the extracellular fluid flow.

Extrusion-assisted Extraction

EAE is a process that involves extruding a by-product solution and extracting the extrudates in water. The stages involved in this traditional extrusion process include heating to high temperatures at high pressure, mechanical mixing, and shearing. This EAE operates by rupturing cell walls and with a thermo-mechanical action, insoluble macromolecules are transformed into soluble ones. This technology has several advantages such as reduction in process time, energy consumption, and solvents; and an increase in extraction yield. However, this method is not suggested for thermo-sensitive compounds and it has been used mainly to extract biomolecules from seafood wastes.

Membrane Separation Technologies

In this method, as the membrane acts as a selective and semi-permeable barrier, the molecules of the sample are isolated depending on their molecular size. Further, molecules and particles with a diameter less than the membrane pores often pass through, while those with a diameter larger than the membrane pores are repelled. On the other hand, at the molecular level, the microporous membranes can segregate particles (*i.e* by nanofiltration and reverse osmosis). The molecules so segregated mostly depend on their chemical composition. MST is primarily used in seafood processing plants to separate and recover biomolecules from the fisheries byproducts.

Combined Extraction Techniques

When a single extraction method is found insufficient to extract all of the desired biomolecules from the source material, a combination of green processing methods (Fig. **9**) for extraction may be required to improve the extraction process. Such combined extraction techniques not only enhance the extraction efficiency but also improve the quality of target compounds.

Major Problems in the Development of New Marine Pharmaceuticals (= Marine Drugs)

a. Bottleneck in the permanent availability of sufficient amounts of organisms.
b. Difficulties in harvesting the organism.
c. Difficulties in the identification of marine species.
d. Limited quantities of bioactive compounds from original source organisms.
e. Complex chemical structures of bioactive compounds.
f. Difficulties in isolation and purification procedures.
g. Difficulties in synthesizing bioactive compounds.

h. Enormous time it takes to reach the market (*i.e.* about 12 years to develop one approved drug from about 5,000-10,000 bioactive compounds) and the cost of drug production.

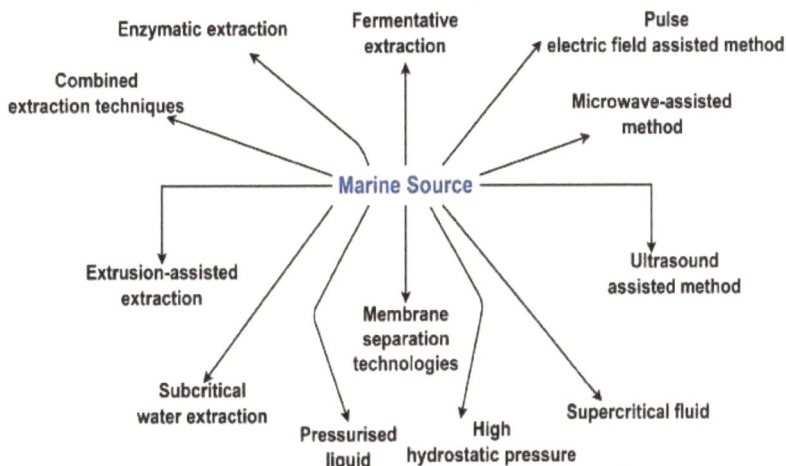

Fig. (9). Green processing methods to extract biomolecules from marine life. Image credit: Ghosh *et al.* (CC as per message received).

How to Address the Supply Problem?

Supply problem is considered to be a critical point in the process of drug development from marine organisms. Permanent availability of sufficient amounts of organisms and compounds without harming the marine environment is the basic need of the marine drug development. Only when the supply is addressed in an economically and ecologically feasible fashion, then only marine drugs can reach the market easily. However, the supply problem can also be solved by processes such as aquaculture (mariculture), marine biotechnology or fermenter cultivation; genetic engineering; enzymatic synthesis or modification, or by chemical synthesis/semi-synthesis/modification as detailed below.

Aquaculture

Aquaculture (mariculture) is the cultivation of organisms in coastal water bodies under controlled conditions following standard methods. Commonly cultivated marine organisms include seaweeds (macroalgae), crustacean shrimp (Arthropoda), mussels (Mollusca), and fishes.

Genetic Engineering

This method involves the transfer of the genetic information for the desired compound into host cells (which can be easily cultivated), thereby obtaining sustainable production of the needed bioactive compound in the host cells. Exact knowledge of the genetic information is the prerequisite in dealing with this method. The techniques associated with this method would allow the isolation and expression of genes of organisms, which cannot be cultivated otherwise. Unfortunately, this approach is only at the research level and not on industrial scale for marketable marine drugs.

Synthesis/semi Synthesis/Modification

Although the total synthesis of the required bioactive compounds is principally possible for many of the hitherto known marine compounds, it is believed to be economically realized only for relatively simple products (*e.g.* analgetic peptide ziconotide). In the semisynthetic production technique, easily available bioactive compounds are transferred by chemical or biochemical processes into the desired product (*e.g.* trabectedin by transformation of cyanosafracin B, a bacterial product). Chemical and/or enzymatic modifications of the naturally available bioactive compound as lead structure can also improve the properties of the product.

Remedial Measures for the Supply of Bioactive Compounds

a. In order to ensure a sustainable supply of drug candidates, marine biotechnology processes *viz.* aquaculture/mariculture/ fermenter cultivation, genetic engineering, enzymatic synthesis, chemical synthesis, or semi-synthesis need to be encouraged.
b. Sufficient investment by pharmaceutical companies.
c. Enhancing the research in pharmaceutical companies with staff with adequate expertise.

CONCLUSION

The presently marketed over half of all drugs are largely based on terrestrial natural products as sources. The largely unexplored marine world which is known to harbor the most pharmaceutical biodiversity could be a unique resource to discover novel drugs. Advancements in technologies such as sampling strategies, total chemical synthesis, biosynthesis, and genetic engineering could pave the way to the success of marine natural products as drug leads. Further, a joint venture between experts in Marine Biology and Pharmaceutical disciplines and drug companies with their financial support would certainly lead to successful marine drug discovery in the future.

CHAPTER 3

Promising Pharmaceutical Compounds of Marine Plants: Their Chemistry and Therapeutic Applications

Abstract: This chapter deals with the promising marine bioactive compounds of marine plants such as, seaweeds, seagrasses, mangroves, and halophytes; and their chemistry and therapeutic applications. Among the different constituents, the seaweeds in general and brown and red algae exhibited a variety of bioactivities followed by mangroves, seagrasses, and halophytes in that order.

Keywords: Halophytes chemical classes of bioactive compounds, Marine plants, Mangroves, Pharmaceutical marine biodiversity, Seaweeds, Seagrasses, Therapeutic activities.

INTRODUCTION

Several types of secondary metabolites have been isolated from plant sources of terrestrial origin and many of them are presently in preclinical trials or clinical trials or they are undergoing further investigation. However, the derivation of bioactive compounds as therapeutic agents from marine plants such as seaweeds. seagrasses, mangroves and halophytes is still in an infant stage due to the absence of an analogous ethno-medical history as compared to that of terrestrial environments; and the relative technical difficulties associated with the collection of the marine plant samples. In the past few decades, considerable efforts have been made, by both academic institutions and pharmaceutical companies to isolate new marine-derived secondary metabolites especially from marine invertebrates. However, marine plants are largely unexplored, and further research is therefore urgently needed in this field.

SEAWEEDS

Seaweeds (also known as macroalgae), which form one of the main ingredients used in East Asian food are multicellular, photoautotrophic organisms and are mainly inhabiting the seas or brackish water environments. Unlike terrestrial

Santhanam Ramesh, Ramasamy Santhanam & Veintramuthu Sankar

plants, these seaweeds are without vascular differentiations, and are distinguished by their coloration present in thallus, *i.e.* red (Rhodophyta), green (Chlorophyta), and brown (Phaeophyceae). Seaweeds are known for their rich health promoting molecules and minerals *viz.* sulphated polysaccharides, polyphenolics, terpenoids, flavonoids, pigments, MUFAs (monounsaturated fatty acids), PUFAs (polyunsaturated fatty acids), and HUFAs (highly unsaturated fatty acids), essential amino acids, vitamins (A, B1, B2, B9, B12, C, D, E, and K), and essential minerals (calcium, iron, iodine, magnesium, phosphorus, potassium, zinc, copper, manganese, selenium, and fluoride). These compounds have been reported to be of great value in the development of novel food products,nutraceuticals and pharmaceuticals. While the nutraceutical products might help prevent health problems, such as cancer, arthritis, diabetes, autoimmune diseases, ocular diseases, and cardiovascular diseases, the bioactive compounds of these organisms possess: anti-cancer, anti-fungal, anti-inflammatory, anti-cholesterol, anti-pruritic, anti-allergic, anti-viral, anti-bacterial, antioxidant, neuroprotective, chemoprotective, immunomodulatory, and hepatoprotective properties [14].

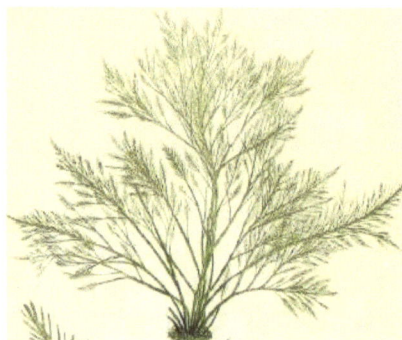

Fig. (1). *Bryopsis* sp.

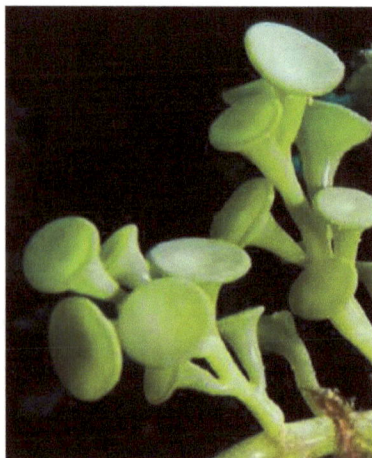

Fig. (2). *Caulerpa racemosa.*

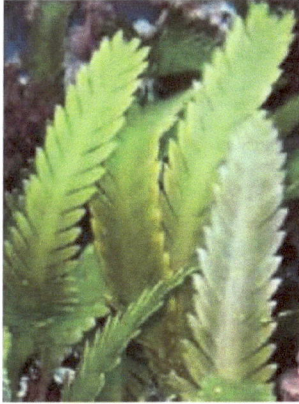

Fig. (3). *Caulerpa scalpelliformis.*

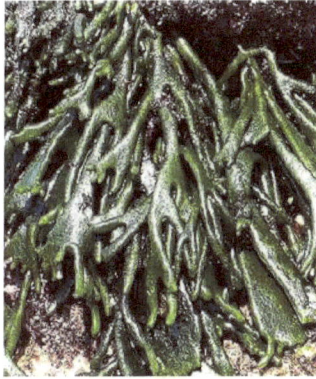

Fig. (4). *Codium decorticatum.*

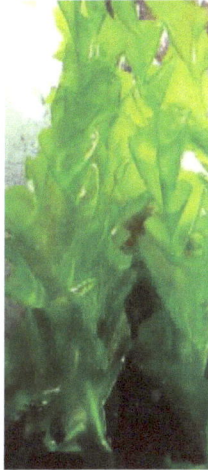

Fig. (5). *Ulva fasciata.*

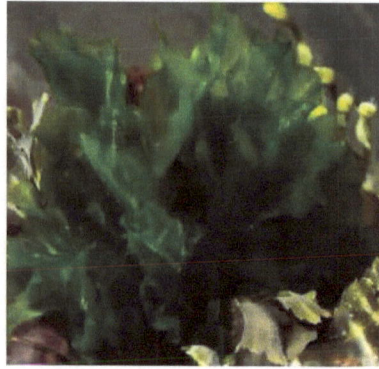

Fig. (6). *Ulva lactuca.*

Pharmaceutically Most Important Seaweed Species

Green Algae

Bryopsis sp.*, Caulerpa racemosa, Caulerpa scalpelliformis, Codium decorticatum, Ulva fasciata* and *Ulva lactuca* (Figs. **1** - **6**).

Image credit: *Bryopsis* sp., Internet Archive, Wikimedia commons; *Caulerpa racemose* and *Ulva lactuca,* Wikipedia;

Brown Algae

Alaria esculenta, Ascophyllum nodosum, Bifurcaria bifurcata, Colpomenia sinuosa, Eisenia bicyclis, Ecklonia cava, Fucus vesiculosus, Ishige okamurae, Laminaria digitata, Laminaria japonica, Sargassum spp.*, Stypodium* sp. and *Undaria pinnatifida* (Figs. **7** - **19**).

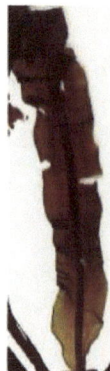

Fig. (7). *Alaria esculenta.*

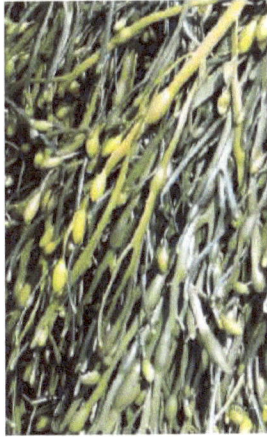

Fig. (8). *Ascophyllum nodosum.*

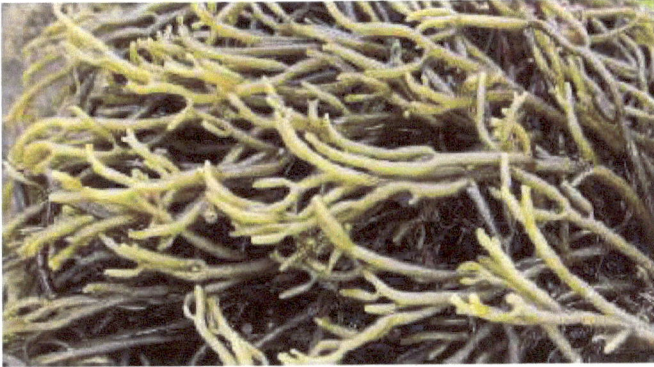

Fig. (9). *Bifurcaria bifurcata.*

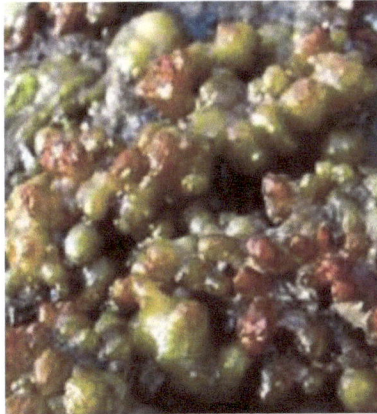

Fig. (10). *Colpomenia sinuosa.*

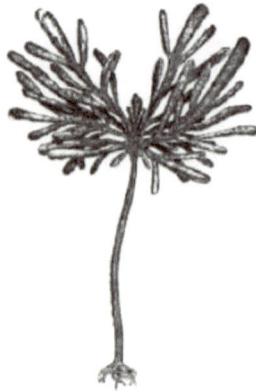

Fig. (11). *Eisenia bicyclis.*

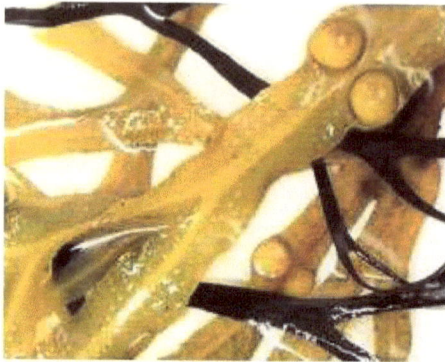

Fig. (12). *Ecklonia cava.*

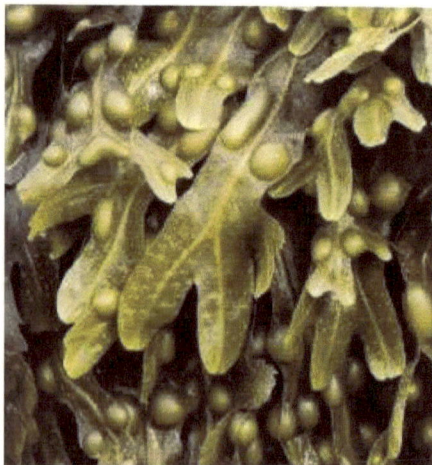

Fig. (13). *Fucus vesiculosus.*

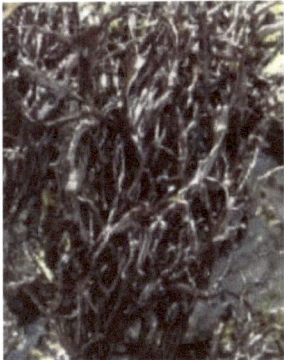

Fig. (14). *Ishige okamurae.*

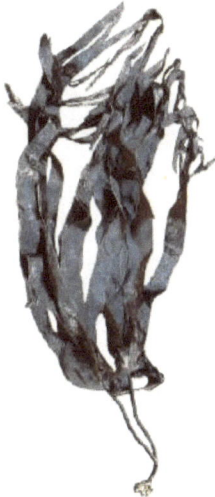

Fig. (15). *Laminaria digitata.*

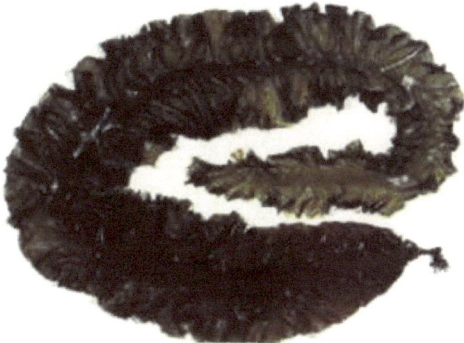

Fig. (16). *Laminaria japonica.*

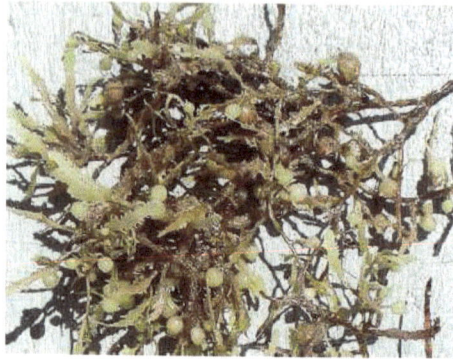

Fig. (17). *Sargassum* sp.

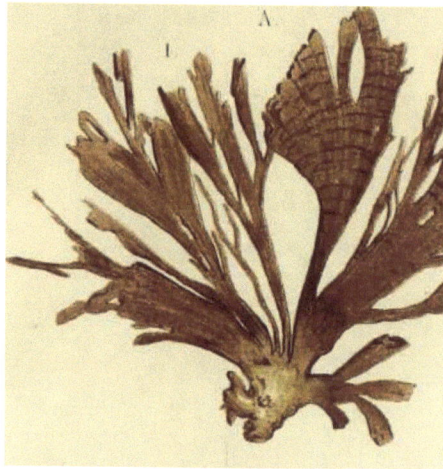

Fig. (18). *Stypodium* sp.

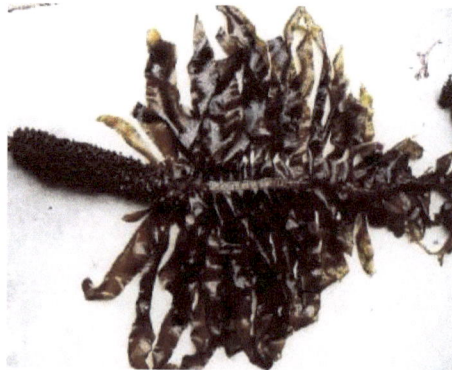

Fig. (19). *Undaria pinnatifida.*

Image credit: *Alaria esculenta, Ascophyllum nodosum, Colpomenia sinuosa Eisenia bicyclis* and *Laminaria digitata:* Wikipedia; Laminaia japonica: FAO; *Sargassum* sp., *Stypodium* sp. and *Undaria pinnatifida:* Wikipedia;

Red Algae

Champia parvula, Chondrus armatus, Chondrus ocellatus, Eucheuma sp., *Gigartina pistillata, Gracilaria* sp., *Grateloupia filicina, Portieria hornemannii* and *Spyridia* sp. (Figs. **20-28**).

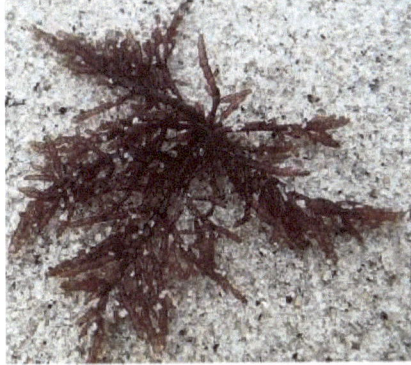

Fig. (20). *Champia parvula.*

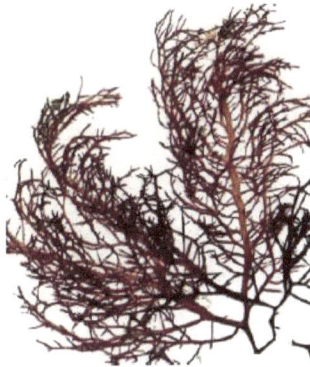

Fig. (21). *Chondrus armatus.*

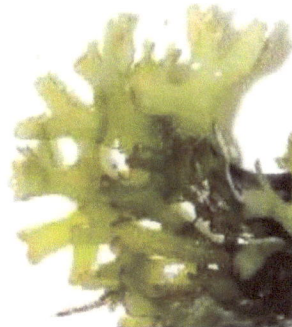

Fig. (22). *Chondrus ocellatus.*

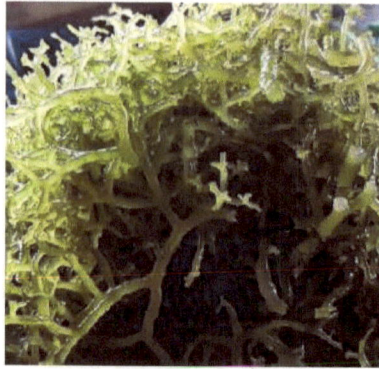

Fig. (23). *Eucheuma* sp.

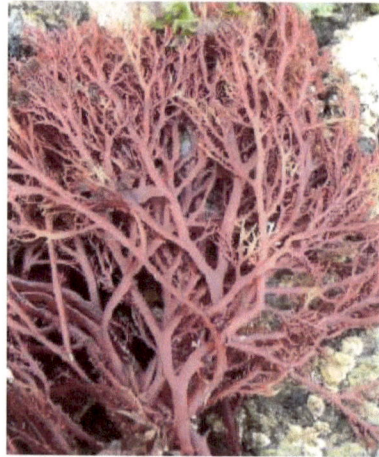

Fig. (24). *Gigartina pistillata.*

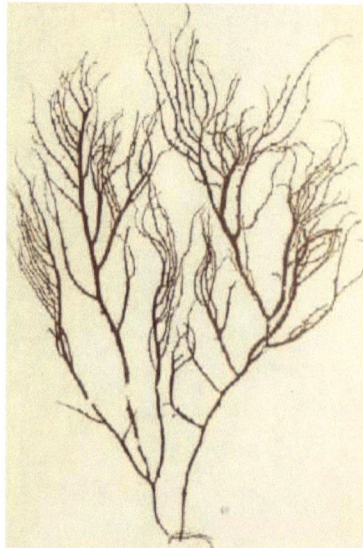

Fig. (25). *Gracilaria* sp.

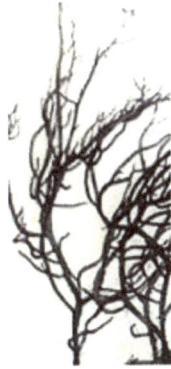

Fig. (26). *Grateloupia filicina.*

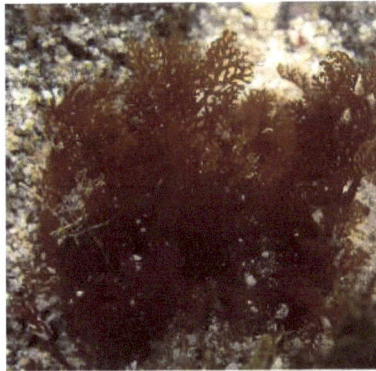

Fig. (27). *Portieria hornemannii.*

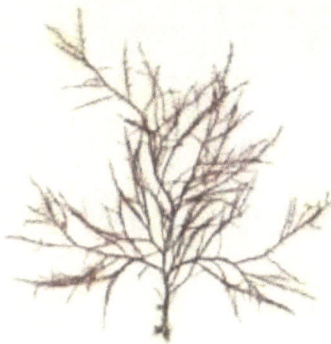

Fig. (28). *Spyridia* sp.

Image credit: *Champia parvula, Eucheuma* sp., *Portieria hornemannii.* and *Spyridia* sp.: Wikimedia commons;

THE BIOACTIVE COMPOUNDS AND THEIR THERAPEUTIC ACTIVITIES OF SEAWEEDS

Anticancer Activity

Green Algae

Bryopsis sp.

A depsipeptide kahalalide F derived from this alga (which is invariably fed by the marine mollusc *Elysia rufescens*) has been reported to show anticancer activity [15].

Caulerpa racemosa var. cylindracea

The sesquiterpene compound *viz.* caulerpenyne derived from this species displayed antiproliferative and apoptotic activity against neuroblastoma. In the model of HSY5Y and Kelly cell lines, an IC_{50} value of 6.02 µM was recorded [15].

Caulerpa racemosa and Caulerpa scalpelliformis

The high contents of phenolic and flavonoid compounds present in these species showed antitumoural activity against human hepatoma cancer cells Huh-7 and human cervical cancer cells HeLa [16].

Codium decorticatum

The dichloromethane and acetone/methanol extracts of this species showed anticancer activity by dramatically inhibiting the expression of the pro-inflammatory cytokine in endothelial cells. Further, the dichloromethane extract of this species displayed cytotoxic activity against the HeLa cell line (cervix cancer cells) by inducing apoptosis at the highest concentrations, thus suggesting this species as the potential candidate in therapeutic use for inflammatory diseases and cancer treatments [16].

Ulva lactuca and Ulva fasciata

The chloroform extracts of these species displayed potent cytotoxic activity against MCF-7, Hela cell lines. Further, the compound extracted from *Ulva lactuca* proved the cytotoxicity activity in fibroblast-like cells (L929) of C3H/HeJ mice connective tissue. On the other hand, the chloroform extract of *Ulva fasciata* extract had strong cytotoxic activity against PC3 and HepG2 cell lines [16].

Ulva rigida

The ethanolic extract of this species when injected in 24 male Wistar rats with induced diabetes mellitus created not only genotoxic and/or cytotoxic effect, but also it is effective in reducing the chromosome damage induced by the diabetes [16].

Brown Algae

Fucus vesiculosus, Alaria esculenta, Ascophyllum nodosum, Laminaria japonica, Sargassum muticum and Bifurcaria bifurcata

The phlorotannin extracts of these species have been reported to dose-dependently reduce the cell proliferation of tumour cell lines like human fibroblast (HFF-1), gastric cancer cells (MKN-28), human colon cancer cells lines (HT-29 cells and Caco-2), human hepatoma (BEL-7402), mouse leukaemia (P388) and mouse teratocarcinoma (ATDC5) [16].

Carpodesmia tamariscifolia (= Cystoseira tamariscifolia)

The acarotenoid metabolite, isololiolide derived from this species displayed anticancer activity against hepatocellular carcinoma by activating Caspase-3; decreasing Bcl-2 levels; and increasing p53 expression and PARP cleavage. The IC_{50} values recorded for Hep G2, AGS and HCT-15 cell lines were 13.2 µM, 32.4 µM, and 23.6 µM, respectively [15].

Colpomenia sinuosa and Sargassum prismaticum

The xanthophyll pigment *viz.* fucoxanthin isolated from these species has been reported to show a reduction in the viability of HCT-116 (colon adenocarcinoma), MCF-7 (breast adenocarcinoma) and HepG-2 (liver adenocarcinoma) cell lines [16].

Eisenia bicyclis

The phlorotannin, phlorofucofuroeckol A derived from this species showed anti-proliferative activity against colorectal adenocarcinoma by regulating transcriptional activity and apoptosis [15].

Ecklonia cava

The phlorotannin, eckol isolated from this species possessed potent anti-proliferative activity against human breast cancer cells MCF-7 [16].

Fucus vesiculosus

At a concentration of 100 ng/mL, the fucoidan derived from this species showed activity against human hepatoma cell line MHCC-97H by inhibiting tumor cell migration [15].

Ishige okamurae

The fucoxanthin isolated from this species showed anticancer activity by inhibiting B16-F10 melanoma cells implanted in albino mice [16].

Laminaria digitata

At a concentration of 25 mg/kg, the polysaccharide laminarin derived from this species showed activity against B16-ovallbumin melanoma tumor which was associated with the inhibition tumor growth and metastasis in mice mode [15].

Laminaria japonica

The fucoxanthin isolated from this species displayed anticancer activity by inhibiting the tumour growth in lung cancer. Further, this compound showed similar effects *in vitro* metastasis models of B16-F10 melanoma cells [16].

Sargassum carpophyllum

Two bioactive sterols derived from this species have been reported to exhibit cytotoxic activity against several cultured cancer cell lines [17].

Sargassum hemiphyllum

At a concentration of 50 mg/mL, the oligo-fucoidan derived from this species showed anticancer activity against HCT116 cell line with tumorigenicity and regulation of apoptosis [15].

Sargassum sp.

At a concentration of 21-33 mg/mL, the fucoidan derived from this alga showed antimetastatic (anti-cancer) activity against SMMC-7721, Huh7, and HCCLM3 liver by deactivating the integrin $\alpha V\beta 3$/SRC/E2F1 signaling pathway [16].

Stypodium zonale

An o-quinone compound stypoldione isolated form this species showed cytotoxicity by inhibiting microtubule polymerization and thus preventing mitotic spindle formation [17].

Undaria pinnatifida

The long chain sulfated polysaccharide, fucoidan derived from this species has shown anticancer activity against Hep G2 cells through oxidative stress and chronic inflammation reduction and the LD50 recorded in this case was 18.01 µg/mL. Further, at a concentration of 10 µg/mL, the anticancer drug, eckol derived from this species showed radioprotective activity against V79-4 cells through the inhibition of cellular DNA damage and membrane lipid peroxidation. Furthermore, the fucoidan derived from the sporophylls of this species showed T-cell mediated and NK cell response in leukemia A20 cells through the tumor destruction by immune response [15]. The fucoxanthins extract from this species showed anticancer activity against human lung adenocarcinoma cell line A549 melanoma Malme-3M and cervix squamous SiHa cells carcinoma by inhibiting their cell growth [16].

Unidentified species of brown Algae

The polyphenolic compound phloroglucinol derived from this unidentified brown alga showed anticancer activity against intraductal carcinoma by decreasing CD44+ cancer cell population and as expression of CSC regulators such as Sox2, CD44, Oct4, Notch2 and β-catenin; and by inhibiting KRAS and its downstream PI3K/AKT and RAF-1/ERK signaling pathway. In the model cell line MCF-7, an IC_{50} value of 50 µM was recorded. Further the fucoidan and phycocolloid, Algasol T331 compounds derived from similar algal species showed anticancer activity [15].

Red Algae

Champia parvula

In vivo tests with its polysaccharides displayed antitumoural effect with sarcoma 180 ascites tumour cells implanted subcutaneously into mice. Further, these polysaccharides showed *in vitro* cytotoxicity against the proliferation of HL-60 (human leukaemia), MDA-MB-435 (melanoma), SF-295 (brain), and HCT-8 (human colon) cell lines. Further, these polysaccharides inhibited sarcoma 180 tumour growth in mice. Furthermore, when these mice were treated simultaneously with both the sulphated polysaccharide and the chemotherapeutic agent fluorouracil (5-FU), the tumour inhibition rate increased significantly. The latter is a very interesting finding to improve the efficacy of anticancer therapy, developing efficient combination of chemotherapeutic drugs, whereas the side effects are reduced [16].

Chondrus armatus

The sulfated polysaccharides *viz.* κ-carrageenan and λ-carrageenan originally derived from this species (and sourced from Sigma-Aldrich) displayed anti-cancer and anti-proliferative activity against cervical carcinoma. While κ-carrageenan delayed cell cycle in G2/M phase in HeLa cell line model with an iC_{50} value of 550.8 µg/mL the λ-carrageenan hindered the cell cycle in both G1 and G2/M phase; and cellular division suppression with an IC_{50} value of 475 µg/mL. Further, λ-carrageenan (sourced from Sigma-Aldrich), when injected every two days intratumorally at a dose of 50 mg/kg in mice, inhibited tumor growth in melanoma B16-F10 and mammary cancer 4T1 by increasing tumor-infiltrating M1 macrophages, and proinflammatory cytokines [15].

Chondrus ocellatus

The extract of this species has shown anti-tumoural activity against H-22 tumour cells implanted on mice. Further, the ingestion of a mixture of ʎ-carrageenan and 5-FU resulted in an enhanced anti-tumour activity. 5-Fu, which is otherwise called as fluorouracil, is one of the most commonly used drugs to treat cancer.

This drug is usually included in chemotherapy treatments due to their suppression of many tumour cells [15,16].

Chondrus, Gigartina, Eucheuma and Iridaea spp

κ-carrageenan of the carrageenans extract from the species of these genera has been reported to significantly prevent *in vitro* growth of fibroblasts, HeLa cells and mammary cells [16].

Gigartina pistillata

The κ/ι hybrid carrageenan derived from the female gametophyte of this species showed anti-tumor and anti-proliferative activity against colorectal adenocarcinoma. In the models of CSC-enriched tumourspheres and HT29, SW620- and SW480- derived tumourspheres, an IC_{50} value of 0.6572 µg/mL was recorded. Further, λ/ξ hybrid derived from the tetrasporophyte of this species showed similar activity with an IC_{50} value of 0.7050 µg/mL. Further, the ι/ε carrageenans extracted from this species demonstrate din vitro potential against colorectal cancer stem cells-like cells [16].

Gracilaria dominguensis

The agar-type polysaccharide extracted from this species possessed potent *in vivo* anti-tumour activity by inducing apoptosis and inhibiting the transplantation of Ehrlich ascites carcinoma in mice. It is also suggested that the agar oligosaccharides of this species may be used as an alternative or complementary drug for people with diseases [16].

Grateloupia filicina

An agaran-type polysaccharide derived from this species displayed anti-angiogenic activity through HUVECs differentiation into capillary-like structures inhibition *in vitro* and reduction of migrated cells. In the model of HUVECs, an inhibitory ratio of 28.6% was recorded [15].

Portieria hornemannii

The methanol extracts of this species showed potent cytotoxic activity against Dalton's lymphoma ascite and Ehrlich ascite carcinoma cell lines with IC_{50} values of 209 μg/mL and 190 μg/mL respectively [17, 18].

Spyridia fusiformis

The methanol extracts of this species showed potent cytotoxic activity against Dalton's lymphoma ascite and Ehrlich ascite carcinoma cell lines with IC_{50} values of 190 μg/mL and 1182 μg/mL, respectively [18].

ANTICANCER COMPOUNDS FROM SEAWEEDS THAT ARE ALREADY IN USE OR IN ADVANCED CLINICAL TRIALS

i. The fucoidan derived from certain species of brown seaweeds has been reported to show chemoprotection. In clinical trials, 92.8% disease control rate has been recorded in patients with colorectal adenocarcinoma. Further it is also known that this compound decreased fatigue and increased longevity of patients who underwent chemotherapy [15].
ii. A depsipeptide. kahalalide F isolated from the species of green seaweeds has been serving as anti-cancer agent in various types of cancers. In the clinical trial relating to hepatocellular carcinoma treatment, this compound induced cell death through oncosis [15].
iii. The phycocolloid, algasol T331 derived from certain species of brown seaweeds has served as radioprotective and post-surgical adjuvant in various types of cancer. In clinical use, this compound has been reported to increase in physical condition performance, in patients undergoing surgery or radiation therapy [15].

Antiviral Activity

Green Algae

Caulerpa brachypus

The different fractions of polysaccharides isolated from this species showed antiviral activity by not only inhibiting the first stages of HSV-1 but also in the penetration into host cells [16].

Caulerpa sp.

The alkaloid compound, caulerpin isolated from this alga demonstrated antiviral effects on bovine viral diarrhea virus. The viability test conducted in Vero cells showed that caulerpin has promising antiviral activity against HSV-1 [16].

Ulva fasciata

The sphingosine derivative produced by this species has shown antiviral activity *in vivo* [17].

Ulva lactuca

The polysaccharide ulvan derived from this species has shown anti-influenza A virus (IAV) activity [16].

Brown Algae

Fucus evanescens

The fucoidan from this species and its derivative have shown antiviral activity against Herpes Simplex Virus type 1 (HSV-1), Herpes Simplex Virus type 2 (HSV-2), enterovirus (ECHO-1) and human immunodeficiency virus (HIV-1). The *in vitro* results displayed the ability of both fucoidans to increase resistance to virus, directly affecting the cell and inhibiting early stage of virus replication [16].

Sargassum patens

The fucoidans of this species showed antiviral activity. *In vivo* studies demonstrated that the intraperitoneal administration of fucoidans in mice protected the animals from lethal intravaginal HSV-2 infection. Further, an increase of anti-HSV activity was detected with the increasing sulphate ester content of polysaccharides of this species. These results suggest the feasibility of inhibiting HSV infection with its polysaccharide which is believed to possess specific structure against the virus [16].

Red Algae

Gigartina skottsbergii

The carrageenans of this species have shown antiviral activity against intraperitoneal murine HSV-1 and HSV-2 infection. Further, its ι- and k-carrageenans expressed their antiherpetic activity. Furthermore, its λ-carrageenan and ι-carrageenan have been reported to serve as potent inhibitors of dengue virus type 2 (DENV-2) and type 3 (DENV-3) [16].

Laurencia obtusa and Pterocladia capillacea

The extracts of this species have shown antiviral activity against Hepatitis C Virus *in vitro* [16].

Schizymenia binderi

By a plaque reduction assay in Vero cells, it was found that the polysaccharide extracted from this species has shown antiviral activity against HSV-1 and HSV-2 [16].

Anti-inflammatory Activity

Green Algae

Caulerpa mexicana

The methanolic extract treatment of this species has been reported to ameliorate ulcerative colitis in mice. This algal treatment has decreased the level of cytokines which is associated with a reduction in tissue damage found in the colon of the animals. This extract therefore appears to be promising for research on metabolites that may be helpful for anti-inflammatory treatment [16].

Caulerpa racemosa

At the concentration of 40 and 4 mg/kg of body weight, the indole alkaloid compound, caulerpin displayed anti-inflammatory activity by reducing leukocyte recruitment *in vitro* on zymosan-induced peritonitis model and *in vivo* on DSS-induced ulcerative colitis mice [16].

Chaetomorpha linum, Ulva intestinalis, Ulva lactuca and Ulva prolifera

The extract of these species showed anti-inflammatory activity by inhibiting the cyclooxygenase-2 (COX-2) which seems to be responsible for inflammation [16].

Codium decorticatum

The dichloromethane and acetone/methanol extracts of this species displayed anti-inflammatory activity by dramatically inhibiting the expression of the pro-inflammatory cytokine in endothelial cells. This species has been suggested to be a potential candidate in therapeutic use for inflammatory diseases [16].

Ulva conglobata

The methanol extracts of this species have shown anti-inflammatory activities in hippocampal neuronal HT22 cells and mouse microglial BV2 cells [16].

Brown Algae

Fucus vesiculosus

The fucoidan extracted from this species has shown anti-inflammatory activity. Its fucoidan-based cream has been reported to dose-dependently inhibit paw edema after topical application and it has the potential to treat pain and inflammatory diseases [16].

Rhizoclonium riparium

The extract of these species showed anti-inflammatory activity by inhibiting the cyclooxygenase-2 (COX-2) which is believed to be responsible for inflammation [16].

Antioxidant Activity

Brown Algae

Colpomenia sinuosa and Sargassum prismaticum

Fucoxanthin isolated from this species has shown *in vivo* antioxidant activity [16].

Cystoseira hakodatensis and Sargassum horneri

The higher total phenolic content and fucoxanthin of these species have shown antioxidant activity [16].

Cystoseira sedoides, Cladostephus spongeosis and Padina pavonica

The phlorotannin-rich fractions derived from these species displayed *in vivo* antioxidant activity. Among these species, *Cystoseira sedoides* recorded strong activity towards radicals which was associated with a reduction of paw edema and ear thickness in a dose-dependent way in mice models [16].

Red Algae

Laurencia dendroidea

The extract of this species has shown antioxidant activities in DPPH, nitric oxide radical scavenging and metal chelating assays [16].

Anticoagulant Activity

Green Algae

Ulva lactuca

The sulphated polysaccharides of this species have been reported to possess anticoagulant potential. Intravenous injection of polysaccharides of this species into the caudal vein of rats inhibited venous thrombus formation. Further, this compound displayed 56% reduction in the weight of the thrombus formed with polysaccharides (20 μg/g of rat weight). This finding makes this species an exciting option for future investigation for anticoagulant drugs [16].

Brown Algae

Fucus vesiculosus

The high molecular weight of fucoidan from this species has elucidated the anti-coagulant bioactivities in several *in vitro* models [16].

Undaria pinnatifida

The anticoagulant activity of fucoidan of this species has been detected in *in vivo* assay, where human volunteers consumed 3 g fucoidan for 12 days of oral administration [16].

Red Algae

Solieria filiformis

The anticoagulant potential of carrageenans of this species has been assessed by both *in vitro* activated partial thromboplastin time (APTT) and prothrombin (PT) tests. These results displayed a considerable reduction and inhibition of thrombin and factor X in blood coagulation and this species is therefore considered a good candidate for the development of anticoagulant natural drugs [16].

Antidiabetic Activity (Alpha-glucosidase Inhibitory Activity and the Anti-hyperglycemic Effects)

Brown Algae

Ecklonia cava

The methanol extract of this species has been reported to possess anti-diabetic activity by significantly reducing the plasma glucose level and increasing insulin concentration in type 1 diabetes mellitus rats. Further, the elevation of plasma ALT (alanine aminotransferase) in the experimental diabetic rats was significantly restored near to normal range by the extract treatment whereas the AST (aspartate aminotransferase) level was not at all altered in these rats throughout the experiment. Furthermore, the typical indications of diabetes, *viz.* polyphagia and polydipsia, were also found to be greatly improved by this extract treatment [19].

Ecklonia stolonifera

The high content of polyphenols *viz.* phlorotannins present in the methanolic extract of this species have shown anti-diabetic activity by strongly inhibiting alpha-glucosidase in non-insulin dependent diabetic mice. While male KK-A(y) mice, a genetically non-insulin dependent diabetic model, showed hyperglycemia with aging, the ingestion of the extract has been reported to suppress the increase in plasma glucose and lipid peroxidation levels in unfasted KK-A(y) mice dose dependently. Further, in KK-A(y) mice, which were fed the extract diet for 4 weeks, the extract moderated the elevation of plasma glucose levels after the oral administration of maltose. These findings suggest that this seaweed species may have beneficial properties in the prevention of diabetes and it could be very useful in the development of an anti-diabetic pharmaceutical and functional food [20].

Ishige okamurae

Obesity has been reported to yield deleterious consequences relating to insulin resistance, which is known to adversely affect blood glucose. The bioactive compounds derived from the extract of this species are known to possess anti-diabetic activity *via* the regulation of glucose homeostasis [21].

Macrocystis pyrifera and Sargassum fusiforme

The polysaccharides of these species have shown anti-diabetic activity in streptozotocin-induced diabetic rats. Oral administration of these polysaccharides has been reported to significantly control the increase of levels of blood glucose, triglyceride and total cholesterol in diabetic rats. It is therefore suggested that the polysaccharides from these species could be promising candidates as natural medicines and functional foods for the improvement of diabetes problems [16].

Undaria pinnatifida

The fucoidan extract of this species has been reported to display significant inhibitory effects against α-glucosidase, suggesting fucoidans from this species could serve as an anti-diabetic agent [16].

Red Algae

Grateloupia lithophila, Spyridia filamentosa, Grateloupia lithophila and Hypnea musciformis

The methanolic extract of these species has shown anti-diabetic property. However, the crude methanolic extract of *Spyridia filamentosa,* showed significant anti-diabetic potential through the inhibition of α-amylase and α-glucosidase [16].

Hypnea valentiae

An iodinated novel nucleoside isolated from this species showed anti-diabetic activity by serving as a potent and specific inhibitor of adenosine kinase [17].

Laurencia dendroidea

The anti-diabetic activity was tested *in vivo* on mice. The extract of this species showed anti-diabetic activity which is associated with a strong inhibition of α-glucosidase [16].

Anti-allergic Effects

Ecklonia stolonifera

Phlorotannins *viz.* phlorofucofuroeckol A isolated from this brown alga have been reported to attenuate allergic reactions and this species may serve as a promising candidate for the design of novel inhibitor allergic reaction. *In vivo* assay on rats fed with this species displayed inhibition of IgE and anti-degranulation of histamine, suggesting that this species might possess anti-allergic effects [16].

AChE and BChE Inhibitory Activity (for the Treatment of Alzheimer's Disease)

Brown Algae

The acetylcholinesterase (AChE) inhibiting agents of brown seaweed species include phlorotannins of *Dictyota humifusa;* phenols in *Cystoseira tamariscifolia, Cystoseira nodicaulis, Ecklonia maxima, Ecklonia stolonifera* and *Ishige okamurae*; ethanol extracts of *Cystoseira usneoides* and *Fucus spiralis*; and dieckol and phlorofucofuroeckol, (phlorotannins) in brown *Eisenia bicyclis* and *Ecklonia* sp.[16]. The ethyl acetate (EtOAc) fraction of the ethanolic extract of Eisenia bicyclis displayed potent inhibitory activities against AChE and BChE with IC_{50} values of 2.8 and 3.5 µg/mL, respectively. It is also suggested that these algae could be used in the future as therapeutic agents for Alzheimer's disease [22].

Brown and Red Algae

Machadoa, *et al.* (2015) reported that the ethanolic extract of the brown alga, *Ecklonia stolonifera* and the methanolic and ethanolic extracts of the brown alga *Ishige okamurae* displayed anti-AChE activity with an IC_{50} value of 100 g/ml (*Ecklonia stolonifera*); and IC_{50} values of 163.1 M and IC_{50} 137. 3 M, respectively (*Ishige okamurae).* However, the extracts of red alga, *Ochtodes secundiramea* showed moderate activity (48.6%), while the other red algal species *viz.Hypnea musciformis* and *Pterocladiella capillace*a extracts had weak activity (7.2 and 5.4%, respectively), at a higher concentration [16].

Angiotensin-converting Enzyme (ACE) Inhibitory Activity (Angiotensin Receptor Blockers for Treating Cardiovascular Disorders)

Brown Algae

Ecklonia cava

The phlorotannins such as dieckol, 2,7-phloroglucinol-6,6-bieckol, phloro-fucofuroeckol A, and pyrogallol-phloroglucinol-6,6- bieckol (PPB) derived from this species inhibited monocyte migration and differentiation to inflammatory macrophages and monocyte associated vascular cell dysfunction. Further, the PPB has been reported to improve blood circulation and significantly reduce blood pressure, serum cholesterol, and lipoprotein levels in vivo. Furthermore, its dieckol promoted vasodilation by regulating blood-flow velocity in a zebrafish model [23].

Ecklonia stolonifera

Phlorotannins, such as Phloroglucinol, eckstolonol, eckol, phlorofucofuroeckol A, and dieckol; polyphenol Triphlorethol-A; and sterol fucosterol derived from this species displayed ACE inhibitory activity with IC_{50} values: phloroglucinol: (N.A.), eckstolonol (410.1 μM), eckol (70.8 μM), phlorofucofuroeckol A (12.7 μM), dieckol (34.3 μM), Triphlorethol-A (700.9 μM) and fucosterol (N.A.) [23].

Antiaging Activity

Cystoseira nodicaulis, Eisenia bicyclis and Ecklonia kurome

The phlorotannins derivatives such as fucophloroethol, fucodiphloroethol, fucotriphloroethol, 7-phloroeckol, phlorofucofuroeckol and bieckol/dieckol derived from *Cystoseira nodicaulis* displayed hyaluronidase activity thereby these compounds serve as potential candidates for the production of anti-aging creams. Similarly, the dieckol, eckol, bieckol, and phlorofucofuroeckol A derived from *Eisenia bicyclis* and *Ecklonia kurome* also displayed potent inhibition towards *hyaluronidase* [16].

Ecklonia cava

The phlorotannins, 7-phloroeckol and dieckol isolated from this brown algae exhibited higher inhibitory activity against tyrosinase, an enzyme linked with the melanin hyperpigmentation of skin [16].

Anti-obesity Activity (Anti-adipogenesis)

Brown Algae

Ecklonia cava

At a concentration of 20 µM, polyphenol, triphlorethol-A and phlorotannins, eckol and dieckol isolated from this species showed anti-obesity activity by decreasing intracellular lipid accumulation and increasing intracellular calcification. Further, at 200 µg/mL, in *in vitro* studies, its dieckol inhibited adipocyte differentiation, intracellular triglyceride accumulation, and lipid accumulation in 3T3-L1 cells. Furthermore, *in vivo* studies, administration of dieckol was found to reduce total cholesterols, triglycerides and low-density lipoproteins in the serum of high-fat diet mice [23].

Ecklonia stolonifera

In *in vitro* studies, the phlorotannins of this species such as phloroglucinol, eckol, dieckol, dioxinodehydroeckol, and phlorofucofuroeckol A showed anti-obesity effects by reducing lipid accumulation and suppressed adipocyte differentiation through inhibiting C/EBPα and PPARγ expression. Further, in *in vivo* studies, these compounds exhibited Cu^{2+}-induced LDL oxidation inhibitory activity with IC_{50} values *viz.* phloroglucinol (87.3 µM), dioxinodehydroeckol (16.6 µM), eckol (7.5 µM), phlorofucofuroeckol-A (4.3 µM), dieckol (3.1 µM), and 7-phloroeckol (9.1 µM) [23].

Eisenia bicyclis

In *in vitro* studies, its phlorotannin compounds *viz.* 6,60 -bieckol, 6,80 -bieckol, 8,80 -bieckol, dieckol, and phlorofucofuroeckol-A displayed anti-obesity effects by suppressing the differentiation of 3T3-L1 adipocyte through the downregulation of adipogenesis and lipogenesis [23].

Ishige okamurae

The bioactive compounds derived from the extract of this species are known to possess anti-obesity and anti-diabetic properties, elicited *via* the regulation of lipid metabolism [21].

Red Algae

Gracilaria lemaneiformis, Kappaphycus alvarezii and Sarconema filiforme

In *in vivo* studies, ingestion of ι-carrageenan derived from *Sarconema filiforme* and κ-carrageenan extracted from *Kappaphycus alvarezii* showed anti-obesity effects by decreasing body weight, systolic blood pressure, abdominal fat, liver fat and plasma total cholesterol concentrations in mice models. Further, the consumption of polysaccharides extracted from *Gracilaria lemaneiformi*s displayed significant anti-obesity activities in obese hamsters, with a decrease in the weight of adipose tissue, body and liver and lower plasma leptin, total cholesterol and triglyceride levels [16].

Antinociceptive Activity

Dichotomaria obtusata

The methanolic extract of this red algae showed antinociceptive activity in the writhing test in mice treated with acetic acid. Treatment of the extract at 12.5 mg/kg reduced the number of writhes in 47.7%, which was subsequently decreased in 80.2% with 100 mg/kg of the extract. It is also interesting to note that the maximum dose of the extract (800 mg/kg) had a very clear antinociceptive effect with a significant reduction of the number of writhes [24].

Neuroprotective Activity

Several species of marine macroalgae have shown neuroprotective activity [25]. The algal species possessing neuroprotective activity along with their compounds and effective concentrations are given below (Table 1).

Table 1. Neuroprotective activity of marine macroalgal species.

Alga/Species	Compound	Chemistry	Effective conc.
Green alga *Caulerpa racemosa*	Racemosins A	Bisindole alkaloid	10μM
Brown algae *Dictyopteris undulata*	Zonarol	p-hydroquinone sesquiterpene	ED50, 0.22 μM
Ecklonia cava	Eckol, dieckol and 8,8′-bieckol	Phlorotannins	1–50 μM
Ecklonia maxima	Eckmaxol	Phlorotannin	20 μm
Ecklonia stolonifera	Fucosterol	Sterol	5–10 μM
Eisenia bicyclis	Phloroglucinol; dioxinodehydroeckol, eckol, phlorofucofuroeckol A, dieckol, and 7-phloroeckol	Phloroglucinol: Polyphenol; Others: Phlorotannins	2.5, 5, 10 and 20 μg/m respectively

(Table 1) cont.....

Alga/Species	Compound	Chemistry	Effective conc.
Padina gymnospora	α-Bisabolol	Sesquiterpene	5 µg/mL
Undaria pinnatifida	Fucoxanthin	Xanthophyll	0.15–1.5 µmol/L
Shige okamurae	Diphlorethohydroxycarmalol	Phlorotannin	50 µM
Red alga *Gracilaria cornea*	Sulfated agaran	Sulfated Polysaccharide	60 µg

Hepatoprotective Activity

Brown Algae

Colpomenia sinuosa and Sargassum prismaticum

The xanthophyll pigment *viz.* fucoxanthin isolated from these species has been reported to show *in vivo* hepatoprotective ability [16].

Turbinaria ornata

At a concentration of 200 mg/kg, the extract of this species showed hepatoprotective activity with a significant reduction of direct bilirubin [26].

Red Algae

Gracilaria crassa and Laurencia papillosa

At a concentration of 200 mg/kg, the extract of *Gracilaria crassa* showed a prominent hepatoprotective activity by showing a marked effect on the serum marker enzymes. Further, the level of the liver enzyme *viz.* serum glutamic pyruvic transaminase was found to be prominently reduced by all extract concentrations than that by standard drug. Further, at the same concentration, the extract of *Laurencia papillosa* was also found to reduce the level of bilirubin equal to that of the standard drug [26].

Antiulcer Activity

Gracilaria crassa and Laurencia papillosa

At 200 mg/kg concentration, the acetone extract of these red algae has been reported to possess antiulcer activity by significantly reducing the total volume of gastric juice, free and total acidity of gastric secretion and Na+ content of gastric juice in experimental rats. Further, the considerable increase in pH level and K+ content indicated good antiulcer activity against gastric pyloric ulcers in these animals. Furthermore, the activities of these extracts were comparable to the performance of the standard drug Ranitidine. It is also worthy of mention that the extract of *Laurencia papillosa* exhibited the highest level of gastric protection activity at all concentrations [26].

Wound Healing Activity

Brown Alga

Turbinaria ornata

At a concentration of 200 mg/kg, the extract of this species displayed weak wound-healing activity when compared to standard drug on the 20th day [26].

Red Algae

Gracilaria crassa and Laurencia papillosa

The extracts of these algae have been reported to show marked wound-healing activity when compared to that of the reference standard and a control group of albino rats. At a concentration of 200 mg/kg, *Gracilaria crassa* displayed wound-healing activity ((249 mm2) on the 6th day of the experiment and this was comparable with that of standard ointment ((243 mm2). Further, the reduction in wound area was significant in rats treated with *Gracilaria crassa* (9 mm2) and *Laurencia papillosa* (10 mm2) at the concentration of 200 mg/kg when compared to the positive control group of animals (5mm2) on the 18th day. Furthermore, on the 20th day, these two extracts at the same concentration showed complete healing at the same concentration in comparison with the standard drug [26].

Immunomodulatory Activity

Green Alga

Ulva conglobata

The methanol extracts of this species have shown immunomodulatory activity by inhibiting iNOS, (inducible nitric oxide synthase) decreasing the production of free radicals and COX-2 (cyclooxygenase-2) expressions in microglia which are a type of neuroglia (glial cell) located throughout the brain and spinal cord. These microglia are considered immune sentinels that are capable of orchestrating a potent inflammatory response [16].

Brown Algae

Undaria pinnatifida, Laminaria japonica, Laminaria cichorioides, Fucus vesiculosus and Fucus evanescens

The fucoidans derived from these algae have been reported to possess immunomodulatory activity. Purified fucoidan of *Undaria pinnatifida* promoted activation of human neutrophils, natural killer cells (NK), and production of pro-inflammatory cytokines (IL-6, IL-8, and TNF-α) and delayed their spontaneous cell death. Similarly, the fucoidan of Fucus vesiculosus enhanced the immune responses of the T helper type 1 (Th1) cells. Further, the fucoidans of *Laminaria japonica, Laminaria cichorioides,* and *Fucus evanescens* activated the immune defense [27].

Ascophyllum nodosum, Macrocystis pyrifera, Undaria pinnatifida, and Fucus vesiculosus

All fucoidans of these species have been reported to possess immunomodulatory activity by increasing the production of IL-6, IL-8, and TNF-α from purified human neutrophils. Further, the fucoidan from *Macrocystis pyrifera* has been reported to be the most promising compound due to its delayed neutrophil apoptosis and potential to enhance T cell immune responses [27].

Red Alga

Gracilaria fisheri

The predominant sulfated galactan, SG-1 of this species showed immunomodulatory activity by activating murine J774A.1 macrophages *via* the dectin-1 signaling pathway. It is also suggested that the sulfated galactans of this species may be of great value for immune-potentiating treatment in humans [28].

SEAGRASSES

Seagrasses are one of the true marine flowering plants (angiosperms) with worldwide distribution. There are 72 species of seagrasses belonging to four families *viz.* Zosteraceae, Hydrocharitaceae, Posidoniaceae, and Cymodoceaceae. The seagrass beds of temperate, subtropical, and tropical seas are found in shallow coastal areas with distribution ranging between 50 and 90 m in depth. These seagrass meadows are known to act as biological indicators as they store carbon, improve water quality and provide food and habitat to other organisms. The seagrass species producing biomedically important compounds are given below.

Biomedically Important Seagrass Families and their Species

Cymodoceaceae

Cymodocea nodosa, Cymodocea rotundata, Cymodocea serrulata, Halodule pinifolia, Halodule uninervis, Syringodium isoetifolium, Syringodium filiforme and *Thalassodendron ciliatum* (Figs. **29 - 36**).

Hydrocharitaceae

Enhalus acoroides, Halophila beccarii, Halophila ovalis, Halophila stipulaceae, Thalassia hemprichii, and *Thalassia testudinum* (Figs. **37 - 42**).

Posidoniaceae

Posidonia oceanica (Fig. **43**).

Zosteraceae

Zostera marina and *Zostera noltei* (Figs. **44** and **45**).

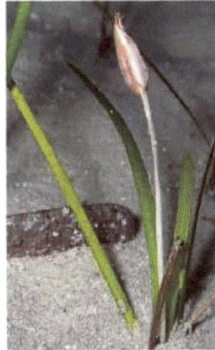

Fig. (29). *Cymodocea nodosa.*

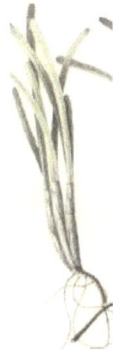

Fig. (30). *Cymodocea rotundata.*

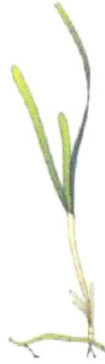

Fig. (31). *Cymodocea serrulata.*

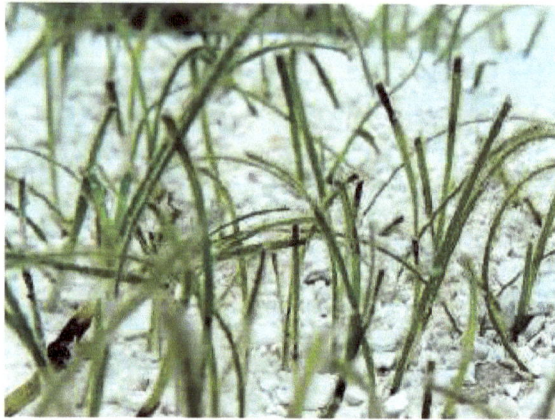

Fig. (32). *Halodule pinifolia.*

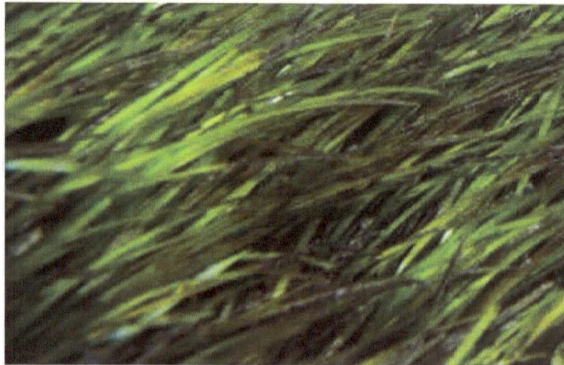

Fig. (33). *Halodule uninervis.*

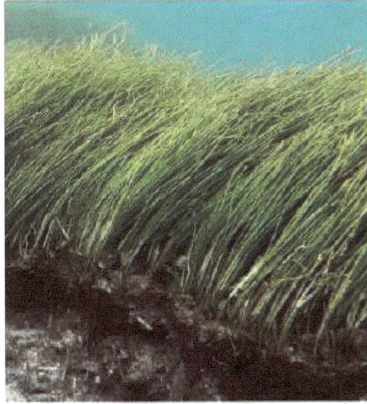

Fig. (34). *Syringodium isoetifolium.*

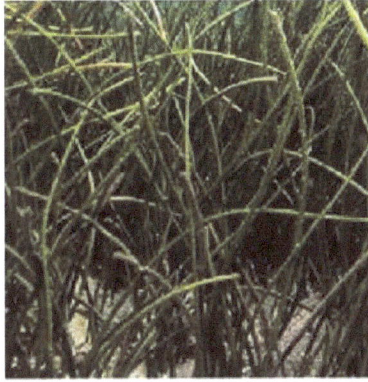

Fig. (35). *Syringodium filiforme.*

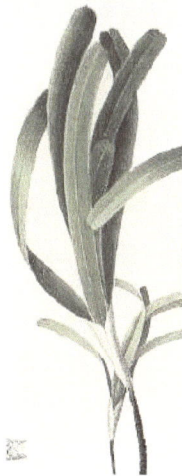

Fig. (36). *Thalassodendron ciliatum.*

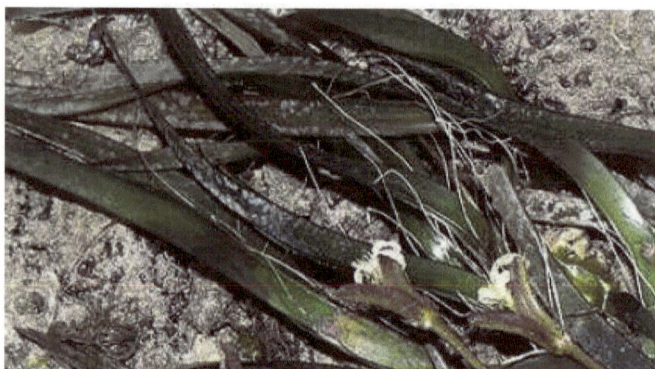

Fig. (37). *Enhalus acoroides.*

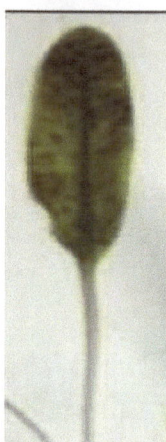

Fig. (38). *Halophila beccarii.*

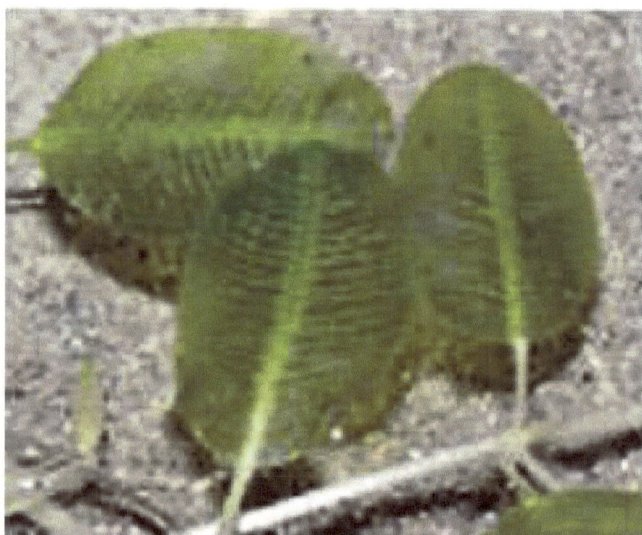

Fig. (39). *Halophila ovalis.*

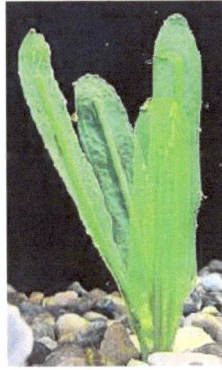

Fig. (40). *Halophila stipulaceae.*

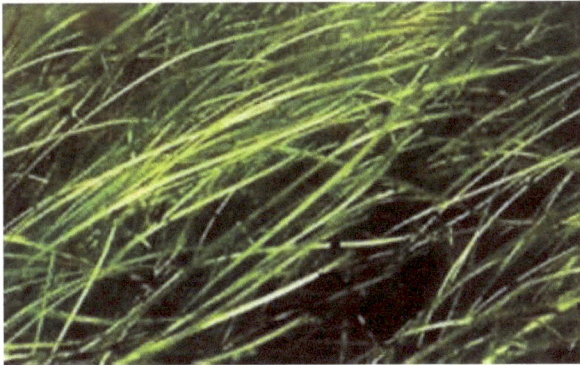

Fig. (41). *Thalassia hemprichii.*

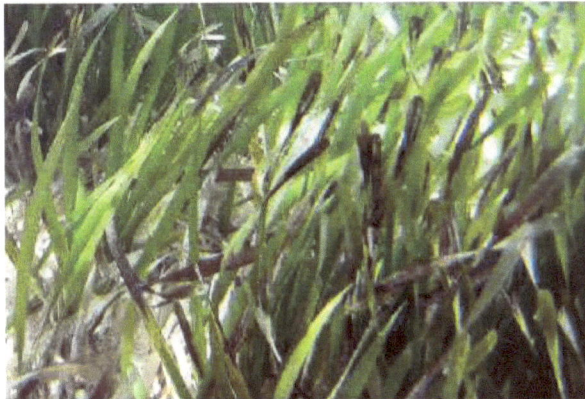

Fig. (42). *Thalassia testudinum.*

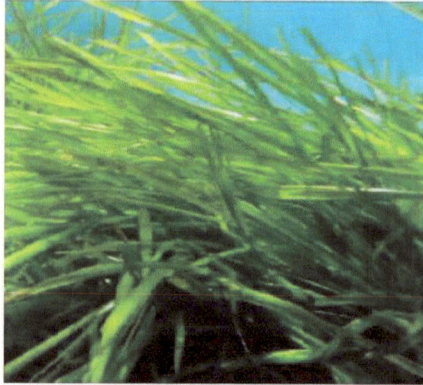

Fig. (43). *Posidonia oceanica.*

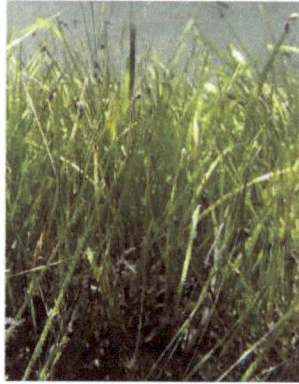

Fig. (44). *Zostera marina.*

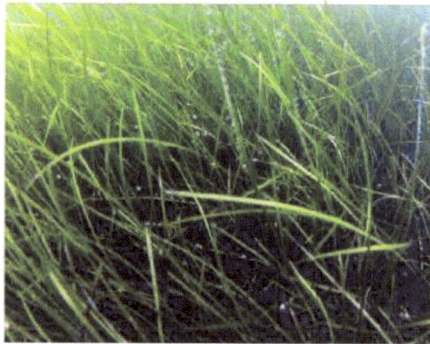

Fig. (45). *Zostera noltei.*

Image credit: *Cymodocea nodosa:* Wikimedia Commons*; Cymodocea rotundata:* Wikispecies; *Halodule uninervis:* Wikimedia Commons*; Syringodium isoetifolium:* Wikimedia Commons*; Thalassodendron ciliatum:* Wikimedia Commons*; Enhalus acoroide:* Wikipedia*; Halophila stipulaceae:* Wikimedia

Commons; *Thalassia testudinu:,* Wikipedia; *Posidonia oceanica:* Wikispecies; *Zostera marina:* Wikimedia commons; *Zostera noltei:* Wikispecies.

Bioactive Compounds of Seagrasses and their Therapeutic Activities

Seagrasses, are also considered to be valuable sources of biologically active, therapeutic compounds such as polyphenols, terpenoids, and halogenated compounds with anticancer (antitumor), cytotoxic, antiviral, antidiabetic, antimalarial, antioxidant, anti-inflammatory, antimicrobial and anti-aging properties. Apart from preventing human diseases, these seagrasses are also used as a remedy for stings of venomous rays and as tranquilizers for babies. In folk medicine, seagrasses were used for the treatment of fevers, stomach problems, wounds, muscle pain, and skin diseases. However, seagrass-derived drugs are yet to be discovered and the reported drug candidates under clinical trials include rutin, ferulic acid, quercetin, gallic acid, azelaic acid, lauric acid, and rosmarinic acid. The anticancer and antioxidant activities of the seagrass extracts are given below (Tables 2 and 3).

Table 2. Anticancer activity of the seagrass extracts [29].

Species	Extract	Cell Line	IC_{50} Value/Action
Cymodocea serrulata	Aqueous	HeL	107.7 µg/mL
Halophila stipulaceae (Leaves)	Ethyl acetate	MG63	29.4 µg/mL
Halophila stipulaceae (Stems)	Ethyl acetate	MG63.	19.1 µg/mL
Halophila stipulaceae (Leaves)	Hexane extract	HCT116.	19.5 µg/mL
Halophila stipulaceae (Stems)	Hexane extract	HCT116.	7.6 µg/mL.
Posidonia oceanica	EtOH/H$_2$O (7:3)	SH-SY5Y	After 7 h treatment with 3 µg/mL, inhibition of 57% cell migration
Posidonia oceanica	Hydrophilic	HT1080	After 12 h treatment with 3 µg/mL, inhibition of 72.3% cell migration
Posidonia oceanica	MeOH/H$_2$O (7:3)	HepG2	24.3 µg/mL
Posidonia oceanica	MeOH/H$_2$O (7:3)	MCF7.	22.6 µg/mL.
Posidonia oceanica	MeOH/H$_2$O (7:3)	HCT116.	22.5 µg/mL
Posidonia oceanica (Leaves)	MeOH/H$_2$O (7:3)	HepG2.	17-28.3 µg/mL
Posidonia oceanica (Leaves)	MeOH/H$_2$O (7:3)	HCT116	27.8 µg/mL
Syringodium filiforme	Chloroform fraction of hydroethanolic	A549	At 100 µg/mL, decreases viability of cell line below 60%
Thalassodendron ciliatum	Methanolic	HCT-116	4.2 µg/mL

(Table 2) cont.....

Species	Extract	Cell Line	IC$_{50}$ Value/Action
Thalassodendron ciliatum	Methanolic	HeLa	9.8 µg/mL.
Thalassodendron ciliatum	Methanolic	HepG2	8.12 µg/mL.
Thalassodendron ciliatum	Methanolic	MCF7	4.12 µg/mL.
Thalassodendron ciliatum	Chloroform fraction of hydroethanolic	A549	20.4 µg/mL.
Thalassodendron ciliatum	Chloroform fraction of hydroethanolic	EA.hy926	248.4 µg/mL
Thalassodendron ciliatum	Hydroethanolic	RKO	174.9 µg/mL
Thalassodendron ciliatum	Hydroethanolic	SW480	58.9 µg/mL
Thalassodendron ciliatum	Hydroethanolic	CT26	115.3 µg/mL
Thalassodendron ciliatum	Hydroethanolic	HepG2.	102 µg/mL
Thalassodendron ciliatum	Hydroethanolic	PC12	135 µg/mL
Thalassodendron ciliatum	Hydroethanolic	Caco2	165 µg/mL
Thalassodendron ciliatum	Hydroethanolic	4T1.	129 µg/mL
Thalassodendron ciliatum	Polyphenol fraction of hydroethanolic	HCT15.	22.47 µg/mL
Thalassodendron ciliatum	Polyphenol fraction of hydroethanolic	HT29	93.1 – 121.7 µg/mL

Table 3. Antioxidant activity of the seagrass extracts [29].

Species.	Compound/ Extract	Inhibition	Conc.
Cymodocea nodosa	Sulfated polysaccharide	82.4%	0.5 mg/mL
Cymodocea rotundata	Aqueous methanol (1:4)	70.3%	---
Cymodocea rotundata	Ethyl acetate	50%	362.6 ppm
Cymodocea rotundata	Methanolic	50%	214.7 ppm
Cymodocea serratula	Aqueous	53.8; 65.7%	100 µg/mL; 600 µg/mL
Cymodocea serratula	Aqueous methanol (1:4)	41.3%	----
Cymodocea serratula	Butanol fraction	82.6%	600 µg/mL
Cymodocea serratula	Ethanolic	61.9%	---
Cymodocea serratula	Ethyl acetate fraction	89.5%	600 µg/mL
Cymodocea serratula	Petroleum ether fraction	27.8%	600 µg/mL
Enhalus acoroides	Aqueous extract	30.7%	200 µg/mL
Enhalus acoroides	Aqueous methanol (1:4)	35.8%	------

(Table 3) cont.....

Species.	Compound/ Extract	Inhibition	Conc.
Enhalus acoroides	Chloroform extract	32%.	200 µg/mL
Enhalus acoroides	Ethanolic extract	30%	200 µg/mL
Enhalus acoroides	Ethyl acetate extract	30.7%	200 µg/mL
Enhalus acoroides	Hexane extract	26.9%	200 µg/mL
Enhalus acoroides	Methanolic extract	50%.	115.8 ppm
Enhalus acoroides	Petroleum ether fraction	33.8%	600 µg/mL
Halophila beccarii	Aqueous, Butanol, Ethyl acetate & Petroleum ether fractions	24.4, 13.9, 84.6, &14.3% & respectively	600 µg/mL
Halophila ovlais	Aqueous, Butanol, Ethyl acetate & Petroleum ether	5.2, 12.2, 6.7 & 4.8% respectively	600 µg/mL
Halodule pinifolia	Aqueous, Butanol, Ethyl acetate & Petroleum ether	22.2, 28.4, 80.3 & 21% respectively	600 µg/mL
Halophila stipulaceae	Ethanolic extract	67.4%	---
Halophila stipulaceae- old & young leaf extract	EtOH/H$_2$O (3:1)	85 & 45%respectively	100 µg/mL
Syringodium filiforme	MeOH/H$_2$O (1:1)	IC$_{50}$: 0.8 mg/mL	---
Syringodium isoetifolium	Acetone extract	45.7%	---
Syringodium isoetifolium	Aqueous fraction	16.2%	600 µg/mL
Syringodium isoetifolium	Aqueous methanol (1:4)	51.6%	----
Syringodium isoetifolium	Butanol fraction	6.2%	600 µg/mL
Syringodium isoetifolium	Ethanolic extract	23.7%	---
Syringodium isoetifolium	Hexane extract	15.2%	--
Syringodium isoetifolium	Methanolic extract	83%	---
Syringodium isoetifolium	Petroleum ether fraction	10.2%	600 µg/mL
Thalassodendron ciliatum	Catechins	50%	3.82 mM
Thalassodendron ciliatum	Methanolic extract	71%	1 mg/mL
Thalassodendron ciliatum	Aqueous fraction	26.6%	600 µg/mL
Thalassodendron ciliatum	Aqueous methanol (1:4)	38.62%	---
Thalassia hemprichii	Aqueous fraction	26.6%	600 µg/mL
Thalassia hemprichii	Aqueous methanol (1:4)	38.6%	-----
Thalassia hemprichii	Butanol fraction	84.9%	600 µg/mL
Thalassia hemprichii	Ethanolic extract	61.6%	-----
Thalassia hemprichii	Ethyl acetate extract	IC$_{50}$: 25.98 µg/mL	----
Thalassia hemprichii	Ethyl acetate extract	50%	250.72 ppm

Bioactivities of the Sea Grass Extracts

The extracts of species of the sea grass have shown anti-inflammatory, antiviral, larvicidal, lipid-reducing, anti-diabetic and anti-aging activities [29]. Such species and their bioactivities are given below.

Anti-Inflammatory Activity

Posidonia oceanica

The ethanolic extract of this species displayed anti-inflammatory activity by reducing the LPS-induced high levels of COX2. Further, this extract has been reported to strongly inhibit the oxidative stress by reducing iNOS and COX-2 levels and affecting the production of both ROS and NO radicals. Furthermore, it inhibited the NF-κB-signaling pathway through the modulation of ERK1/2 and Akt intracellular cascades.

Syringodium filiforme and Thalassia testudinum

The palmitoleic acid derived from these species displayed significant anti-inflammatory activity by inhibiting the LPS-induced release of TNF-α, IL-1β, IL-6, MIP-3α, and l-selectin. Further, this compound showed strong anti-inflammatory activity through MAPK and NF-κB-signaling pathways. Furthermore, the stearic acid of these species reduced considerably the inflammatory response by inhibiting neutrophil migration, and subsequent reduction of TNF-α and IL-1β.

Halophila ovalis

The methanolic extract of this species showed 50% inhibition of the proliferation of peripheral blood mononuclear cells at the concentration of 78.7 μg/mL.

Thalassodendron ciliatum

At a concentration of 20 mg/kg, its extract displayed significant anti-inflammatory activity in the carrageenan-induced rat paw edema test.

Antiviral Activity

Posidonia oceanica

At a concentration of 100 μg/mL, the MeOH/H$_2$O (7:3) extract of this species displayed antiviral activity against H5N1 virus with 45% inhibition.

Thalassodendron ciliatum

At a concentration 20 µg/mL, the methanolic extract of this species displayed antiviral activity against Hepatitis A (HAV) and herpes simplex (HSV-1) viruses with 100% inhibition.

Thalassia hemprichii

At a concentration of 23 µg/mL, the methanolic extract of this species displayed antiviral activity against HCV virus with 50% inhibition.

Unidentified species of Zosteraceae family

The polyphenol complex derived from this seagrass showed activity against tick-borne encephalitis (TBE). At 100 µg/mL concentration, this complex suppressed accumulation of the pathogen in the cell culture.

Anti-Dengue Activity (Larvicidal Activity)

Cymodocea serrulata

The EtOH/water (3:1) extract of the leaves of this species displayed larvicidal activity of the mosquito *Aedes. Aegypti* with an LC_{50} value of 0.08 µg/mL. On the other hand, its 70% ethanol recorded an LC_{50} value of 42.9 µg/mL.

Enhalus acoroides

The distilled water extract of this species displayed larvicidal activity of the mosquito *Aedes. Aegypti* with an LC_{50} value of 0.085 µg/mL.

Halophila ovalis

The distilled water extract of this species displayed larvicidal activity of the mosquito *Aedes. Aegypti* with an LC_{50} value of 0.07µg/mL.

Halodule pinifolia

The 70% ethanol extract of the root of this species displayed larvicidal activity of the mosquito *Aedes. Aegypti* with an LC_{50} value of 22 µg/mL.

Syringodium isoetifolium

The EtOH/water (3:1) extract of the leaves and root of this species displayed larvicidal activity of the mosquito *Aedes. Aegypti* with LC_{50} values of 0.062 µg/mL. and 0.0604 µg/mL, respectively.

Thalassia hemprichii

The ethanolic extract of this species displayed larvicidal activity of the mosquito *Aedes. Aegypti* with an LC_{50} value of 201.7μg/mL.

Thalassia testudinum

70% ethanol extract of this species displayed larvicidal activity of the mosquito *Aedes. Aegypti* with an LC_{50} value of 44.8 μg/mL.

Lipid-Reducing Activity

Thalassia hemprichii

The ethanolic extract treated alloxan-induced diabetic mice showed lipid-reducing activity with the considerable reduction in their LDL and VLDL cholesterol levels.

Halophila stipulacea

Both the ethyl acetate and methanolic extracts of this species displayed lipid-reducing activity by inhibiting the acetyl-CoA carboxylase and PPARα agonists in the 48 h test using the zebra fish Nile red fat metabolism assay. The IC_{50} values recorded for these two extracts were 2.2 μg/mL and 1.2 μg/mL, respectively.

Anti-diabetic Activity

Syringodium filiforme and Thalassia testudinum

The compounds 52 and 53 derived from these species possess the potential for the treatment of type 2 DM by increasing GLUT4 expression and translocation.

Halophila stipulacea

At doses of 100 and 200 mg/kg/day, the extracts of this species displayed 9- and 13-fold increases in serum NO, respectively, and this is largely due to the improvement of glucose uptake by the body tissues through the restoration of liver GLUT-2. Further, these extracts have also been reported to reduce oxidative stress status which is due to the release of free radicals and dyslipidemia under diabetic conditions.

Thalassia hemprichii

Intraperitoneal administration of the ethanolic extract of this species for 15 days led to a significant increase in body weight.

Significant reversion of alloxan-mediated bodyweight reduction has also been observed by this treatment.

Halophila beccarii

The methanolic extract of this species displayed a 50% inhibition of α-amylase and α-glucosidase at 270 µg/mL and 100 µg/mL, respectively. Further, this treatment also regulated the glucose movement out of the cells and gained glucose by facilitating diffusion into the bloodstream, thereby the post-postprandial glucose levels are controlled.

Halodule uninervis

Administration of the methanol extract of this species at the concentration of 250 mg/kg reduced glucose levels by 30% after 6 h and by 62% on the 18th day. Further, in the Streptozotocin-induced diabetic rats, treatment of the extract at 150 mg/kg reduced the glucose levels by 25% after 6 h and 53% on the 18th day.

Posidonia oceanica

The hydroalcoholic extracts of the leaves of this species showed strong *in vitro* activity against human serum albumin glycation.

Hepatoprotective Activity

Thalassia hemprichii

The ethanolic extract of this species displayed hepatoprotective activity by reducing the levels of SGPT and SGOT in alloxan-induced diabetic mice.

Halodule uninervis

In treated rats with the concentrations of 150 and 250 mg/kg of the methanolic extract of this species, there was a significant improvements in their hepatic and renal function.

Cymodocea rotundata

In paracetamol-induced rat, the administration of 280 mg/kg ethanolic extract of the rhizome of this species significantly reduced their SGPT and SGOT levels.

Thalassodendron ciliatum

The hydro-methanolic extract of this species has been reported to improve histopathological changes in the liver through the stimulation of the Nrf2/ARE pathway which was associated with a decrease in lipid peroxidation, nitric oxide, alanine aminotransferase, and aspartate aminotransferase levels in thioacetamide - induced liver failure; inducing antioxidant defense enzymes superoxide dismutase and elevation of GSH (non-enzymatic antioxidant glutathione).

Anti-Aging Activity

Posidonia oceanica

The ethanolic extract of this species showed an increase in lipolysis at a concentration range of 10–200 µg/mL; and a significant increase in collagen production in fibroblasts at 5 and 10 µg/mL. Further, this extract has been reported to induce 20% tyrosinase inhibition at 5 µg/mL and 45% inhibition at 1000 µg/mL.

MANGROVES

Mangroves, the most ecologically productive and diverse wetland ecosystems occupy about 25% of the world's coastline and are found distributed among 112 countries and territories worldwide with about 181,000 sq. km. They are also considered to be a potential coastal resource providing valuable products and a unique range of ecological services. The mangrove species are generally categorized as true mangrove (strict mangrove or obligate mangrove) and mangrove associates. While the true mangroves include 'exclusive' species which are confined to the mangrove environment, mangrove associates (semi-mangrove, back mangrove) are nonexclusive' species that are mainly distributed in a terrestrial or aquatic habitat but also occur in the mangrove ecosystem. According to some researchers, true mangroves possess the following characteristics: (i) occur only in mangrove environment and not extending into terrestrial communities; (ii) taxonomic isolation from terrestrial relatives; (iii) morphological specialization (aerial roots, vivipary); and (iv) physiological mechanism for salt exclusion and/or salt excretion [30]. True mangroves are however, confined to intertidal mangrove habitats where the salinity ranges from 17.0 to 36.6 ppt. Species of these mangroves largely include the genera of the families such as Avicenniaceae, Bombacaceae, Combretaceae, Maliaceae, Myrtaceae, Myrsinaceae, Pellicieraceae, Plumbaginaceae, Rhizophoraceae, Rubiaceae, and Sonneratiaceae.

Pharmaceutically Important Species of Mangroves

Aegiceras corniculatum, Avicennia germinans, Avicennia marin, Bruguiera cylindrica, Bruguiera gymnorhiza, Bruguiera sexangular, Ceriops decandra, Ceriops tagal, Excoecaria agallocha, Kandell candel, Rhizophora apiculata, Rhizophora mucronata, Rhizophora apiculata, Rhizophora stylosa, Sonneratia caseolari and *Xylocarpus moluccensis* (Figs. **46 - 61**).

Pharmaceutical Importance of True Mangroves

Owing to their unique adaptations to live in extremely harsh environmental conditions, these mangrove plants are known to synthesize some bioactive compounds with unusual activities. Such metabolites belong to chemical classes like alkaloids, carbohydrates, flavonoids, carotenoids, aliphatic alcohols, amino acids, hydrocarbons, fatty acids, phenolic compounds, tannins, saponins, terpenes, *etc.* According to available reports, a total of 349 metabolites have so far been isolated from the species of mangrove ecosystems and among them, 200 metabolites have been exclusively derived from true mangrove plants [31]. The mangrove plant *Acanthus ilicifolius* which is used in the treatment of rheumatic pain, asthma, and paralysis has a rich source of long-chain alcohols and triterpenes with analgesic and anti-inflammatory activities. Its steroid, stigmasterol has shown hypercholesterolemic effects. Further, species of the families Avicenniaceae, Rhizophoraceae, and Sonneratiaceae have been reported to be rich in tannins; *Acrosticum aureum* and *Rhizophora apiculata* possess terpenoids, steroids, and novel terpenoid ester; *Rhizophora mucronata* is a rich source of alkaloid rhizophorin; and *Avicenniaalba* is a rich source of naphthoquinones. The bark extracts of *Bruguiera sexangular* containing the alkaloid compound, brugin have been reported to be active against tumors, *viz.* Sarcoma 180 and Lewis Lung Carcinoma. Further, brugin is also largely used as a central nervous system depressant. Although several secondary metabolites have been isolated from mangroves, only a few of them have been used in drug discovery research with clinical trials. For example, the extracts of *Rhizophora mangla* have shown clinical application in combating diabetes. Similarly, several clinical trials made on the extracts of *Avicennia africana, Bruguiera sexangular,* and *Excoecaria agallocha* have shown potential anti-cancer, anti-viral, and anti-HIV activities [32]. These reports suggest that the chemical compounds isolated from the mangrove plants are very important from human health perspective and further research is required to explore the chemical diversity of this ecosystem.

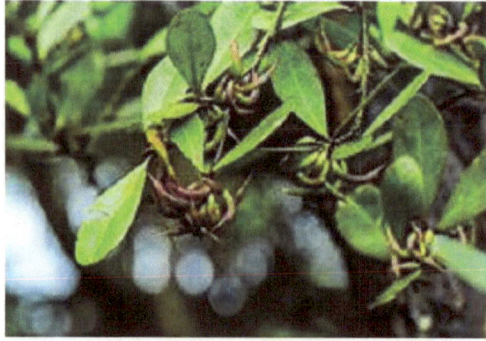

Fig. (46). *Aegiceras corniculatum.*

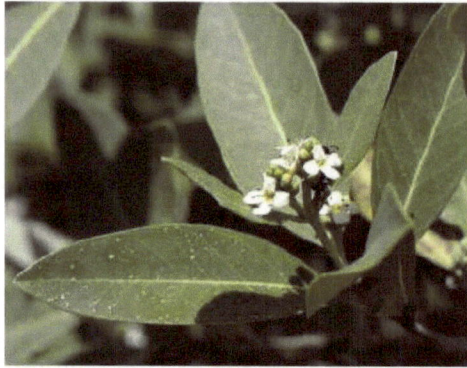

Fig. (47). *Avicennia germinans.*

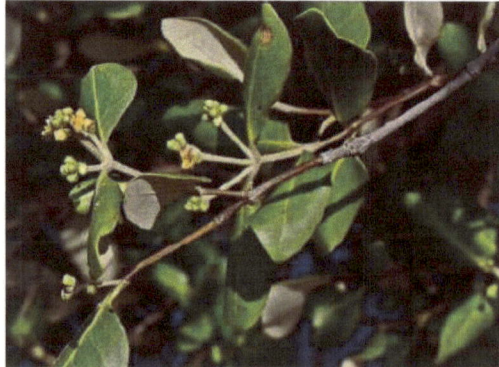

Fig. (48). *Avicennia marina.*

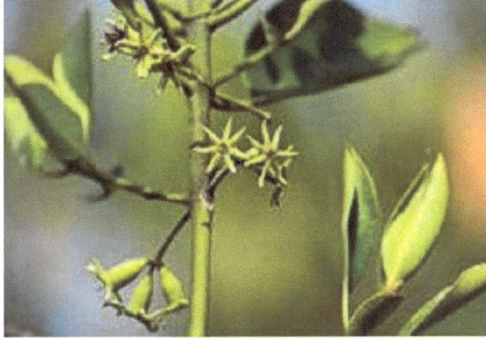

Fig. (49). *Bruguiera cylindrica.*

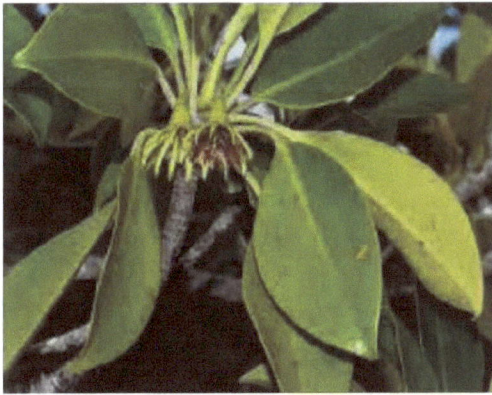

Fig. (50). *Bruguiera gymnorhiza.*

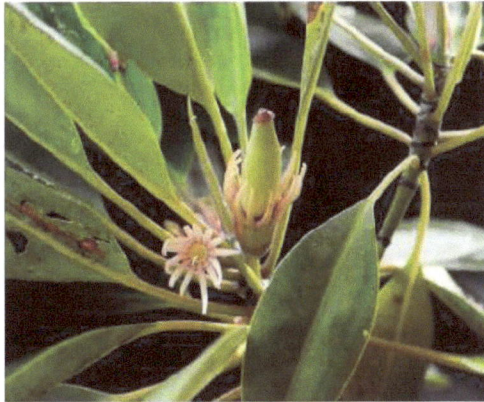

Fig. (51). *Bruguiera sexangular.*

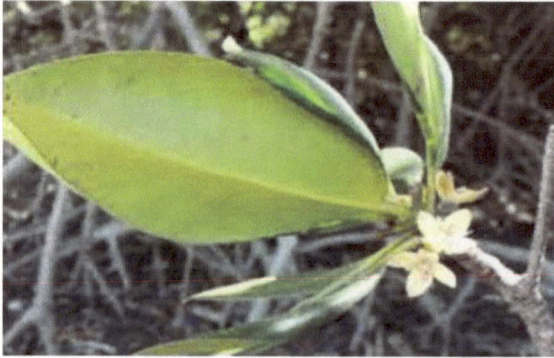

Fig. (52). *Ceriops decandra.*

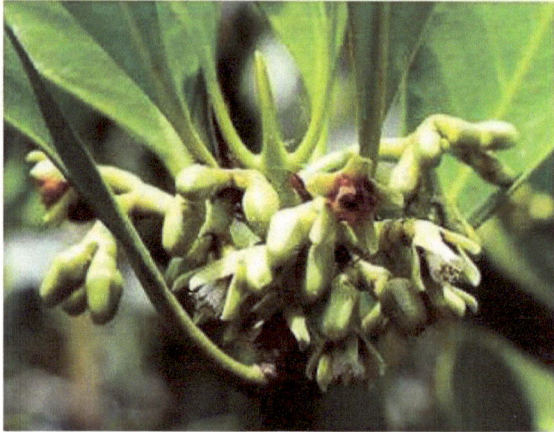

Fig. (53). *Ceriops tagal.*

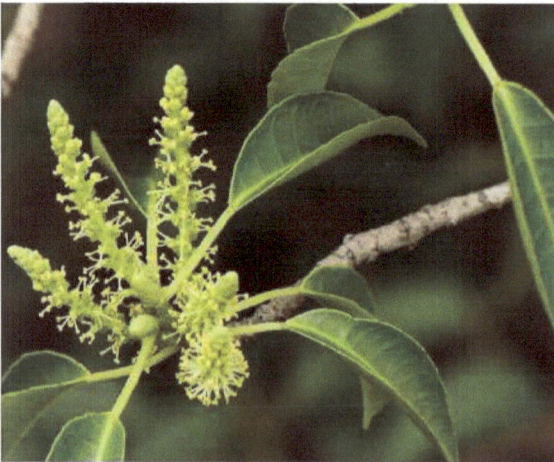

Fig. (54). *Excoecaria agallocha.*

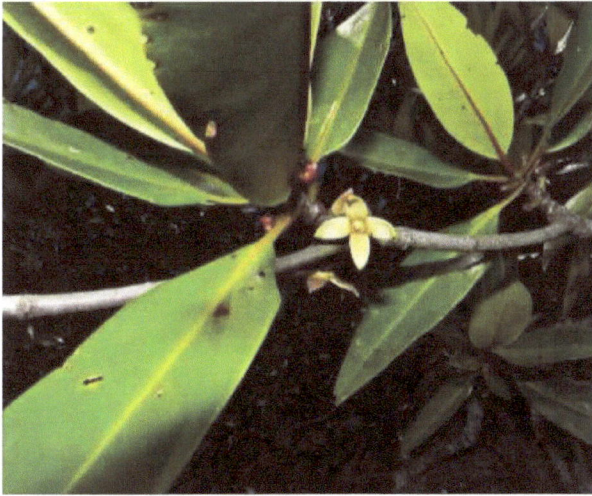

Fig. (55). *Rhizophora apiculata.*

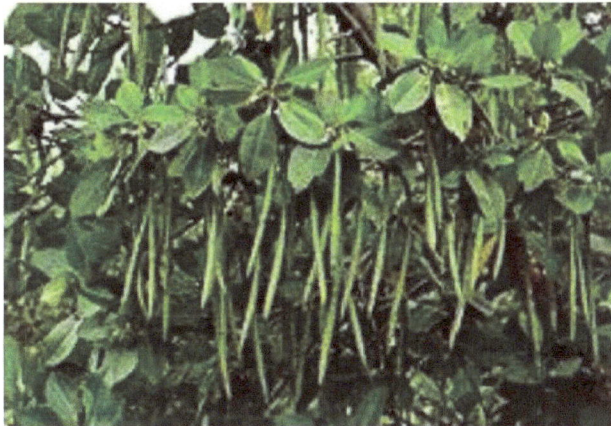

Fig. (56). *Rhizophora mucronata.*

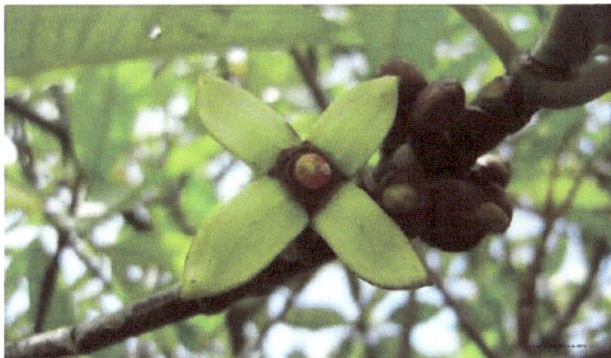

Fig. (57). *Rhizophora apiculata.*

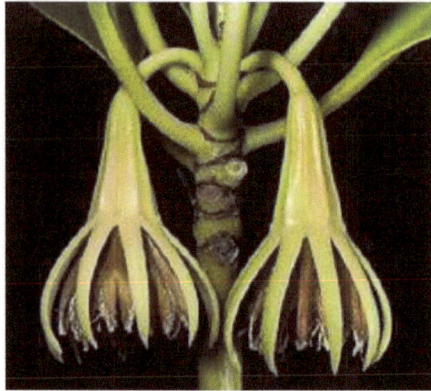

Fig. (58). *Rhizophora stylosa.*

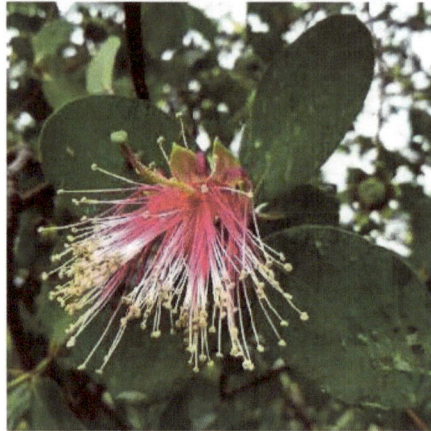

Fig. (59). *Sonneratia caseolaris.*

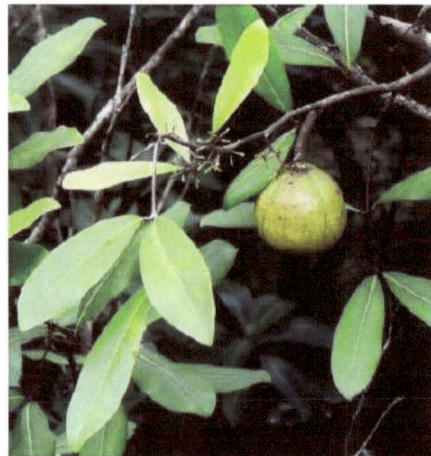

Fig. (60). *Xylocarpus moluccensis.*

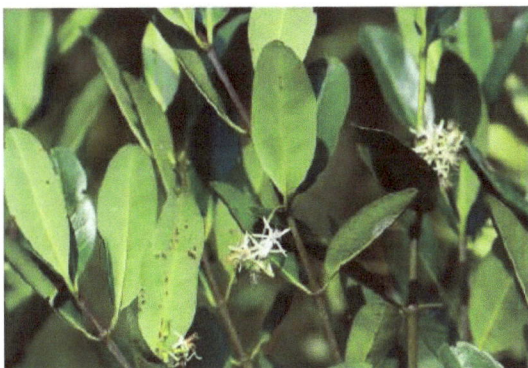

Fig. (61). *Kandella candel.*

Image credit: *Aegiceras corniculatum:* Wikipedia; *Avicennia germinans:* Wikipedia; *Avicennia marin:* Wikipedia; *Bruguiera cylindrica:* Wikipedia; *Bruguiera sexangular:* Wikipedia; *Ceriops decandra,:* Wikipedia; *Ceriops tagal:* Wikipedia; *Excoecaria agallocha:* Wikimedia commons; *Kandella candel:* Wikimedia commons ;*Rhizophora. apiculata:* Wikimedia commons; *Rhizophora. mucronata:* Wikipedia; *Rhizophora. apiculata:* Wikipedia; *Rhizophora stylosa,:* Wikipedia; *Sonneratia caseolaris:* Wikimedia commons; *Xylocarpus moluccensis:* Wikipedia;

The bioactive compounds of mangroves and their therapeutic activities as reported by Dahibhate, *et al.* [32] are given below.

THE BIOACTIVE COMPOUNDS OF MANGROVES AND THEIR THERAPEUTIC ACTIVITIES

Anticancer Activity

Plant-derived secondary metabolites have been reported to show promising anticancer activity and some of these potential compounds can be used in the development of potential drugs for treating breast cancer. Recent research findings have reported that true mangrove plant species such as *Aegiceras corniculatum, Excoecaria agallocha, Rhizophora stylosa, Sonneratia paracaseolaris, Xylocarpus genus, Ceriops tagal,* and *Bruguiera cylindrica* are capable of yielding novel anticancer compounds

Aegiceras corniculatum

A triterpene, saponin, aegicoroside A derived from the leaves of this species has shown anticancer activity by inhibiting the growth of human cancer cell line such as MCF7, HCT116, B16F10 and A549.

Avicennia alba

The extract of the leaves of this species has been reported to show high anticancer activity against HeLa cell lines.

Bruguiera gymnorrhiza

The methanolic extract of the leaves of this species has shown cytotoxic activity.

Excoecaria agallocha

Two beyerene-type diterpenoids *viz.* Excoecarin L and Excoecarin O derived from the extracts of the twigs and leaves of this species have shown weak cytotoxic activity against two human cancer cell lines KB and LU-1.

Heritiera littoralis

The Methanolic extract of the leaves of this species has shown cytotoxic activity.

Rhizophora stylosa

The cycloartane glucoside compound rhizostyloside isolated form this species has shown cytotoxicity against human cancer cell line such as, KB, LU-1, SK-Mel-2. Further this compound has been reported to activate caspase 3/7 in LU-1 cell line.

Sonneratia paracaseolaris

The aerial part of this species has yielded five triterpenoids *viz.* paracaseolins A-E. Among these compounds, paracaseolin D showed significant cytotoxic activity against A549 cell line.

Xylocarpus granatum

The limonoids named thaixylogranins A-H derived from the seeds of this species demonstrated weak cytotoxicity against the MDA-MB-231 cell line. Further, apotirucallane protolimonoid compounds *viz.* xylogranatumines A-G were isolated from the twigs and leaves of this species. Among these compounds, xylogranatumine F, was found to display *in vitro* cytotoxic activity against A549 cell line. Furthermore, among the tetranortriterpenoid compounds, xylomexicanins E-H of this species, Xylomexicanin E exhibited moderate cytotoxic activity against the cell lines A 549 and RERF.

Xylocarpus spp

The unidentified species of Xylocarpus have been reported to yield alkaloids *viz.* granatoine and xylocarpin L; and limonoids like, thaixylomolins D-F, granatumins V-Y, Andhraxylocarpins A-E, granatumins H-I, hainangranatumins A-J, and Godavarin K. These compounds have shown various bioactivities.

Ceriops tagal

Two new phenylpropanoid compounds *viz.* tagalphenylpropinoidin A and tagalphenylpropinoidin B isolated from the stem and twig of this species have shown anti-tumor activity against MCF-7 and HL-60 cell lines. Further, two dolabranediterpenes namely tagalenes J and K of this species displayed cytotoxic activity against MCF-7, SW480, HepG2, HeLa, PANC-1 and A2058 cell lines. Furthermore, four diterpenes *viz.* tagalons A-D have also been derived from this species and among them, tagalons C and D displayed selective cytotoxicity against the human breast cancer MT-1 cell line. The dolabrane dinorditerpene, compound *viz.* tagalsine X isolated from the leaves of this species however did not show obvious inhibitory activity against four human carcinoma cell lines namely CNE-2, HCT-116, HepG2 and A549. Further, this compound has also yielded diterpenes tagalenes G-I and tagalsin L-N, the bioactivities of which are yet to be known.

Bruguiera cylindrica

The compound, β-Taraxeryl-trans-pchlorocinnamate isolated from this species displayed cytotoxic activity against mouse neuroblastoma Neuro 2A cell line.

Anti-inflammatory and Antioxidant Activities

Avicennia marina

A caffeic acid derivative *viz.* maricaffeolylide A and a megastigmane derivative, maricyclohexene derived from the fruit of this species have shown antioxidant activity.

Bruguiera gymnorhiza

8-hydroxyquercetagetin glycoside compound *viz.* brugymnoside A isolated from this species has shown antioxidant activity.

Excoecaria agallocha

Six ent-kauranediterpenoids named agallochaols K-P and an atisane-type diterpenoid agallochaol Q have been obtained from the stems and twigs of this mangrove species. Among these compounds, agallochaols K, O, P and Q displayed anti-inflammatory activity by suppressing the expression of TNF-α and IL-6. Further, these compounds have been reported to block NF-κB activation while agallochaols K and Q blocked AP-1 activation. Furthermore, the diterpenes excolides A-B and agallochaexcoerins D-F derived from the stem of this species have shown various pharmacological properties.

Kandella candel

A sesquiterpene glycoside, kandelside and three megastigman glycoside compounds have been derived from this species. Among these compounds, one megastigman glycoside compound displayed strong anti-inflammatory activity by inhibiting the production of pro-inflammatory cytokines IL-6, and tumor necrosis factor a (TNF-a) in lipopolysaccharide (LPS)-stimulated bone marrow-derived dendritic cells.

Rhizophora mucronata

Two pentacyclic triterpenoids *viz.* olean18(19)-en-3b-yl-(3,6-dimethyl-3E,6Z-dienoate) and (13a)-27-frido-olean-14(15)- en-(17a)- furanyl-3b-ol have been isolated from this species. Among these compounds, the furanyl oleanene displayed significant anti-oxidative activity than prenylated oleanane.

Rhizophora annamalayana

The ethyl acetate extract of the leaves of this species have shown anti-inflammatory activity.

Xylocarpus granatum

A flavanol derivative dihydrocaffeic acid-(3→8)- epicatechin derived from this mangrove species displayed antioxidant activity with its ability to scavenge DPPH radicals.

Xylocarpus moluccensis

An andirobin, thaimoluccensin A, two phragmalin-type limonoids, thaimoluccensins B and C and a lmonoid, 7-deacetylgedunin have been isolated from this species. Among these compounds, only 7- deacetylgedunin displayed anti-inflammatory activity by strongly inhibiting nitric oxide production from activated macrophages. Further among limonoids, thaixylomolins A-C isolated from the seeds of this species, only thaixylomolin B displayed inhibitory activity against nitric oxide production in lipopolysaccharide and IFN-γ-induced RAW264.7 murine macrophages.

Antiviral Activity

Sonneratia paracaseolaris

The triterpenoid compound *viz.* paracaseolin A derived from this species displayed significant anti-H1N1 virus activity.

Rhizophora mucronata

The stilt root extract of this species has shown insecticidal activity against the dengue vector Aedes aegypti.

Antiulcerogenic Activity

Xylocarpus moluccensis

The limonoids xyloccensins X,Y derived from this species have shown antiulcerogenic activity which is believed to be due to its antisecretory activity.

Halophytes

The present world population has been reported to reach 9.7 billion by 2050, and there are serious concerns about the strength of agriculture to produce sufficient food for the growing population. It is also estimated that food production needs to go up by about 60 percent through an increase in crop yields per unit area to meet the future demand. Further, the presently grown major cereal crops such as rice, barley, wheat and corn are unable to withstand scarce water resources especially in marginal environments which are most vulnerable to climate change. Keeping these in view, there is an urgent need to identify alternative plant species so as increase agricultural productivity in areas where growing traditional crops has become difficult and uneconomical. It is, therefore, necessary to identify the potential of food plants which can grow in salty soils or waters (*i.e.*, halophytes) to produce food for human consumption. The halophyte genera (glassworts) such as *Salicornia* and *Sarcocornia* (Family: Amaranthaceae) are unique plant species which are able to grow in the salt marshes along the coastline due to the development of adaptive mechanisms and responses that allow them to counteract the extreme adversity inherent to their biotope. The species of these halophytes are known for their biotechnological and biomedical potential. The succulent young shoots of these species that are sold as "Samphire" or "Sea asparagus" have become an important source of forage and their edible oils and by-products which are rich in protein and carbohydrates serve as food supplements for humans. The shoots of these species are also rich in minerals and bioactive compounds which include phenolic compounds, l-ascorbic acid, *etc.* The genetic make-up of these halophytes has been reported to determine their physiological tolerance to high salinity and their production of bioactive compounds. The main pigments associated with the reddish colour of the shoots of these halophytes are betacyanins and other phenolic compounds which have displayed anti-stress and antioxidant properties. Though reports are available on the bioactivities of *Salicornia ambigua, Salicornia europaea* (Fig. **62**), *Salicornia freitagii,* and *Salicornia patula,* the taxonomic status of species other than *Salicornia europaea* is questionable as per the WoRMS.

The pharmaceutical compounds and their bioactivities of the different species of halophytes are given below.

Salicornia ambigua (=Sarcocornia ambigua)

The flavonoids kaempferol, quercetin, gallic acid and other hydroxybenzoic acids have been reported to be the major phenolic compounds in this species. The shoot extract of this species showed antioxidant activity, the values of which ranged between 3.4 and 4.9 mmol TEAC 100 g− 1 fw [33]. Owing to its rich bioactive compounds, the shoot of this species has the potential for use as additives in the food industry.

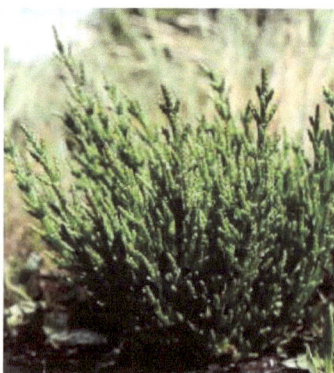

Fig. (62). *Salicornia europaea.* Image credit: Wikimedia commons.

Salicornia europaea (=Salicornia herbacea)

The tungtungmadic acid (3-caffeoyl-4 dihydrocaffeoyl quinic acid) of this species has been reported to possess higher antioxidative activity [34]. As this species possesses antioxidative and whitening effects on skin, it would be a good candidate for skin rejuvenating agent. An aqueous extract treatment of this species to B16 melanoma cells decreased the synthesis of melanin and inhibited tyrosinase activity. Further, this had potent antioxidative capacity and protected human dermal fibroblasts from tert-butyl hydroperoxide (tbOOH)-induced oxidative stress in a dose-dependent manner [35]. Its hydroalcoholic extract of the edible part of this species displayed antioxidant activity. Further its extract at a concentration of 50ug induced antibacterial activity against the pathogenic bacterium Bacillus subtilis with an MIC value of 1mg/ml. Furthermore, the methanol extract of this species displayed potential protective effect against TNFα-induced inflammatory alterations on the HT-29 human colonic adenocarcinoma cell line [36]. The methanol extract of this species showed antibacterial activity against the pathogenic Escherichia coli with an MIC value of 0.9 mg/ml. Further, this extract displayed the highest mean inhibition zones diameter of 3.8 mm against Bacillus subtilis. It is also suggested that the extract and oil of this species can be used as potential bioactive and antimicrobial agents for pharmaceutical and cosmetics applications [37].

Salicornia freitagii

The phenolic compounds vanillic acid and p-coumaric acid present in the extracts of this species showed maximum DPPH radical scavenging activity. Further, these extracts also showed high antiproliferative activity against HT-29 (IC_{50} 1.67 mg/ml) and Caco-2 (IC_{50} 3.03 mg/ml) cells for 72 h. [38].

Salicornia patula

The methanol extract of this edible, euhalophyte species has been reported to possess five phenolic acids *viz.* caffeic, coumaric, veratric, salicylic, and transcinnamic; four flavonoids namely quercetin-3-O-rutinoside, kaempferol/ luteolin, apigenin 7-glucoside, and pelargonidin-3-O-rutinoside; fatty acids such as palmitic, oleic, linoleic and stearic; and flavonoids such as apigenin--glucoside and pelargonidin 3-O-rutinoside. Among these compounds, the flavonoids displayed prebiotic properties [39]. Its consumption both as an additional ingredient or in a traditional way make this euhalophyte a functional food.

CONCLUSION

In recent years, several anticancer investigations have been made with the bioactive compounds derived from the various classes of seaweeds. Several such compounds have shown potential anticancer effects by inducing cancer cell death through a number of signaling pathways. Further, many of these compounds have been reported to inhibit angiogenesis by antagonizing the interaction of VEGF with its receptor. However, the anticancer activity of several species of the easily available seaweeds is yet to be carried out and intensive research on this aspect would yield novel anticancer drugs with few or no side effects.

CHAPTER 4

Promising Pharmaceutical Compounds of Marine Sponges: Their Chemistry and Therapeutic Applications

Abstract: This chapter deals with the promising bioactive compounds of the marine sponge species belonging to the classes Calcarea and Demospongiae. Further, the chemical classes and the bioactivities of these secondary metabolites are dealt with.

Keywords: Ara-C, Bioactivities, Calcarea, Demospongiae, Marine sponges, Secondary metabpolites, Vira-A.

INTRODUCTION

Marine invertebrates, due to their high genetic richness, have been reported to be an important and major source of bioactive compounds that can find applications in various fields like pharmaceutics, nutraceuticals, cosmetics, *etc.* Among the most studied marine invertebrates for pharmaceutically important compounds, the marine sponges with their 8500 species ranked first in both diversity and number of compounds [11]. These sponges are also well known for harboring substantial amounts of symbiotic microorganisms, including bacteria, fungi, and microalgae. For example, many of the structurally diverse and bioactive secondary metabolites originally derived from sponge extracts are known to be produced by such microorganisms [40]. Thus the sponge holobiome is considered as the source of the rich chemical diversity. As a source of various secondary metabolites, they possess significant applicability in biomedical research. Though considerable research has been done on this promising biopharmaceutical potential, it is still vastly unexplored.

MARINE SPONGE SPECIES YIELDING PROMISING BIOACTIVE COMPOUNDS

1. Leucetta chagosensis; 2. Agelas sp.; *3. Axinella* sp.; *4. Cymbastela* sp.; *5. Chondrosia* sp.; *6. Spirastrella* sp.; *7. Aplysilla* sp.; *8. Cacospongia* sp.; *9. Dactylospongia elegans; 10. Dysidea* sp.; *11. Hyrtios erectus; 12. Ircinia* sp.; *13. Lendenfeldia* sp.; *14. Psammocinia* sp.; *15. Scalarispongia scalaris; 16.* Smenos-

Santhanam Ramesh, Ramasamy Santhanam & Veintramuthu Sankar

pongia aurea; 17. *Spongia* sp.*; 18. Arenosclera brasiliensis;.19. Callyspongia (Callyspongia) siphonella; 20. Haliclona* sp.; *21. Neopetrosia* sp.; *22. Niphates olemda.*

Class: Calcarea: *Leucetta chagosensis* (Fig. **1**) and *Leucetta microraphis.*

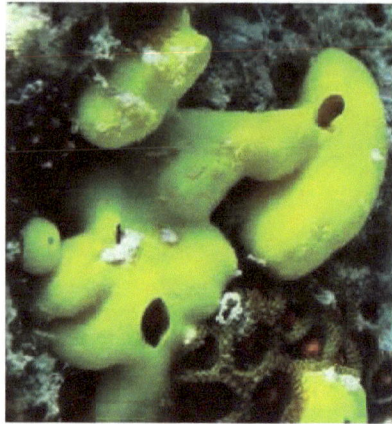

Fig. (1). *Leucetta chagosensis.*

Class: Demospongiae:

Order: Agelasida: *Agelas oxeata (= Agelas mauritiana)* (Fig. **2**)

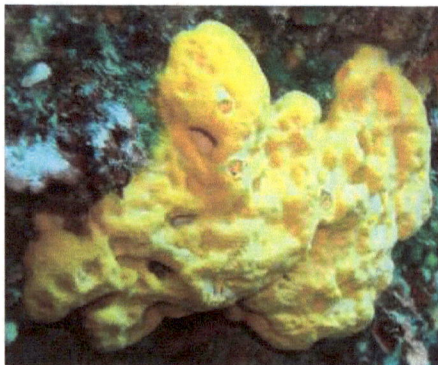

Fig. (2). *Agelas* sp.

Order: Axinellida: *Axinella brevistyla, Axinella infundibuliformis, Axinella* sp. (Fig. **3**), *Cymbastela cantharella, Cymbastela* sp. (Fig. **4**), and *Lithoplocamia lithistoides.*

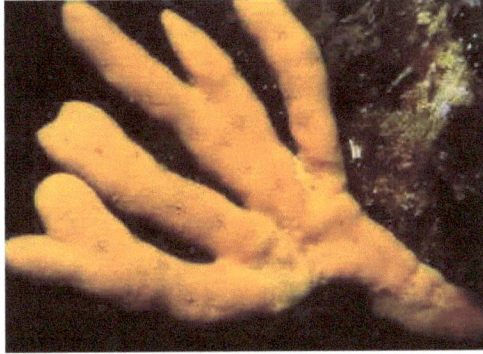

Fig. (3). *Axinella* sp.

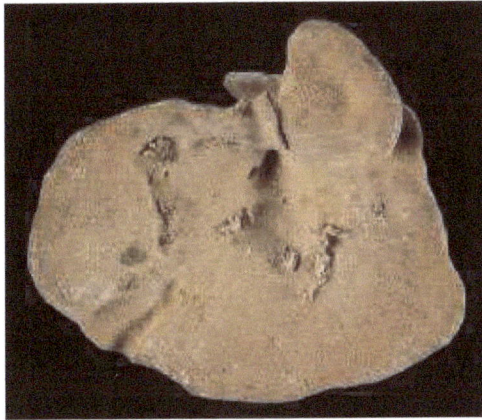

Fig. (4). *Cymbastela* sp.

Order: Bubarida: *Lipastrotethya* sp.

Order: Chondrosiida: *Chondrosia corticata.* (Fig. **5**)

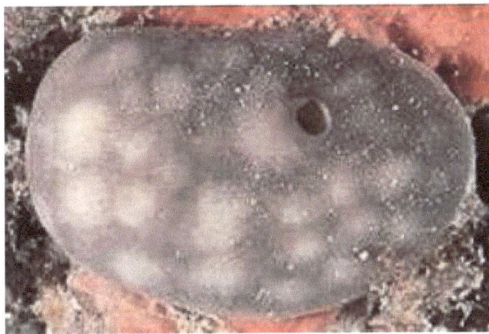

Fig. (5). *Chondrosia* sp.

Order: Clionaida: *Spirastrella pachyspira.*(Fig. **6**).

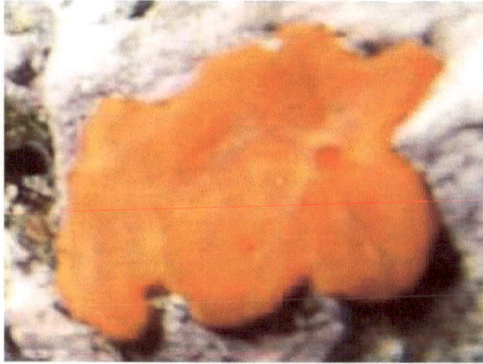

Fig. (6). *Spirastrella* sp.

Order: Dendroceratida: *Aplysilla glacialis* (Fig. **7**)

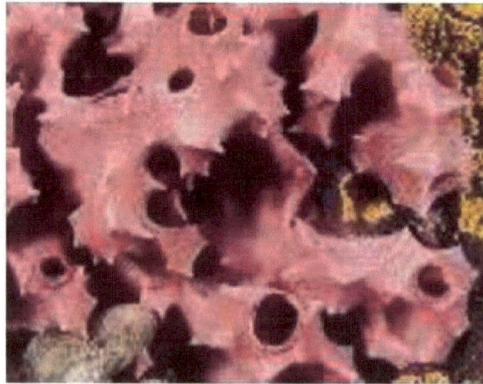

Fig. (7). *Aplysilla* sp.

Order: Dictyoceratida: *Cacospongia mycofijiensis, Cacospongia* sp. (Fig. **8**), *Candidaspongia* sp., *Coscinoderma mathewsi, Dactylospongia elegans* (Fig. **9**), *Dysidea etheria. Dysidea* sp. (Fig. **10**), *Fascaplysinopsis reticulata, Hyrtios erectus* (Fig. **11**)., *Ircinia ramosa, Ircinia* sp. (Fig. **12**), *Lendenfeldia chondrodes, Lendenfeldia* sp. (Fig. **13**), *Psammocinia* sp. (Fig. **14**), *Sarcotragus* sp., *Scalarispongia scalaris* (Fig. **15**), *Smenospongia aurea,* (Fig. **16**) and *Spongia* sp. (Fig. **17**).

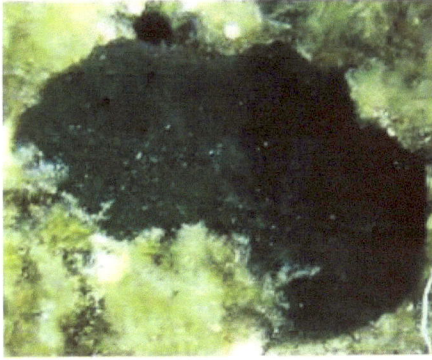

Fig. (8). *Cacospongia* sp.

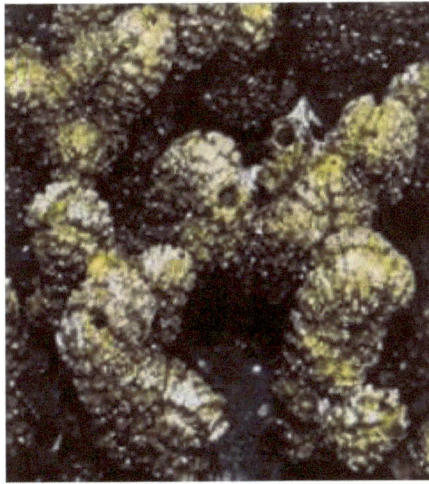

Fig. (9). *Dactylospongia elegans*.

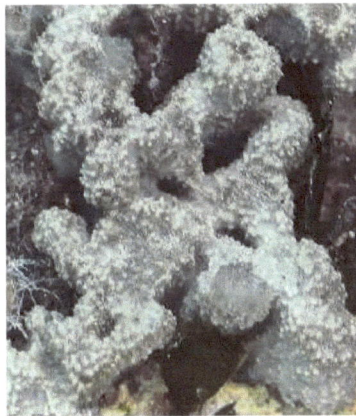

Fig. (10). *Dysidea* sp.

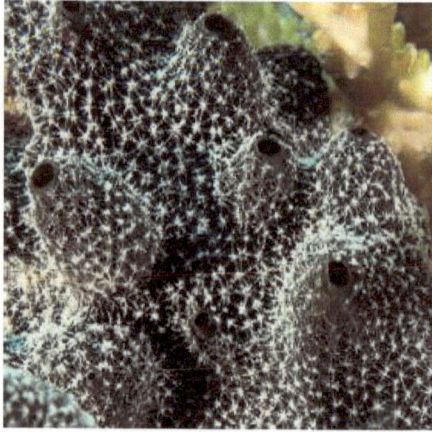

Fig. (11). *Hyrtios erectus*.

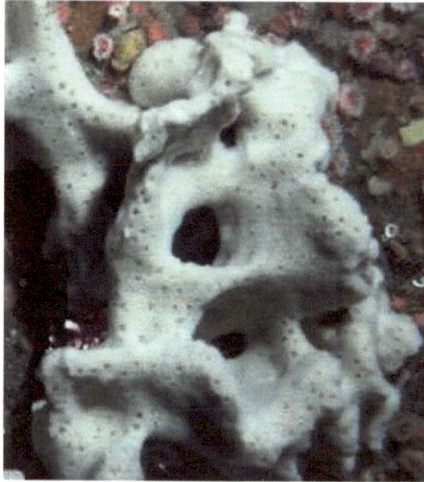

Fig. (12). *Ircinia* sp.

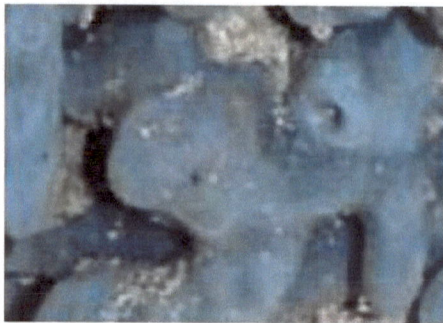

Fig. (13). *Lendenfeldia* sp.

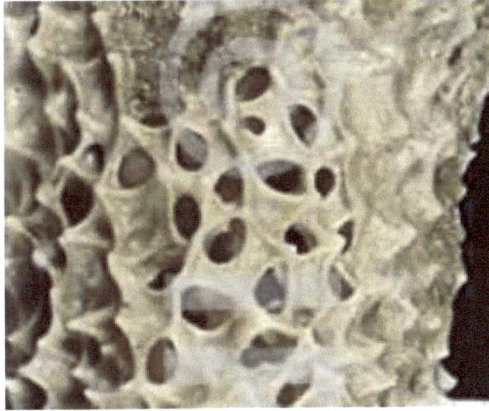

Fig. (14). *Psammocinia* sp.

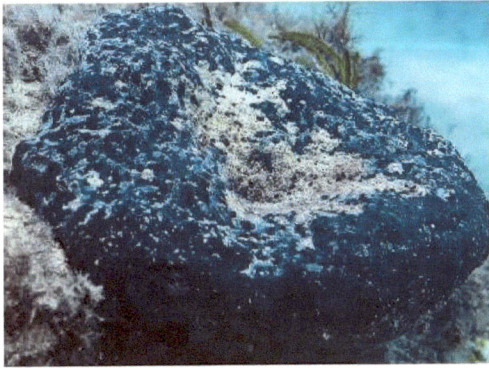

Fig. (15). *Scalarispongia scalaris*.

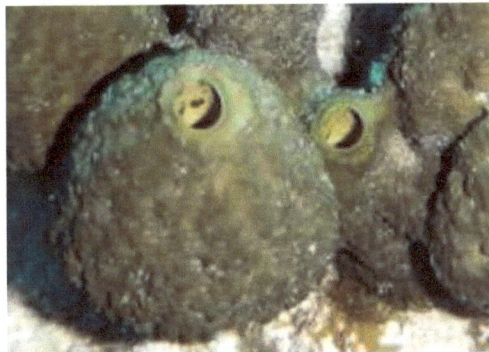

Fig. (16). *Smenospongia aurea*.

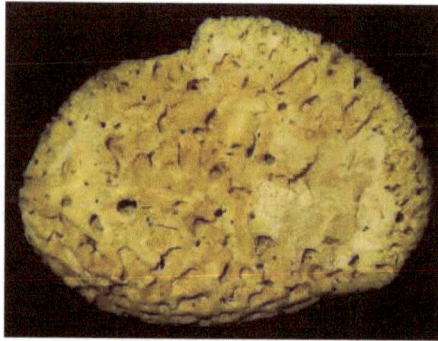

Fig. (17). *Spongia* sp.

Order: Haplosclerida: *Arenosclera brasiliensis,* (Fig. **18**), *Callyspongia (Callyspongia) siphonella* (Fig. **19**).

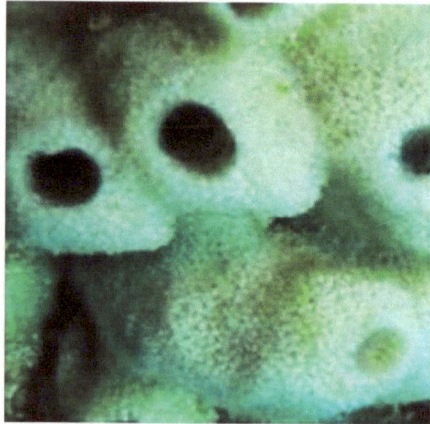

Fig. (18). *Arenosclera brasiliensis*.

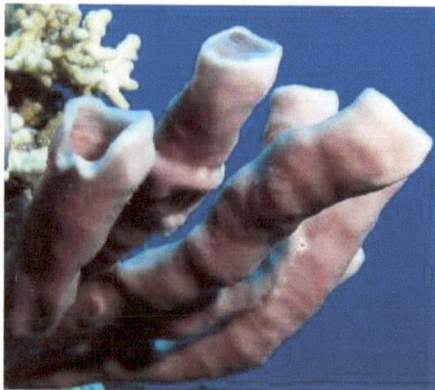

Fig. (19). *Callyspongia (Callyspongia) siphonella*.

Haliclona (Soestella) mucosa, Haliclona sp. (Fig. **20**), *Neopetrosia chaliniformis,*
Neopetrosia sp. (Fig. **21**), *Niphates olemda* (Fig. **22**), *Oceanapia incrustata,*
Oceanopia sp. (Fig. **23**), *Pachychalina alcaloidifera, Petrosia* sp. Fig. **24**),
Siphonochalina sp. (Fig. **25**) and *Xestospongia* sp. (Fig. **26**).

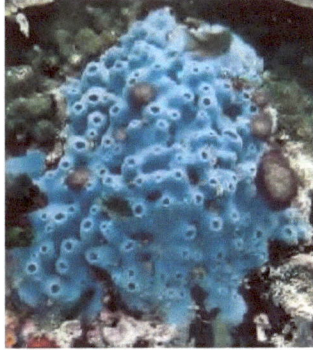

Fig. (20). *Haliclona* sp.

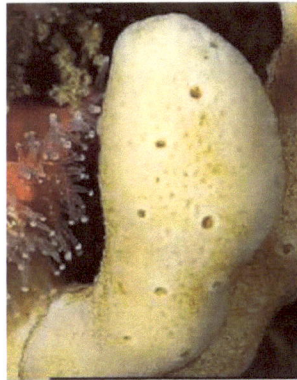

Fig. (21). *Neopetrosia* sp.

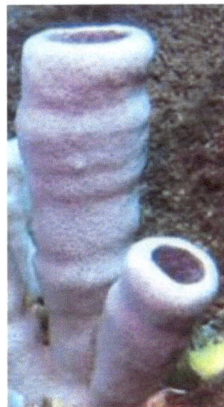

Fig. (22). *Niphates olemda.*

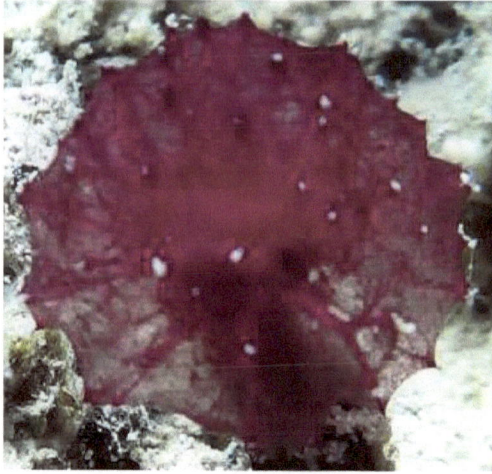

Fig. (23). *Oceanapia* sp.

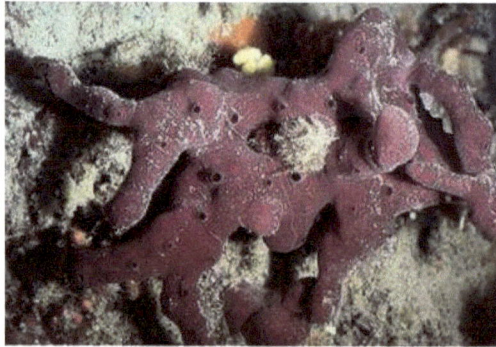

Fig. (24). *Petrosia* sp.

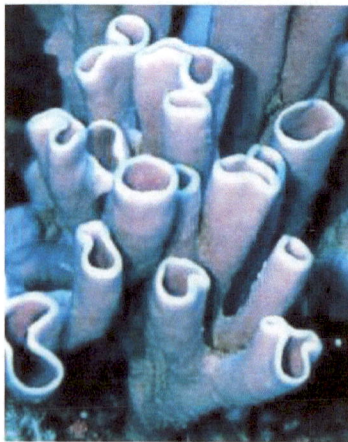

Fig. (25). *Siphonochalina* sp.

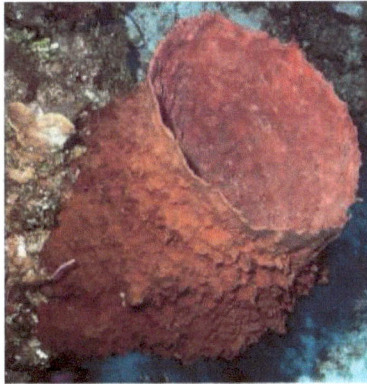

Fig. (26). *Xestospongia* sp.

Order: Poecilosclerida: *Batzella* sp., *Crambe crambe* (Fig. **27**), *Diacarnus megaspinorhabdosa, Forcepia* sp. (Fig. **28**), *Kirkpatrickia variolosa, Latrunculia (Latrunculia) brevis,* Lantrunculia sp. (Fig. **29**), *Monanchora arbuscula* (Fig. **30**), *Mycale hentscheli, Mycale* sp. (Fig. **31**), and *Negombata magnifica* (Fig. **32**).

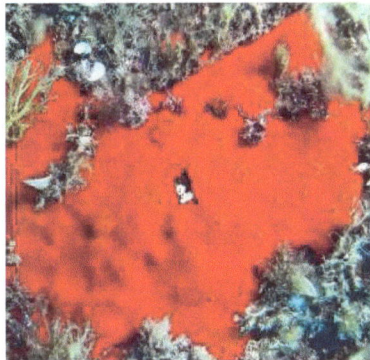

Fig. (27). *Crambe crambe.*

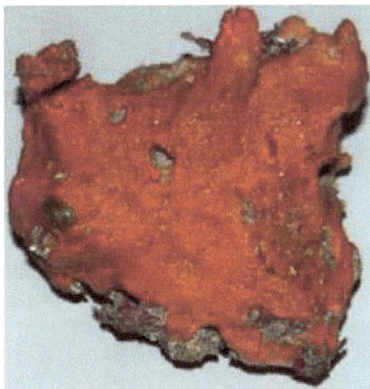

Fig. (28). *Forcepia* sp.

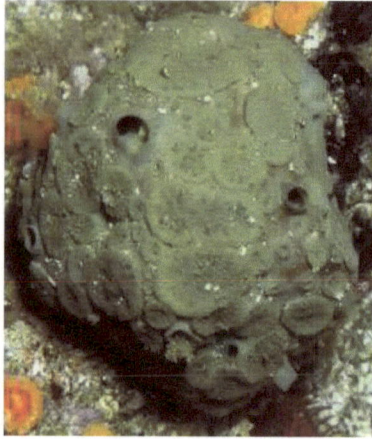

Fig. (29). *Latrunculia* sp.

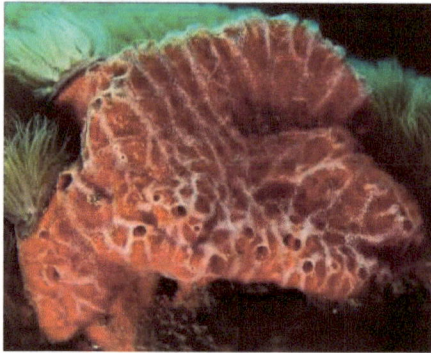

Fig. (30). *Monanchora arbuscula.*

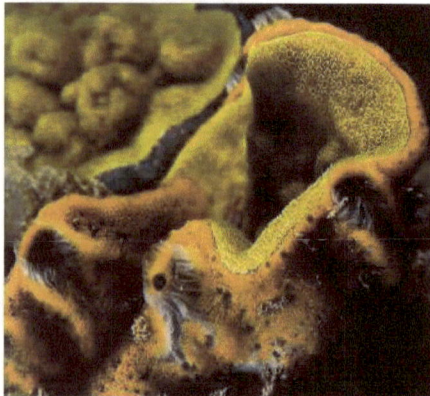

Fig. (31). *Mycale* sp.

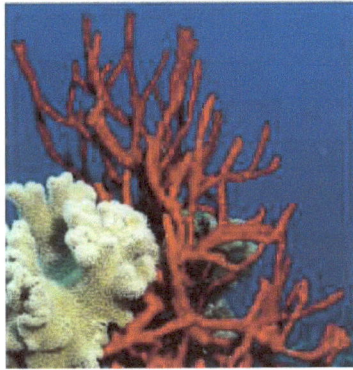

Fig. (32). *Negombata magnifica.*

Order: Scopalinida: *Stylissa flabeliformis.,* Stylissa sp. (Fig. **33**).

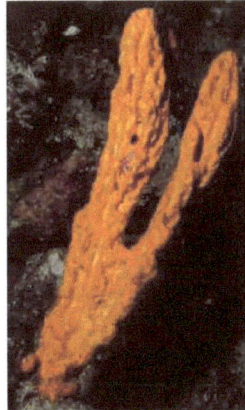

Fig. (33). *Stylissa* sp.

Order: Suberitida: *Halichondria (Halichondria) okadai, Halichondria* sp. (Fig. **34**) and *Aaptos aaptos,* and *Aaptos* sp. (Fig. **35**).

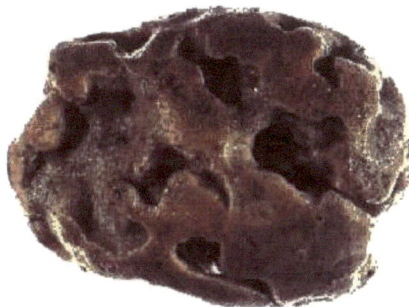

Fig. (34). *Halichondria* sp.

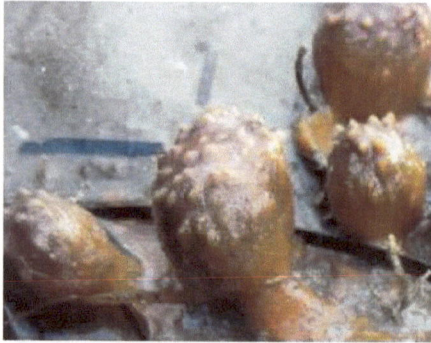

Fig. (35). *Aaptos* sp.

Order: Tethyida: *Hemiasterella vasiformis, Hemiasterella* sp. (Fig. **36**) and *Tectitethya crypta* (Fig. **37**).

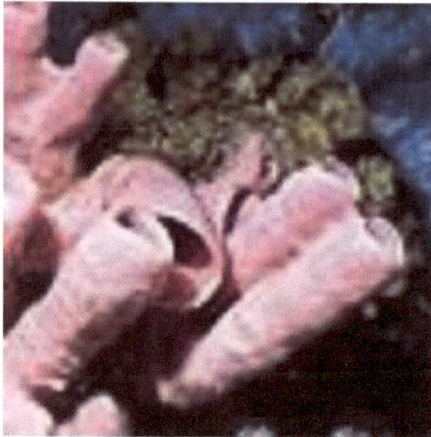

Fig. (36). *Hemiasterella* sp.

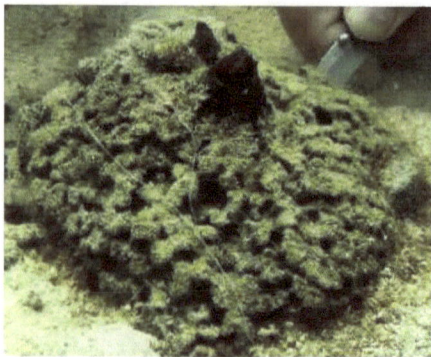

Fig. (37). *Tectitethya crypta.*

Order: Tetractinellida: *Amphibleptula* sp., *Discodermia calyx, Discodermia* sp. (Fig. **38**), *Geodia japonica, Geodia* sp. (Fig. **39**), *Jaspis stellifera, Jaspis* sp. (Fig. **40**), *Leiodermatium* sp. (Fig. **41**) , *Pachastrissa* sp., *Pachymatisma johnstonia* (Fig. **42**), *Rhabdastrella globostellata* (Fig. **43**) and *Stelletta* sp.

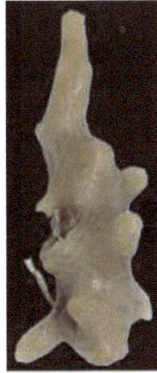

Fig. (38). *Discodermia* sp.

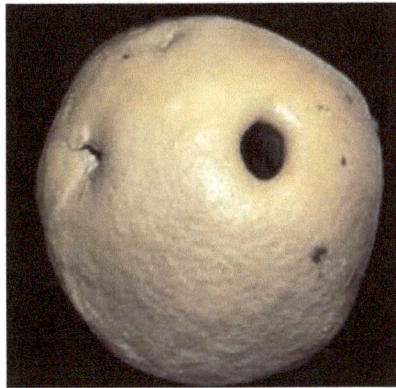

Fig. (39). *Geodia* sp.

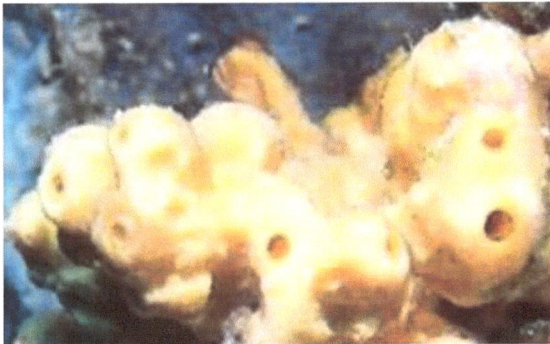

Fig. (40). *Jaspis* sp.

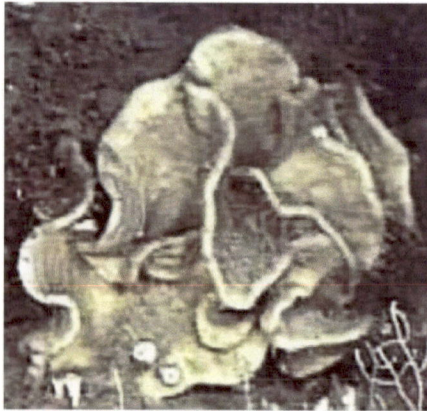

Fig. (41). *Leiodermatium* sp.

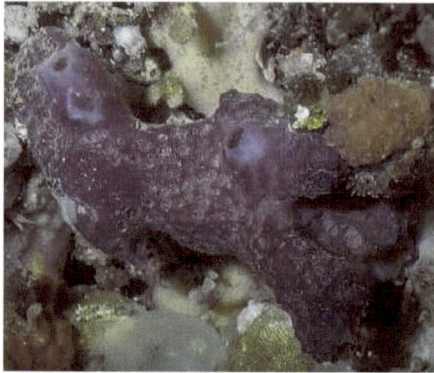

Fig. (42). *Pachymatisma johnstonia.*

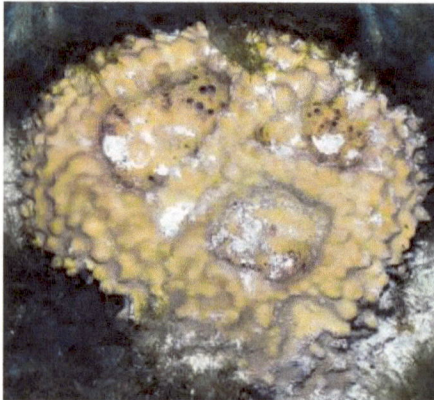

Fig. (43). *Rhabdastrella globostellata.*

Order: Trachycladida: *Trachycladus spinispirulifera* (Fig. **44**).

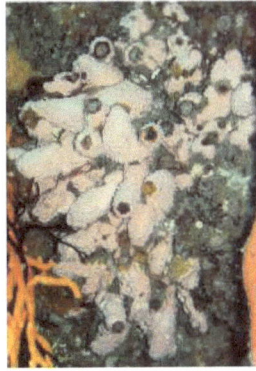

Fig. (44). *Trachycladus spinispirulifera.*

Order: Verongiida: *Aplysina aerophoba* (Fig. **45**), *Ianthella* sp. (Fig. **46**), and *Pseudoceratina purpurea*, *Pseudoceratina* sp. (Fig. **47**).

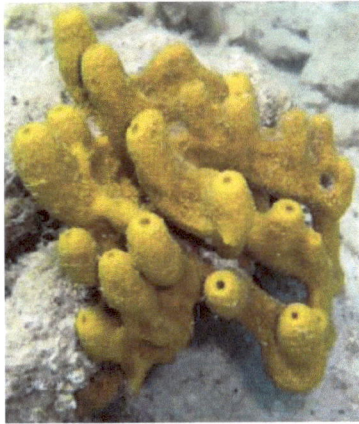

Fig. (45). *Aplysina aerophoba.*

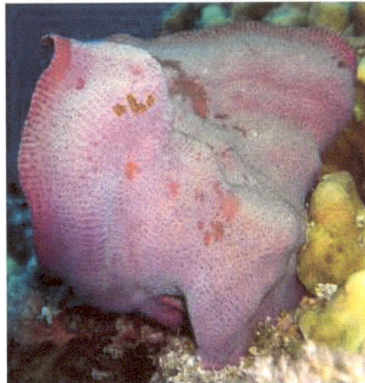

Fig. (46). *Ianthella* sp.

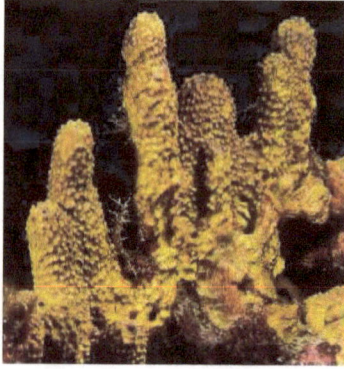

Fig. (47). *Pseudoceratina* sp.

Class: Hexactinellida: *Aphrocallistes Beatrix* (Fig. **48**).

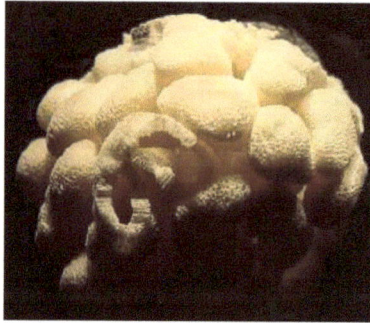

Fig. (48). *Aphrocallistes beatrix.*

Class: Homoscleromorpha: *Plakinastrella* sp. and *Plakortis angulospiculatus,* and *Plakortis* (Fig. **49**).

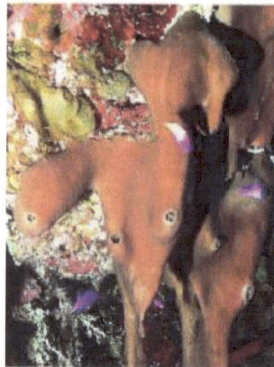

Fig. (49). *Plakortis* sp.

Image credit: *Leucetta chagosensis:* Wikipedia; *Agelas* sp.: Wiki species; *Axinella* sp.: Wiki species; *Cymbastela* sp.: Wikipedia; *Chondrosia* sp:. Wikipedia commons; *Spirastrella* sp.: Wikipedia commons; *Cacospongia* sp.: Wikipedia; *Dysidea* sp.: Wikipedia; *Ircinia* sp. : Wikipedia; *Scalarispongia scalaris:* Wikipedia commons; *Spongia* sp.: Wikipedia; *Callyspongia (Callyspongia) siphonella:* Wikipedia; *Haliclona* sp.: Wikipedia; *Petrosia* sp.: Wikipedia; *Xestospongia* sp.: Wikipedia; *Crambe crambe:* Wikipedia; *Forcepia* sp.: Wikipedia commons; *Latrunculia* sp.: Wikipedia commons; *Monanchora arbuscula:* Wikipedia; *Mycale* sp:. Wikipedia; *Negombata magnifica:.* Wikipedia; *Stylissa* sp.: Wikipedia; *Halichondria* sp:. Wikipedia; *Aaptos* sp.: Wikipedia; *Tectitethya crypta:* Wikipedia; *Discodermia* sp.: Wikipedia; *Geodia* sp.: Wikipedia; *Leiodermatium* sp. Wikipedia; *Pachymatisma johnstonia:.* Wikipedia commons; *Rhabdastrella globostellata:* Wikipedia; *Trachycladus spinispirulifera:* Wikipedia; *Aplysina aerophoba:.* Wikipedia; *Ianthella* sp.: Wikipedia; *Pseudoceratina* sp.: Wikipedia; *Aphrocallistes Beatrix:* Wikipedia; *Plakortis* sp.: Wikipedia;

Anticancer Activity

Class: Calcaea; Order: Clathrinida; Family: Leucettidae.

Leucetta chagosensis

The alkaloid naamidine A derived from this species has been reported to induce cell death, which is accompanied by the disruption of the mitochondrial membrane potential, and cleavage and activation of caspases 3, 8, and 9. Further, naamidine A-induced cell death is believed to be caspase-dependent [41]. Further, its imidazole alkaloid compound, naamine D has been reported to serve as nitric oxide (NO) synthetase inhibitor [42]. The concentration of nitric oxide plays an important role in tumorogenesis. At a low concentration, the NO has been reported to cause tumor progression.

Leucetta microraphi

The compound, leucettamol A served as an active inhibitor of ubiquitin E2 enzymes Ubc13 and Uev1A. This inhibiting compound is presumed to be a potential anti-cancer agent that upregulates the activity of the tumor suppressor p53 protein [43].

Class: Demospongiae; Order: Agelasida; Family: Agelasidae.

Agelas mauritiana

Its galactosylceramide compound agelasphin (KRN7000) has been reported to serve as NKT cell activator [42]. NKT cell activation leads to rapid production of inflammatory cytokines and modulates the function of several effectors and regulatory immune cells.

Order: Axinellida; Family: Axinellidae.

Axinella brevistyla

The organic compound girolline isolated from this species has been reported to initiating G2/M cell cycle arrest in cancer cells [43].

Axinella infundibuliformis

Axinelloside A, a sulfated lipopolysaccharide isolated from this sponge species has been reported to inhibit telomerase activity with an IC_{50} of 400 nM [44]. Telomerase activity is readily detected in most cancer biopsies.

Family: Axinellidae.

Cymbastela cantharella

The organic compound, girolline isolated from this species has been reported to induce G2/M cell cycle arrest in several tumor cell lines [43].

Family: Raspailiidae.

Lithoplocamia lithistoides

The polyketide compounds PM050489 and PM060184 derived from this sponge species induced apoptosis of A549 cancer cell line at a concentration of 0.25 and 0.001 uM, respectively. Further, its PM060184 also showed similar activity on HCT116 cancer cell line at a concentration of 0.01 uM and on MDA-MB-231 subcutaneous xenografts at a concentration of 16 mg/kg [45].

Order: Bubarida; Family: Dictyonellidae.

Lipastrotethya sp.

The extract of this sponge has shown anti-proliferative effect on wild-type p53 (WT) or p53 knockout (KO) HCT116 cells [46].

Order: Chondrosiida; Family: Chondrosiidae.

Chondrosia corticata

The macrolide, (19Z)-Halichondramide isolated from this sponge species induced apoptosis of A549 cancer cell line at a concentration range of 0.025–0.1 uM [45].

Order: Clionaida; Family: Spirastrellidae.

Spirastrella pachyspira

The ethyl acetate extracts of this species have been reported to display antiproliferative/cytotoxic properties and the LD50 of the extracts was found to be 2000 mg/kg b.wt [47].

Order: Dendroceratida; Family: Darwinellidae.

Aplysilla glacialis

The glaciasterols A and B, 9,11- Secosterol of this sponge species displayed anticancer activity. The concentrations of these metabolites producing this activity are not known [42].

Order: Dictyoceratida; Family: Dysideidae.

Candidaspongia sp.

The polyketide candidaspongiolide induced apoptosis of U251 and HCT116 cell lines at a concentration range of 0.05–0.10 uM [45].

Dysidea etheria

The extracts of this species have been reported to inhibit Cdc25 protein phosphatase which is associated with cancer cell proliferation [43].

Family: Irciniidae.

Ircinia ramosa

Irciniastatin A (= psymberin,) a pederin-type natural product isolated from this marine sponge species has been reported to induce apoptosis of lurkat cancer cell line at a concentration of 0.01 uM [45].

Ircinia sp.

The extracts of this species have been reported to inhibit Cdc25 protein phosphatase which is associated with cancer cell proliferation [43].

Psammocinia sp.

The compound, irciniastatin A (= psymberin) which belongs to the pederin natural product family, of this species induced apoptosis of Jurkat cancer cell line at a concentration of 0.01 uM. Further, its furanosesterterpene compounds *viz.* (8E,13Z,20Z)-strobilinin and (7E,13Z,20Z)-felixinin (1:1) induced apoptosis of HeLa cancer cell line at a concentration range of 10-50 uM [45].

Sarcotragus sp. 1

The difurano sesterterpene compound, ircinin-1 derived from this species induced apoptosis of SK-MEL-2 cancer cell line at a concentration range of 25-50 uM [45].

Sarcotragus sp. 2

The triterpenoid hydroquinones, adociasulfates derived from this sponge acted as Kinesin motor protein inhibitors [42]. Kinesin motor proteins are implicated in the proliferation of cancer cells through mitosis.

Family: Spongiidae.

Coscinoderma mathewsi

Coscinosulfate, a metabolite isolated from this sponge species has been reported to show inhibitory activity towards Cell division cycle 25 A (Cdc25A), which plays a key role in cancer cell proliferation [43].

Spongia sp. 1

The furanoditerpenoid compound spongiatriol isolated form this sponge induced apoptosis of cancer cell lines such as AsPC-1, PANC-1, MIA PaCa-2 and BxPC-3 at a concentration of 6.8uM [45].

Spongia sp. 2

An antimitotic macrolide (polyketide) dictyostatin-1 isolated from this sponge induced apoptosis of A549 cancer cell line at a concentration range of 0.01–1 uM [45].

Family: Thorectidae.

Cacospongia mycofijiensis

The macrolide, laulimalide produced from this sponge species has been reported to induce apoptosis of MDA-MB-435, A-10 and SK-OV-3 cell lines [45].

Dactylospongia elegans

Smenospongine, a sesquiterpene aminoquinone isolated from this marine sponge species

induced apoptosis of U937 and HL-60 cancer cell lines; and K562 cell line at a concentration range of 3-15 uM [45].

Dactylospongia metachromia, (= Hippospongia metachromia)

The compound, ilimaquinone produced by this species induced apoptosis of HCT116 and PC-3 cancer cell line at a concentration range of 2.5–10uM and 2-10 uM, respectively [45].

Fascaplysinopsis reticulata

The alkaloid compound, 3-bromofascaplysin of this species served as an inhibitor of the activating enzyme MALME-3M with an IC_{50} value of 0.45um [48].

Fascaplysinopsis sp. 1

The macrolide salarin C isolated from this marine sponge induced apoptosis of K562 cancer cell line at a concentration range of 0.01–0.2uM [45].

Fascaplysinopsis sp. 2

The indole alkaloid Fascaplysin, pentacyclic alkaloid, Camptothecin and 10-hydroxycamptothecin derived from this species of this marine sponge induced apoptosis of NCI-H417 cancer cell line at a concentration range of 0.5– 2uM [45].

Fasciospongia cavernosa

The sesterterpene compound cacospongionolide induced apoptosis of Hela and T47D cancer cell lines at a concentration of10 µg/mL [45].

Hyrtios erectus

This marine sponge yielded a pentacyclic nitrogen-containing scalarane; 24-methoxypetrosaspongia C and scalaranes *viz.* sesterstatin 3, 12-deacetyl-12--pi-scalaradial and 12-deacetyl-12,18-di-epi-scalaradial. All these compounds displayed growth inhibitory activity on hepatocellular carcinoma (HepG2), colorectal carcinoma (HCT-116) and breast adenocarcinoma cells (MCF-7) [49].

Its macrocyclic lactone polyether compound, Spongistatin 1 induced apoptosis of Jurkat and L3.6pl cancer cell lines at a concentration of 0.0002 uM and at a concentration range of 0.00001–0.01 uM respectively [45].

Hyrtios reticulatus

The alkaloid compound, hyrtioreticulins A of this species showed activity against (E1) with an IC_{50} value of 0.75 ug/mL [48].

Hyrtios sp.

The sesterterpenoid compound, heteronemin of this species induced apoptosis of K562, DU145, PC-3, LNCaP, T24 and A498 cancer cell lines at a concentration of 1.4–5.6 uM, 0.01–1 μg/mL, 0.01–1 μg/mL, 0.01 μg/mL, 0.1–0.8 μg and 0.5–3 uM, respectively [45].

Lendenfeldia chondrodes (= Fasciospongia chondrodes)

The polyhomeotic-like protein 1 (PHC-1) isolated from this species induced apoptosis of K562 cancer cell line at the concentration range of 0.1–5 μg/mL [45].

Scalarispongia scalaris (= Cacospongia scalaris)

The scalarane sesterterpenoid compound scalaradial derived from this species induced apoptosis of HeLa and T47D cell lines at a concentration of 10 μg/mL [45].

Smenospongia aurea

The chlorinated peptide/polyketide hybrids *viz.* smenamides A, B derived from this sponge species have induced apoptosis of Calu-1 cell line at a concentration range of 0.05-0.1 uM [45].

Order: Haplosclerida; Family: Callyspongiidae.

Arenosclera brasiliensis

The tetracyclic alkylpiperidine alkaloids, haliclonacyclamine E and arenosclerins (A, B and C) derived from this species have shown cytotoxicity against HL-60, L929, B16, and U138 cells [50].

Callyspongia (Callyspongia) siphonella (= Siphonochalina siphonella)

A sipholane triterpene, sipholenol-A derived form this sponge species induced apoptosis of PC-3 cell line at a concentration of 7.9 uM [45].

Callyspongia sp.

The polyacetylenediol, callyspongidiol derived from this sponge species induced apoptosis of HL-60 cancer cell line at a concentration range of 31.0–77.5 uM [45].

Siphonochalina sp.

The sipholane triterpene compounds sipholenol A, L derived from this sponge have been reported to induce apoptosis of HepG2 and HCT-116 cell lines. The concentrations for compound A were 17.18 and 14.8 uM, respectively; and for L, 24 and 19.8 uM, respectively [45].

Family: Chalinidae.

Haliclona (soestella) mucosa

The hydroquinone panicein A and an anthracycline-group antibiotic doxorubicin of this marine sponge induced apoptosis of MEWO cell line at a concentration of 10 uM and 2 uM, respectively. Further, these compounds showed similar activity on A375 cancer cell line at a concentration of 25 uM and 1.5 uM, respectively [45].

Haliclona sp.

The triterpenoid hydroquinones, adociasulfates derived from this sponge acted as Kinesin motor protein inhibitors [42]. Kinesin motor proteins are implicated in the proliferation of cancer cells through mitosis.

Haliclona (Reniera) sp. (= Prianos sp.)

The pyrrolophenanthroline alkaloid, discorhabdin D derived from this species displayed strong anticancer activity against many cancer cell lines such as human colon cancer, adenocarcinoma, and leukemia [42].

Family: Niphatidae

Niphates olemda

A diterpene compound, niphateolide isolated from this species possessed antitumor activity by serving as p53-Hdm2/Mdm2 interaction inhibitor [43].

Pachychalina alcaloidifera

The alkaloid compounds *viz.* haliclonacyclamine F, arenosclerins (D and E), madangamine F, and ingenamine G derived from this species showed cytotoxic activities against SF 295, MDA-MB-435, HCT-8, and HL-60 cells [50].

Family: Petrosiidae.

Neopetrosia chaliniformis (= Xestospongia exigua)

The pentacyclic polyketide halenaquinone isolated from this sponge species has been reported to inhibit phosphoinositide 3-kinase (PI3K) and induce apoptosis in PC12 adrenal phaeochromocytoma cells [51].

Petrosia sp.

A polyacetylene compound, dideoxypetrosynol A. isolated from this species induced apoptosis of SK-MEL-2 and U937 cancer cell lines at concentration ranges of 0.1–0.3 µg/mL and 0.2–1 µg/mL respectively [45].

Xestospongia sp.

The bishydroquinone, renieramycin M derived from this sponge induced apoptosis of H460 and U373MG cancer cell lies at concentration ranges of 5-40 and concentration of 0.0031uM. Further, its steroid, aragusterol A showed similar activity with A549 cancer cell line at the concentration range of 1-10UM [45].

Family: Phloeodictyidae

Oceanapia incrustata (= Rhizochalina incrustata)

The glycosphingolipid, rhizochalin (= rhizocalinin) of this species has been reported to induce apoptosis of several cancer cell lines such as HL-60, HT-29, THP-1, PC-3, DU-145, 22Rv1 and VCaP at concentration ranges of 10-25, 1-6, 1-10, 0.5-4, 0.5-4, 0.5-4 and 0.5-4 uM, respectively [45].

Oceanapia sagittaria

The pentacyclic alkaloids, kuanoniamine A and C of this sponge species have been reported to be potent growth inhibitor of all the tumour and non-tumour cell lines. On the other hand, kuanoniamine C was less potent but it showed high selectivity toward the estrogen dependent (ER+) breast cancer cell line (Kijjoa *et al.*, 2007). Further these compounds have also induced apoptosis of MCF-7 cancer cell line at the concentration ranges of 0.5-2.5 and 1.0 – 2.5 uM, respectively [45].

Order: Poecilosclerida; Family: Chondropsidae

Batzella sp.

The pyrroloquinoline alkaloids, batzelline A and B, isobatzelline A, C, D and secobatzelline A and B of this marine sponge showed apoptosis inducing activity of AsPC-1 cancer cell line at a concentration of 5 or 25 μg/mL [45].

Family: Coelosphaeridae

Forcepia sp.

The polyketide macrolide Lasonolide A of this sponge induced apoptosis of several cancer cell lines such as CA46, Ramos, Daudi, HL-60, MDA-MD-231, MCF-7, HCT-116, and HT-29 at a concentration of 0.1 μg/mL [45].

Family: Crambeidae.

Crambe crambe

The pentacyclic guanidine derivatives crambescidins 800,816 and 830 isolated from this sponge species induced apoptosis of HepG2 cancer cell line at a concentration range of 0.5–2.5 uM. Further, Crambescidins 14 of this species is believed to act as a Ca^{2+}/channel blocker [45]. Ca^{2+}/channel blocker helps in lowering blood pressure by preventing calcium from entering the cells of the heart and arteries.

Crambe tailliezi

A purified high molecular weight compound, P3 derived from the extract of this species induced apoptosis and decreased proliferation and mitotic index of human osteosarcoma U-2 OS cells [51].

Monanchora arbuscula

The alkaloids, 8bβ-hydroxyptilocaulin and ptilocaulin derived from this species displayed cytotoxicity against HL-60, MDA-MB-435, HCT-8, and SF-295 cells; and these compounds also induced apoptosis of these cancer cell lines [50].

Monanchora pulchra

This species has been reported to yield several anticancer alkaloid compounds such as monanchocidin A -C, ptilomycalin A, monanchomycalin B, normonanchocidin D, urupocidin A and pulchranin A. All these compounds induced apoptosis of HeLa cancer line with concentration ranges from 0.5 to 58 uM [45].

Monanchora unguiculata

Crambescidin 800, an organic heteropentacyclic guanidine alkaloid isolated from this sponge species induced apoptosis of K562 cancer cell line at a concentration range of 0.15- 1.5 uM [45].

Family: Hymedesmiidae.

Kirkpatrickia variolosa

The alkaloid compound, variolin B, which was isolated from this sponge species displayed pro-apoptotic activity and inhibited Cyclin-Dependent Kinase.

(CDK) activity [44].

Family: Latrunculiidae.

Latrunculia (latrunculia) brevis

The pyrrolophenanthroline alkaloid, discorhabdin D derived from this species displayed strong anticancer activity against many cancer cell lines such as human colon cancer, adenocarcinoma, and leukemia [42].

Family: Mycalidae.

Mycale hentscheli

A macrocyclic lactone peloruside A induced apoptosis of H441 and MCF-7 cancer cell lines at the concentration ranges of 0.01-1 and 0.025-0.1 uM [45].

Mycale sp.

The macrodiolide Pateamine and mycalamide A derived from this sponge species induced apoptosis of 32D cancer cell line at a concentration of 0.1 uM [45].

Family: Podospongiidae.

Diacarnus megaspinorhabdosa

The terpenoid compounds sigmosceptrellin B and diacarperoxide B of this species showed activity against L5178Y cell line with IC_{50} values of 0.55ug/mL and 0.88ug/mL, respectively [48].

Negombata magnifica

An actin binding macrolide and toxin latrunculin A produced by this sponge species induced apoptosis of MKN45 and NUGC-4 cancer cell lines at a concentration of -10 and a concentration range of 0.01-10 uM, respectively [45].

Order: Scopalinida; Family: Scopalinidae.

Stylissa flabeliformis

The alkaloid compound debromohymenialdisine of this sponge species induced apoptosis of MCF-7 cancer cell line at a concentration range of 2- 5uM [45].

Stylissa massa (= Hymeniacidon aldis)

Pyrrole-guanidine alkaloid, debromohymenialdisine derived from this sponge species acted as Protein kinase C inhibitor which has application in cancer therapy [42].

Stylissa sp.

The peptide compound, stlissamide X of this species showed activity against HeLa cells with an IC_{50} value of 0.1uM [47].

Order: Suberitida; Family: Halichondriidae.

Halichondria (halichondria) okadai

Its polyether macrolide compound halichondrin B has shown anticancer activity. This compound has yielded a synthetic analog *viz.* eribulin mesylate. Eribulin has been approved by the US Food and Drug Administration (FDA) and the European Medicines Agency (EMA) as late-line therapy for metastatic breast cancer patients who were previously treated with an anthracycline and a taxane [52].

Family: Suberitidae.

Aaptos aaptos

The benzonaphthyridine alkaloid, isoaaptamine produced by this species acted as protein kinase C inhibitor which blocks early T-cell activation, by blocking the protein kinase [42].

Its compound aaptamine helps in inducing apoptosis of NT2 and HepG2 cell lines at a concentration range of 1-50 uM and 50–100 uM, respectively [45].

Aaptos suberitoides

The alkaloid compound, delaaptamine of this species showed activity against L5178Y marine leukemia cell line with an IC_{50} value of 0.9uM [48].

Its compound aaptamine induced apoptosis of MG63 and K562 cell lines at a concentration range of 30 µg/mL and 20-100 uM, respectively [45].

Aaptos sp.

Its alkaloid compounds aaptamine and demethyl(oxy)aaptamine induced apoptosis of THP-1 cell line at a concentration range of 10-25 uM [45].

The alkaloid compound isoaaptamine of this unidentified species showed activity against P338 cell line with an IC_{50} value of 0.28 ug/mL [48].

Order: Tethyida; Family: Hemiasterellidae.

Hemiasterella vasiformis var., minor (= Hemiasterella minor)

The tripeptides, hemiasterlin, hemiasterlin A and B produced by this species induced apoptosis of MCF7cancer cell line at a concentration range of 0.0005–0.01 uM [45].

Family: Tethyidae.

Tectitethya crypta (= Cryptotheca crypta)

The compounds C-nucleosides isolated from this sponge species formed the basis for the synthesis of cytarabine, the first marine anticancer agent developed for clinical use.

Cytarabine is presently used in the routine treatment of leukaemia and lymphoma. Further, gemcitabine, its fluorinated derivative has also been approved for treating pancreatic, breast, non-small-cell lung and bladder cancer [53].

Order: Tetractinellida; Family: Ancorinidae.

Jaspis stellifera

Stellettin B, an isomalabaricane triterpenoid isolated from this marine sponge induces apoptosis of K562, A549 and SF295 cancer cell lines at a concentration range of 0.012-0.054 uM, 0.02-1uM and 0.04-1uM, respectively [45].

Jaspis sp.

The somalabaricane-type triterpene jaspolide B isolated from this species induced apoptosis of Bel-7402, at a concentration of 0.5uM; HepG2 cancer cell line at a concentration range of 10-20uM; B16 cell line at a concentration of 5 uM; and Bel-7402 and HepG2 cell lines at a concentration of 20 uM [45].

Rhabdastrella globostellata

The compounds 13E,17E-globostellatic acid X methyl ester and rhabdastrellic acid-A isolated from this sponge species induced apoptosis of HUVEC cell line at a concentration range of 1-10 um; and these compounds showed similar activity with the HL-60 cell line [45].

Stelletta sp.

An acetylenic acid *viz.* (Z)-stellettic acid C isolated from this sponge induced apoptosis of U937 cell line at a concentration range of 17.2–103.3uM [45].

Family: Azoricidae.

Leiodermatium sp.

The polyketide-derived macrolide, leiodermatolide isolated from this sponge induced apoptosis of AsPC-1, BxPC-3 and MIA PaCa-2 cell lines at a concentration of 0.01 uM. Further, this compound showed similar activity with cancer cell lines *viz.* PANC-1, A549 and U2OS at concentration ranges of 0.01–0.1, 0.01–1 and 0.018-0.23 uM, respectively [45].

Family: Calthropellidae.

Pachastrissa sp.

An anhydrophytosphingosine derivative *viz.* jaspine B (= pachastrissamine) of this species has been reported to induce apoptosis of HaCaT cell line at a concentration of 5 µg/mL [45].

Family: Geodiidae.

Geodia japonica

An isomalabaricane triterpene geoditin A derived from this species induced apoptosis of HL-60 and HT-29 cell lines at a concentration range of 1.6 to 25 µg/mL and 5–30uM, respectively. Further, its triterpenoid stellettin A showed similar activity at a concentration of 4 µg/mL [45].

Geodia tylastra (= Geodia corticostylifera)

The cyclodepsipeptides geodiamolide A, B, H and I derived from this sponge species induced apoptosis of T47D and MCF7cancer cell lines at a concentration of 50 ng/mL [45].

Pachymatisma johnstonia

A glycoprotein, named pachymatismin, isolated from this sponge species induced apoptosis of cancer cell lines *viz.* DU145 and NSCLC-N6 and NSCLC-N6 subcutaneous xenografts at concentration ranges of 4–16uM, 2–20 µg/mL and 0.5–5 mg/kg, respectively [45].

Family: Scleritodermidae.

Amphibleptula sp.

The macrocyclic peptide, microsclerodermin A of this marine sponge induced apoptosis of AsPC-1, BxPC-3 and PANC-1 cell lines at a concentration of 2.4 uM [45].

Family: Theonellidae.

Discodermia calyx

The marine toxin calyculin A isolated from this sponge species induced apoptosis of MDA-MB-468, MCF-7 and MDA-MB-231 cancer cell lines at a concentration of 0.01uM [45].

Discodermia dissoluta

The linear tetraene lactone, discodermolide of this sponge species helps in the stabilization of microtubules [42]. Microtubule inhibitors comprise a highly effective class of anti-cancer drugs and they have been commonly applied in the treatment of hematopoietic and solid tumors.

(+)-Discodermolide of this species induced apoptosis of MCF-7 and CA46 cell lines at a concentration range of 0.01–1 uM; and A549 at a concentration range of 0.07–0.166 uM [45].

Order: Trachycladida; Family: Trachycladidae.

Trachycladus spinispirulifera (= spirastrella spinispirulifera)

The macrocyclic lactone polyether compound, spongistatin 1 isolated from this species has induced apoptosis of MCF-7 cell line at a concentration range of 0.0002–0.0005uM [45].

Order: Verongiida; Family: Aplysinidae

Aplysina aerophoba

The brominated alkaloid, isofistularin-3 of this species induced apoptosis of Raji and U937 cell lines at a concentration of 50 uM [45].

Family: Ianthellidae.

Ianthella sp.

The tribrominated compound bastadin 6 derived from this species induced apoptosis of HUVEC cancer cell line at a concentration range of 0.01–1uM. Further, its other compounds *viz.* Petrosterol-3,6-dione, 5α,6α-epoxy-petrosterol and petrosterol have shown apoptosis of HL-60 cancer cell line at a concentration of 19.9, 21.3 and 21.5 uM, respectively [45].

Family: Pseudoceratinidae.

Pseudoceratina purpurea (= Dendrilla verongiformis)

The alkaloids, dictyodendrins A-E isolated from this species have been reported to serve as telomerase inhibitors at a concentration of 50 microg/mL [54]. By inhibiting telomerase, these compounds enhance tumor cell senescence and apoptosis.

Pseudocerarina sp. (= Psammaplysilla sp.) 1

The phenolic natural product psammaplin A derived from this sponge has been reported to induce apoptosis of human endometrial Ishikawa cell line. Further, an alkaloid compound of this sponge *viz.* psammaplysene A showed similar activity with Ishikawa and ECC1 cell lines at a concentration of 1 uM [45].

Pseudoceratina sp. (= Psammaplysilla sp.) 2

A dibromotyrosine derivative, (1'R,5'S,6'S)-2-(3',5'-dibromo-1',6'-dihydrxy-4'-oxocyclohex-2'-enyl) acetonitrile isolated from this sponge induced apoptosis of K562 cell line at a concentration range of 7.7-30.8uM [45].

Class: Hexactinellida; Order: Sceptrulophora; Family: Aphrocallistidae.

Aphrocallistes beatrix

An adenine-substituted bromotyramine metabolite *viz.* aphrocallistin induced apoptosis of Panc-1 cell line at a concentration of ≤46.5 uM [45].

Class: Homoscleromorpha; Order: Homosclerophorida; Family: Plakinidae.

Plakinastrella sp.

The alkylphenol, elenic acid isolated from this sponge showed anticancer activity by inhibiting topoisomerase II [42].

Plakortis angulospiculatus

The polyketide, plakortide P isolated from this species has been reported to display potent cytotoxicity in the NCI human cancer cell line [55].

Wilke *et al.* (2021) reported that its two dihydrofurans (6-desmethyl--ethylspongosoritin A and Spongosoritin A) and 3 6-membered peroxides (plakortides) have shown cytotoxicity against HCT-116 and PC-3M cell lines [50].

Plakortis halichondrioides

The polyketides plakortide O and plakortide P displayed potent cytotoxicity in the NCI human cancer cell line [55].

Antiviral Activity

Phylum: Porifera; Class: Demospongiae; Order: Agelasida; Family: Agelasidae.

Agelas flabelliformis

The compounds, 4-α-methyl-5 α-cholest-8-en-3 β-ol and 4,5-dibromo-2-pyrrolic acid isolated from this species acted against SARS-CoV-2 proteases [56].

Agelas oroides

The pyrrole-imidazole alkaloid taurodispacamide A, isolated from this species displayed inhibitory activity to IL-2 production and acted against SARS-CoV-2 proteases [56].

Order: Axinellida; Family: Axinellidae.

Axinella cf. corrugaata

Coumarin derivatives such as esculetin-4-carboxylic acid methyl ester and esculetin-4-carboxylic acid ethyl ester isolated from this marine sponge displayed significant inhibitory activity to SARS-coronavirus Mpro [56].

Family: Stelligeridae.

Paratimea sp. (= Halicortex sp.)

The bromoindole alkaloid, dragmacidin F of this species displayed *in vitro* antiviral activity against HIV-1 and HSV-1 with an EC_{50} of 0.9 μM and 96 μM respectively [57].

Order: Dendroceratida; Family: Darwinellidae.

Dendrilla membranosa

The terpene dihydrogracilin A isolated from this species is a potent IL-6 and acted against SARS-CoV-2 proteases [56].

Family: Dysideidae.

Dysidea avara and Dysidea cinerea

The sesquiterpene hydroquinone compounds avarol and avarone have been extracted from Disidea avara. At a concentration of 0.1 μg/mL, avarol displayed a dose-dependent inhibitory effect on acquired immune deficiency syndrome (AIDS) and human T-lymphotropic retrovirus (HTLV III)/lymphadenopathy-associated virus in human H9 cells *in vitro*. Further, avarol or its derivatives have been reported to inhibit reverse transcriptase which is known to play an important role in the inhibition of cyclooxygenase and 5'-lipoxygenase, thus reducing significantly the levels of prostaglandin E2 and leukotriene B4 *in vitro* in the HIV-1 infected monocytes besides modulating the expression of genes in HIV-infected cells. A structurally similar compound *viz.* avarone produced by this species also exhibited similar antiviral activity.

Several new derivatives of avarol extracted from the Red Sea sponge, Dysidea cinerea have shown antiviral activities [57]. Its avarol boosted the humoral immune response upon exposure to SARS-coronavirus viral infection [56].

Dysidea sp.

Its immunosuppressive compounds like 3-polyoxygenated sterol have been reported to block the activity of the cytokine IL-8, which is believed to be responsible for the development of severe respiratory distress syndrome associated with SARS-coronavirus [56].

A sesquiterpene quinone, puupehedione isolated from this marine sponges has been reported to modulate the immune response of T-cells and served as protease inhibitors of the SARS-coronavirus [56].

Family: Spongiidae.

Hippospongia metachromia

A bioactive sesquiterpene, ilimaquinone isolated from this sponge species showed potential inhibitory activity against SARS-CoV-2 proteases [56].

Family: Thorectidae.

Cacospongia mycofijiensis

The terpenoid T3, isolated from this marine sponge, displayed potential inhibition activity against SARS CoV-2 Mpro [56].

Hyrtios sp.

A sesquiterpene quinone, puupehedione isolated from this marine sponges has been reported to modulate the immune response of T-cells and served as protease inhibitors of the SARS-coronavirus [56].

A sesquiterpene quinone, puupehedione isolated from this marine sponges has been reported to modulate the immune response of T-cells and served as protease inhibitors of the SARS-coronavirus [56].

Order: Haplosclerida; Family: Chalinidae.

Haliclona sp.

The alkaloid, manzamine A of Haliclona sp. has been reported to display anti-HIV-1 activity [57].

Family: Petrosiidae.

Acanthostrongylophora sp.

The alkaloid, manzamine A of Acanthostrongylophora sp., exhibited anti-HIV-1 activity with an EC_{50} value of 4.2 µM [56]. Its alkaloid compounds 8-hydroxymanzamine A, 6-deoxymanzamine X, and neokauluamine of this unidentified species showed anti-HIV-1 activity with EC_{50} values of 0.6, 1.6, and 2.3 µM, respectively [57].

Neopetrosia contignata (= Petrosia contignata)

The sterol, contignasterol, derived from this marine sponge, has been reported to downregulate the production of IL-6 and served as protease inhibitors- of SARS-coronavirus [56].

Family: Phloeodictyidae.

Pachypellina sp.

The alkaloid, manzamine A of this unidentified species showed anti-HIV-1 activity with a minimal effective concentration of 0.05 µg/mL [57].

Order: Poecilosclerida; Family: Desmacididae.

Desmapsamma anchorata

A chimyl alcohol (1-O-hexadecylglycerol), isolated from this sponge species displayed potential inhibition activity to SARS-CoV-2 by binding to Mpro SARS-coronavirus [56].

Family: Hymedesmiidae.

Hamigera tarangaensis

At a concentration of 132 µg per disk, its phenolic macrolides displayed 100% *in vitro* virus inhibition against both the herpes and polio viruses [57].

The naphthalene derivative, hamigeran-b, isolated from this marine sponge, served as the inhibitor of Mpro of SARS-CoV and SARS-CoV-2 [56].

Family: Hymedesmiidae.

Phorbas sp.

The terpenoid compounds alotaketals and ansellones isolated from this sponge exhibited antiviral activity [11].

Family: Mycalidae.

Mycale sp. 1

The nucleosides Mycalamide A, B have been isolated from this unidentified species.The crude extract containing 2% mycalamide A acted against A59 corona virus. Further, at a concentration of 5 ng/disc, this compound also inhibited the Herpes simplex type I and Polio type I viruses. Mycalamide B also had similar activities but it was found to be more potent than mycalamide A, as it was active at even a concentration of 1–2 ng/disc [57]. The nucleoside analogues mycalisine A, and B of this species displayed significant inhibition activity to SARS-coronavirus Mpro [56].

Mycale sp. 2

The macrodiolide pateamine A isolated from this sponge exhibited selective inhibition activity on the production of IL-2 and served as protease inhibitors of SARS-coronavirus [56].

Order: Scopalinida; Family: Scopalinidae.

Stylissa carteri

The alkaloid compound, oroidin isolated from this species displayed antiviral (HIV-1) activity [42].

Order: Suberitida; Family: Halichondriidae.

Halichondria (Halichondria) semitubulosa (= Pellina semitubulosa)

The immune-stimulant, lectin isolated from this marine sponge enhanced the production of IL-1 and IL-2 at 0.3 and 10.0 pg/ml and served as protease inhibitors- of SARS-coronavirus [56].

Hymeniacidon sp.

An octa-peptide hymenistatin I, isolated from this sponge displayed humoral and cellular immunosuppressive activity and served as protease inhibitors of the SARS-coronavirus [56].

Family: Suberitidae.

Aaptos sp.

The alkaloid compound, 4-Methylaaptamine of this species has been reported to inhibit 76% of HSV-1 replication in Vero cells at a concentration of 2.4 μg/mL Further, this compound showed anti-HSV-1 activity in Vero cells even 4 h after infection with an EC_{50} of 2.4 μM [57].

Order: Tethyida; Family: Tethyidae.

Tectitethya crypta (= Tethya crypta)

It has been reported to produce arabinose sugar containing nucleosides spongothymidine and spongouridine. The synthetic analogue of spongouridine yielded the first antiviral drug *viz.* Vidarabine or Ara-A which was approved by the US FDA although its marketing was later stopped as it was found to be more

toxic and less efficient. This drug was used for the treatment of herpes encephalitis and the other herpes infections [57].

Order: Tetractinellida; Family Ancorinidae.

Stelletta clavosa

The peptides Mirabamides E-H derived from this species showed antiviral activity [11].

Stelletta sp.

The peptides stellettapeptin A, B derived from this sponge exhibited HIV inhibitory activity [11].

Family: Geodiidae.

Erylus goffrilleri

The penasterol disaccharide Eryloside E, isolated from this sponge sponge, displayed specific immunosuppressive activity against SARS-coronavirus at IC_{50} 1.3 μg/ml [56].

Geodia microspinosa (= Sidonops microspinosa)

The cyclic depsipeptide, microspinosamide derived from this species showed potent anti-HIV activity in C EM-SS target cells at a concentration of 0.2 μg/mL

Further, both the aqueous and organic extracts of this species have been reported to exhibit anti-HIV activity [57].

Family: Theonellidae.

Siliquariaspongia mirabilis

The new cyclic depsipeptides Mirabamides A,C and D isolated from this species displayed antiviral (HIV-1) activity [42].

Theonella mirabilis and Theonella swinhoei

The cyclic depsipeptides, Papuamide A, B, C, and D produced by these species have shown anti-HIV and cytotoxic activities. At an effective concentration of 3.6 ng/mL, these compounds displayed significant anti-HIV activity. On the other hand, at a concentration of 40 and 20 fold higher than papuamides A and B, papuamides C and D were found to be less potent with 30% and 55% inhibition. respectively [57].

The tetrapeptides pseudotheonamide C and D, isolated from the sponge Theonella swinhoei displayed inhibitory activity against TMPRSS2 which is a human serine protease enzyme used by the SARS-coronavirus for its activation and cell entry [56].

Order: Verongiida; Family: Ianthellidae.

Ianthella quadrangulata

The polyketide iso-iantheran A isolated from this sponge species has been reported to activate the P2Y11 receptor which is a regulator of human immune responses [56].

Antimalarial Activity

Phylum: Porifera; Class: Demospongiae; Order: Agelasida; Family: Agelasidae.

Agelas gracilis

Derivatives of plakortin *viz.* gracilioetheres A–C derived from this species have sown antimalarial activity against *Plasmodium falciparum*. Among these compounds, gracilioether B showed significant activity with an IC_{50} value of 1.41 μM [10].

Agelas mauritiana

Three diterpene alkaloids *viz.* agelasine J, agelasine K, and agelasine L, isolated from this species have shown *in vitro* antimalarial activity against *Plasmodium falciparum* [58].

Agelas oroides

The pyrrole-imidazole-related alkaloid, (E)-oroidin of this species possessed significant activity against *Plasmodium falciparum* strains *in vitro* with an IC_{50} value of 10 µM [10].

Agelas sp.

A new glycosphingolipid isolated from this sponge displayed anti-plasmodial activity in the low micromolar range *viz.* IC_{50} of 0.53 µM [10].

Order: Axinellida; Family: Axinellidae.

Pipestela hooperi (= Cymbastela hooperi)

The alkaloid compound, manzamine A isolated from this species has shown antimalarial activity against *Plasmodium falciparum* and *Plasmodium berghei* with an IC_{50} value of 4.5 ng/ml; a tetracyclic diterpene, diisocyanoadociane of this species has shown similar activity with an IC_{50} value of 0.005 µg/ml; and a macrolide, halichondramide of this species had the said activity with an IC_{50} value of 0.002 µg/ml [42].

Order; Biemnida; Family: Biemnidae.

Biemna laboutei

The guanidine alkaloids ptilomycalin F and fromiamycalin isolated from this species showed antimalarial activity with IC_{50} values of 0.23 and 0.24 µM, respectively [10].

Order: Bubarida; Family: Dictyonellidae.

Acanthella sp.

The isonitril-containing kalihinane diterpenoid, Kalihinol A isolated from this species has shown antimalarial activity against *Plasmodium falciparum* with an IC_{50} value of 0.0005 µg/ml [42].

Order: Dictyoceratida; Family: Spongiidae.

Coscinoderma sp.

The sterol compounds (24S)-5α,8α-epidioxy-24-methylcholesta-6-en-3β-ol and 5α,8α-epidioxy-24-methylcholesta-6,9(11), 24(28)-trien-3β-ol isolated from this sponge displayed antimalarial activity against the resistant strain of *Plasmodium falciparum* (Dd2) [10].

Hyattella sp.

The bromotyrosine alkaloid psammaplysin H displayed antiplasmodial activity against 3D7 line of *Plasmodium falciparum* with an IC_{50} value of 0.41 μM [10].

Family: Thorectidae.

Fascaplysinopsis reticulata

The indole alkaloids, (E)-6-bromo-2'-demethyl-3'-N-methylaplysinopsin and (Z)-6-bromo-2'-demethyl-3'-N-methylaplysinopsin of this species displayed antiplasmodial activity [10].

Hyrtios erectus

Alkaloids containing β-carboline ring of this species showed antiplasmodial activity against *Plasmodium falciparum*.

Further, terpene compounds *viz.* smenotronic acid, ilimaquinone and pelorol isolated from this species has shown similar activity with IC_{50} values ranging from 0.8 to 3.51 μM [10].

Order: Haplosclerida; Family: Chalinidae.

Haliclona sp.

The alkaloid compound, manzamine A isolated from this species has shown antimalarial activity against *Plasmodium falciparum* and *Plasmodium berghei* with an IC_{50} value of 4.5 ng/ml [42].

Family: Petrosiidae.

Acanthostrongylophora ingens

The manzamine alkaloids manzamine A and 8-hydroxymanzamine A isolated from this species displayed anti-plasmodial activity against *Plasmodium berghei* with IC_{50} values ranging between 0.010 and 0.060 µM [10].

Xestospongia sp. 1

The pentacyclic quinone alkaloid, xestoquinone of this species has shown moderate antiplasmodial inhibitory activity on *Plasmodium falciparum* protein kinases (PfPK5 and Pfnek-1); and slightly inhibited this parasite *in vivo* [10].

Xestospongia sp. 2

Sterols without peroxide *viz.* kaimanol and saringosterol isolated from this sponge have been reported to show antimalarial activity by reducing the parasite development expressively with IC_{50} values of 359 and 0.250 nM, respectively [10].

Order: Poecilosclerida; Family: Acarnidae.

Zyzzya sp.

The alkaloid tsitsikammamine C isolated from this species has been reported to show potent *in vitro* antiplasmodial activity against resistant strains of *Plasmodium falciparum* (3D7 and Dd2) with IC_{50} values of < 100 nM [10].

Family: Podospongiidae.

Diacarnus levii

The alkaloid compound, manzamine A isolated from this species has shown antimalarial activity against *Plasmodium falciparum* and *Plasmodium berghei* with an IC_{50} value of 4.5 ng/ml [42].

Diacarnus erythraeanus

The norsesterterpene compound, sigmosceptrellin B isolated from this species has shown antimalarial activity against *Plasmodium falciparum* with an IC_{50} value of 1200 ng/ml [42].

Diacarnus megaspinorhabdosa

Norditerpene and norsesterterpene peroxide metabolites isolated from this species showed antimalarial activity [10].

Family: Tedaniidae.

Tedania (Tedania) brasiliensis

A bromopyrrole alkaloid pseudoceratidine of this species showed antiplasmodial potential with an IC_{50} value of 1.1 µM [10].

Order: Suberitida; Family: Halichondriidae.

Axinyssa djiferi

The glycosphingolipids, axidjiferoside A-C isolated from this sponge species displayed significant antimalarial activity [10].

Hymeniacidon sp.

A diterpene alkaloid isolated from this species *viz.* monamphilectine A containing a distinct β-lactam core showed significant antiplasmodial activity (Aguiar *et al.*, 2021). Further its β-lactam compound, monamphilectine. A isolated from this

species has shown similar activity against *Plasmodium falciparum* with an IC_{50} value of 0.6 µM [42].

Spongosorites sp.

An indole alkaloid, nortopsentin A of this species showed significant antiplasmodial activity with an IC_{50} value of 0.46 µM [10].

Order: Tetractinellida; Family: Geodiidae.

Penares nux (= Pachastrissa nux)

The olyketides *viz.* Trisoxazole macrolides isolated from this species have shown antimalarial activity [10].

Order: Verongiida; Family: Aplysinellidae.

Aplysinella strongylata

The bromotyrosine alkaloid psammaplysin H displayed antiplasmodial activity against 3D7 line of *Plasmodium falciparum* with an IC_{50} value of 0.41 µM [10].

Family: Aplysinidae.

Verongula sp.

The bromotyrosine alkaloid psammaplysin H displayed antiplasmodial activity against 3D7 line of *Plasmodium falciparum* with an IC_{50} value of 0.41 µM [10].

Family: Pseudoceratinidae.

Pseudoceratina purpurea

A bromopyrrole alkaloid pseudoceratidine of this species showed antiplasmodial potential with an IC_{50} value of 1.1 µM [10].

Pseudoceratina sp.

The bromotyrosine alkaloid psammaplysin H displayed antiplasmodial activity against 3D7 line of *Plasmodium falciparum* with an IC_{50} value of 0.41 µM [10].

Plakinastrella sp.

Class: Homoscleromorpha; Order: Homosclerophorida; Family: Plakinidae

The macrolides and polyketides (with skeletons containing endoperoxides) isolated from this sponge have shown antimalarial activity [10].

Plakortis simplex

Order: Homosclerophorida

A series of polyketides with endoperoxides isolated from this species have shown antiplasmodial activity with IC_{50} values ranging from 0.39 to 6.18 µM [10].

Plakortis halichondrioides

The endoperoxide derivatives (lactones) isolated from this species have shown antimalarial activity with IC_{50} values ranging from 0.756 to 15.1 µM (Aguiar *et al.*, 2021). Further, the polyketide plakortide O methyl ester, of this species showed similar activity against *Plasmodium falciparum* [55].

Plakortis lita

The tricyclic alkaloids with thiazine-fused quinone, thiaplakortones A–D isolated from this species displayed antimalarial potential in the nanomolar range (IC_{50} < 651 nM) with moderate toxicity [10].

Plakortis simplex

The cycloperoxidase compounds, plakortin and dihydroplakortin isolated from this species have shown antimalarial activity against *Plasmodium falciparum* with IC_{50} values of 1263 and 1117 nM respectively [42].

Antidiabetic activity

Phylum: Porifera; Class: Demospongiae; Order: Agelasida; Family: Agelasidae.

Agelas mauritianus

The a synthetic glycolipid *viz.* α-galactosylceramide (α-GalCer) derived from this sponge species showed antidiabetic activity by inducing protection of pancreatic β cells [59].

Agelas oroides

The extracts of this species have shown α-Glucosidase Inhibitory Activity and at an extract concentration of 3000 μg/mL, the percentage of inhibition was 7.6 [60].

Order: Axinellida; Family: Axinellidae.

Axinella cannabina

The extracts of this species have shown α-Glucosidase Inhibitory Activity and at an extract concentration of 3000 μg/mL, the percentage of inhibition was 6.6 [60].

Axinella polypoides

The extracts of this species have shown α-Glucosidase inhibitory activity and at an extract concentration of 3000 μg/mL, the percentage of inhibition was 5.2 [60].

Order: Bubarida; Family: Dictyonellidae.

Dictyonella incisa

The extracts of this species have shown α-Glucosidase Inhibitory Activity and at an extract concentration of 3000 μg/mL, the percentage of inhibition was 16.8 [60].

Order: Clionaida; Family: Clionaidae.

Cliona viridis

The extracts of this species have shown α-Glucosidase inhibitory activity and at an extract concentration of 3000 μg/mL, the percentage of inhibition was 7.5 [60].

Order: Dictyoceratida; Family: Dysideidae.

Dysidea avara

The extracts of this species have shown α-Glucosidase Inhibitory Activity and at an extract concentration of 3000 μg/mL, the percentage of inhibition was 94.7 [60]. It is one of the most active sponge species and its sesquiterpenoid hydroquinone, avarol and quinone avarone displayed strong inhibitory activities against α-glucosidase enzyme with percentage values of 86.2% and 78.9%, respectively [59].

Dysidea villosa

The compound, dynosine of this sponge species showed antidiabetic activity by activating the insulin receptor by modifying its phosphorylation (by PTP1B inhibition) [59].

Dysidea sp.

The terpene dysidine isolated from this sponge showed antidiabetic activity by inhibiting the enzyme,protein-tyrosine phosphatase 1B (PTP1B). Further this terpene has been reported to strongly promote membrane translocation of the glucose transporter 4 (GLUT4) in CHO-K1 (from Cricetulus griseus ovary) and 3T3-L1 (from Mus musculus embryo) cells which indicate the involvement of GLUT4 in the promotion of glucose uptake [59]. Two sesquiterpene quinones derived from this sponge displayed positive PT1B1 inhibitory action, with IC_{50} values of 6.7 μM and 9.98 μM, respectively [61].

Lamellodysidea herbacea

Six polybromodiphenyl ether derivatives derived from this sponge species displayed *in vitro* PTP1B1 inhibitory action with IC_{50} values varying from 0.6 μM to 1,7 μM [61].

Family: Irciniidae.

Ircinia dendroides

A sesquiterpene named palinurin of this species displayed antidiabetic activity by inhibiting the enzyme GSK-3β [59].

Ircinia incisa

The extracts of this species have shown α-Glucosidase Inhibitory Activity and at an extract concentration of 3000 µg/mL, the percentage of inhibition was 6.3 [60].

Ircinia oros

The extracts of this species have shown α-Glucosidase Inhibitory Activity and at an extract concentration of 3000 µg/mL, the percentage of inhibition was 7.8 [60].

Ircinia variabilis

The extracts of this species have shown α-Glucosidase Inhibitory Activity and at an extract concentration of 3000 µg/mL, the percentage of inhibition was 4.3 [60].

Sarcotragus spinulosa

The extracts of this species have shown α-Glucosidase Inhibitory Activity and at an extract concentration of 3000 µg/mL, the percentage of inhibition was 2.6 [60].

Family: Spongiidae.

Hippospongia lachne

Two sesterpenoids derived from this sponge species showed antidiabetic activity by inhibiting PT1B1 with IC_{50} values of 5.2 µM and 8.7 µM, respectively [61].

Spongia sp. (= Euryspongia sp.)

The sesquiterpenes euryspongin A, derived from this sponge displayed antidiabetic activity by inhibiting protein tyrosine phosphatase IB (PTBIB) [62]. Its sesquiterpene, dehydrourysspongin A displayed *in vitro* PT1B1 inhibitory action with an IC_{50} value of 3.6 µM [61].

Order: Haplosclerida; Family: Callyspongiidae.

Callyspongia truncata

The polyacetylenic acid, callyspongynic acid, isolated from tis sponge species displayed antidiabetic activity by inhibiting α-glucosidase [59].

Family: Petrosiidae.

Petrosia (petrosia) ficiformis

The extracts of this species have shown α-Glucosidase Inhibitory Activity and at an extract concentration of 3000 μg/mL, the percentage of inhibition was 7.4 [60].

Family: Petrosiidae.

Xestospongia muta

The aqueous extracts of this sponge showed antidiabetic activity by inhibiting the dipeptidyl peptidase IV activity in *in vitro* models [59].

Family: Phloeodictyidae.

Siphonodictyon coralliphagum (= Aka coralliphaga)

The bacteria associated with this sponge species have shown antidiabetic activity by inhibiting β- glucosidase [62].

Order: Poecilosclerida; Family: Hymedesmiidae

Hemimycale arabica

A phenylmethylene hydantoins derived from this sponge species showed antidiabetic activity by inhibiting Glycogen synthase kinase-3 beta, (GSK-3β) [59].

Family: Mycalidae

Mycale sp.

The sterols derived from this sponge *viz.* hydroperoxyl sterols, epidioxy sterols and fucosterols displayed *in vitro* PTP1B1 inhibitory action [61].

Order: Verongiida; Family: Aplysinidae

Aplysina aerophoba

The extracts of this species have shown α-Glucosidase Inhibitory Activity and at an extract concentration of 3000 μg/mL, the percentage of inhibition was 7.8 [60].

Antitubercular Activity

Phylum: Porifera; Class: Demospongiae; Order: Agelasida; Family: Agelasidae.

Agelas sp.

The alkaloid compounds, 2-Methoxy-3-oxoaaptamine, 2,3-dihydro-2-3-dioxoaaptamine, demethyl(oxy)aaptamine, 3-aminodemethyl(oxy)aaptamine, and 3-(methylamino)demethyl(oxy)aaptamine were isolated from this marine sponge. Among them, 2-Methoxy-3-oxoaaptamine displayed antimycobacterial activity against *Mycobacterium smegmatis* (in both active-growing and dormancy-inducing hypoxic conditions) with an MIC value of 6.25 µg/ml, and the remaining compounds demonstrated antimycobacterial activities under hypoxic condition with MIC values of 1.5–6.25 µg/ml [63].

Order: Dictyoceratida; Family: Thorectidae.

Hyrtios aeticulatus

The sesquiterpene, heteronemin derived from this species displayed antitubercular activity [63].

Order: Haplosclerida; Family: Callyspongiidae.

Arenosclera brasiliensis

The alkyl pepridine alkaloid arenosclerins A?C derived from this sponge species displayed antimycobacterial (antitubercular) activity against Mycobacterium tuberculosis at a concentration of 16 µg/ml [42].

Callyspongia (cladochalina) aerizusa

The cyclic peptides callyaerin A, B. – derived from this sponge species displayed strong anti-tubercular (Mycobacterium tuberculosis) activity with MIC90 values of 2 and 5 µM, respectively [63].

Family: Chalinidae.

Haliclona sp.

The alkaloid compounds Haliclocyclamines A–C isolated form this species exhibited antitubercular activity [11].

Family: Petrosiidae.

Acanthostrongylophora sp.

The alkaloid compound, 6-hydroxymanzamine E isolated from this sponge species displayed antimycobacterial activity against Mycobacterium tuberculosis at a concentration of 0.9 µg/ml [42].

Order: Suberitida; Family: Halichondriidae.

Halichondria (halichondria) panicea

The alkaloid compounds, (10E,12Z)-Haliclonadiamine, halichondriamines A and B, haliclonadiamine, and papuamine derived from this marine sponge exhibited antimycobacterial activities with inhibition zones of 7–16 mm at 10 µg/disc [64].

Order: Tetractinellida; Family: Ancorinidae.

Jaspis splendens

The bengamides P and Q derived from this species exhibited antitubercular activity. The compound P recorded MIC90 (µg/mL) values of 2.1 and 1.0 for 7 and 14 days, respectively; and the corresponding values for the compound Q were 62.5 and 31.3, respectively [65].

Class: Homoscleromorpha; Order: Homosclerophorida; Family: Plakinidae

Corticium sp.

The lipid, plakinamine N derived from this species has been reported to show antitubercular activity [11].

Antiparasitic Activity

Phylum: Porifera; Class: Desmospongiae; Order Agelasida; Family: Agelasidae.

Agelas sp.

The bicyclic diterpenoids agelasine B,F derived from this sponge displayed potent antiprotozoal activity against *Trypanosoma brucei* with IC_{50} values of 8.4 and 3.3 µg/mL [64].

Chondrosia reniformes

Order: Chondrosiida; Family: Chondrosiidae.

The acetone extracts of this sponge species showed antiprotozoal activity against *Trypanosoma cruzi* epimastigotes, amastigotes and Trypomastigote with an IC_{50} value of 28.6,82.6 and 0.6 lg/mL respectively [66].

Dysidea avara

Order: Dictyoceratida Family: Dysideidae

The acetone extracts of this sponge species showed antiprotozoal activity against *Trypanosoma cruzi* epimastigotes, amastigotes and Trypomastigote with an IC_{50} value of 23.4,40.3 and 1.1 lg/mL respectively [66].

Sargotragus spinosulus (= Ircinia spinosula

Order: Dictyoceratida; Family: Irciniidae.

The aqueous extracts, ethyl acetate extract and dichloromethane extract of this sponge species showed antiprotozoal activity against Leishmania major Promastigotes stages with IC_{50} values of 264.67, 16.09 and 47.38 lg/mL, respectively [66].

Sarcotragus sp.

The aqueous extract, ethyl acetate extract and dichloromethane extract of this sponge species showed antiprotozoal activity against Leishmania major promastigotes stages with IC_{50} values of 3.02, 8.49 and 1.39 lg/mL, respectively [66].

Amphimedon viridis

Order: Haplosclerida; Family: Niphatidae.

The organic extracts and aqueous extracts of this sponge species showed antiprotozoal activity against *Trypanosoma cruzi* trypomastigotes with IC_{50} values of 10.8 lg/mL and 0.6 lg/mL, respectively. Further, its organic extracts and aqueous extracts showed activity against *Trypanosoma cruzi* amastigotes with IC_{50} values of 44.85 lg/mL and 21.37 lg/mL, respectively [66].

Monanchora arbuscula

Order: Poecilosclerida; Family: Crambeidae.

The alkaloid compounds such as monalidine A, batzelladines D, F and L; and norbatzelladine L derived from this marine sponge displayed antiprotozoal activities against *Trypanosoma cruzi* and *Leishmania infantum* with IC_{50} values ranging from 2.0 to 8.0 µM [67].

Crella (crella) sp.

Order: Poecilosclerida; Family: Crellidae

The steroids norselic acids A–E isolated from this sponge showed antiprotozoal activity by inhibiting the growth of the Leishmania parasite at low micromolar levels [67].

Pandaros acanthifolium

Order: Poecilosclerida Family: Microcionidae.

The steroidal glycosides pandarosides E-G, and IJ derived from this sponge species displayed antiprotozoal activity. However, the methyl ester of pandaroside G showed potent activity against *Trypanosoma brucei* rhodesiense with an IC_{50} value of 0.038 µM; and against *Leishmania donovani* with an IC_{50} value of 0.051 µM [67].

Mycale (Zygomycale) angulosa (= Mycale angulosa)

Order: Poecilosclerida; Family: Mycalidae

The acetone extracts of this sponge species showed antiprotozoal activity against *Trypanosoma cruzi* epimastigotes, amastigotes and Trypomastigote with an IC_{50} value of 67.3, 55.5 and 3.8 lg/mL, respectively [66].

Negombata corticata

Order: Poecilosclerida; Family: Podospongiidae.

The dichloromethane extract of this sponge species showed antiprotozoal activity against *Leishmania donovani* promastigotes stages with an IC_{50} value of 74 38 lg/mL [66].

Order: Petrosida.

Petrosid Ng5 Sp5

The alkaloid compounds *viz*. Ingamine A, 22(S)-hydroxyingamine A and dihydroingenamine D derived from this marine sponge strain Petrosid Ng5 Sp5 displayed moderate antileishmanial activities against *Leishmania donovani* promastigotes [67].

The organic extract of this sponge species showed antiprotozoal activity against *Leishmania donovani* promastigotes stages with an IC_{50} value of 1.19 lg/mL [66].

Tethya ignis

Order: Tethyida; Family: Tethyidae

The acetone extracts of this sponge species showed antiprotozoal activity against *Trypanosoma cruzi* epimastigotes, amastigotes and Trypomastigote with an IC_{50} value of 124.7, 7.2 and 6.3 lg/mL, respectively [66].

Tethya rubra

The acetone extracts of this sponge species showed antiprotozoal activity against *Trypanosoma cruzi* epimastigotes, amastigotes and Trypomastigote with an IC_{50} value 109.9, 44.5, and 33.3 lg/mL, respectively [66].

Cardiotropic (Anti-cardiovascular) Activity

Phylum: Porifera; Class: Demonspongiae; Order: Dictyoceratida; Family: Dysideidae.

Lamellodysidea chlorea

The peptide compound, dysinosin A derived from this sponge species showed inhibitory activity on the coagulation factor VIIa and thrombin with Ki (inhibitory constant which is the concentration of the inhibitor that is required in order to decrease the maximal rate of the reaction by half) value of 0.108 and 0.452 μM, respectively. Similarly, its dysinosins B–D inhibited the coagulation factor VIIa with Ki values of 0.090, 0.124, and 1.320 μM, respectively; and thrombin at Ki values of 0.170, 0.550, and >5.1 μM, respectively [67].

Order: Suberitida; Family: Halichondriidae.

Halichondria (Halichondria) okadai

The cyclic aza polyketide, halichlorine derived from this species has been reported to act as vascular cell adhesion molecule (VCAM 1) inhibitor [42].

Order: Tetractinellida; Family: Geodiidae.

Eryltus formosus

The penasterol disaccharide eryloside F derived from this sponge species showed inhibitory activity on human platelet aggregation *in vitro* as a thrombin receptor antagonist. The IC_{50} values of this compound inhibited SFLLRN and U-46619-induced platelet aggregation were at 0.3 and 1.7 µg/mL, respectively [67].

Family: Theonellidae.

Theonella swinhoei

The peptides, pseudotheonamides A1, A2, B2, C and D and dihydrocyclotheonamide A derived from this marine sponge demonstrated selective serine protease inhibitory activity *viz.* inhibition of thrombin with IC_{50} values of 1.0, 3.0, 1.3, 0.19, 1.4, and 0.33 µM, respectively [67].

The peptides, cyclotheonamide A, E; and cyclotheonamide E2, E3 derived from this marine sponge showed significant inhibition activity against serine protease inhibitors *viz.* thrombin and trypsin with IC_{50} values of 23 and 16 nM (A); 2.9 and 30 nM (E); 13 and 55 nM (E2); and 9.5 and 52 n (E3), respectively [67].

Theonella sp.

The peptide, nazumamide A derived from this marine sponge exhibited the inhibition of thrombin with an IC_{50} value of 4.63 µM [67].

The cyclic pentapeptide, cyclotheonamide A isolated from this sponge displayed inhibitory activity of serine protease, which is implicated in major cardiovascular diseases such hypertension and congestive heart failure [42].

CONCLUSION

Among the marine invertebrates, the pharmaceutical contribution of sponges is very significant as they rank first in the quantum of bioactive compounds with several bioactivities including antitumor activity. The symbiotic microorganisms such as bacteria, fungi and microalgae harbored by these sponges are believed to be largely responsible for the latter. However, intensive research on these microorganisms is lacking and large scale investigations on this aspect would address the limitations regarding sustainable supply of marine drugs.

CHAPTER 5

Promising Pharmaceutical Compounds of Marine Cnidarians: Their Chemistry and Therapeutic Applications

Abstract: This chapter deals with the promising secondary metabolites of the different constituents of marine cnidarians *viz.* hydrozoan medusae, scyphozoan medusae and soft corals and their bioactivities. Among the chemical classes of compounds, terpenoids ranked first and cytotoxicity of these compounds was the major activity.

Keywords: Bioactivities, Hydrozoan medusae, Marine cnidarians, Scyphozoan medusae, Soft corals, Secondary metabolites.

INTRODUCTION

Marine invertebrates are known to be potential sources of secondary metabolites and their pharmaceutical and therapeutical applications attract scientific and economic interest worldwide. Among these organisms, cnidarians are ranked second in the chemical diversity and quantity of marine bioactive compounds. The phylum Cnidaria has about 11,000 described species including the classes Hydrozoa (hydroids), Scyphozoa (jellyfish), Cubozoa (box jellies), and Anthozoa (sea anemones, corals, sea pens).

Among these classes of Cnidaria, the class Anthozoa has the maximum number of species over 7500 valid species (about two-thirds of all known cnidarian species) in its 10 orders [68]. However, the order Alcyonacea (soft corals) and Gorgonacea (sea fans) have been reported to contribute with the maximum number of promising bioactive secondary metabolites although other orders, such as Scleractinia (hard corals), and Actiniaria (sea anemones) have also yielded substantial number of promising compounds [69]. Asian countries such as Taiwan, Japan, and China, have been reported to possess more number of cnidarian species for the extraction of marine natural products.

Santhanam Ramesh, Ramasamy Santhanam & Veintramuthu Sankar

Hydroids (Hydrozoa)

The marine hydroids of the phylum Cnidaria inhabit mostly marine environments, though some have invaded freshwater habitats. These organisms are either solitary or colonial, and there are about 3,700 described species. It is also reported that through evolution, many hydroids have suppressed the medusa and retained their sessile hydroid colonies. Studies relating to the bioactive compounds of marine hydroids are still in the infant stage and very few reports are available on anticancer properties of these animals.

Biopharmaceutically Important Marine Hydrozoans

Abylopsis sp. (Fig. **1**), *Aegina citrea* (Fig. **2**), *Aeginura grimaldii* (Fig. **3**), *Arctapodema* sp, *Colobonema sericeum* (Fig. **4**), *Crossota* sp. (Fig. **5**), *Halecium beanie, Halecium muricatum* (Fig. **6**), *Halicreas minimum* (Fig. **7**), *Macrorhynchia philippina* (Fig. **8**), *Pantachogon haeckeli,* and *Thuiaria* sp. (Fig. **9**).

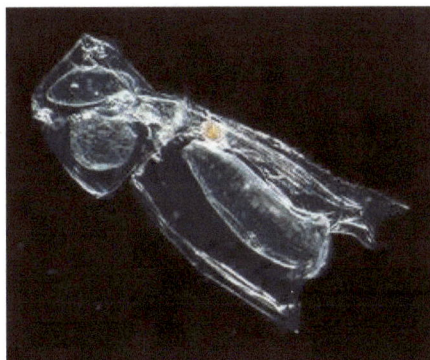

Fig. (1). *Abylopsis* sp.

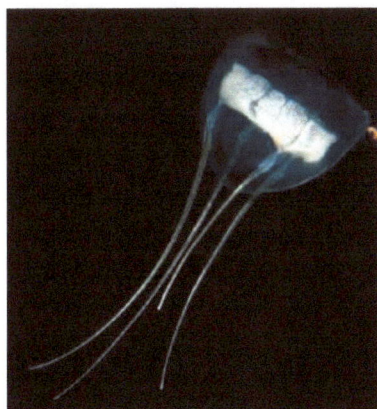

Fig. (2). *Aegina citrea.*

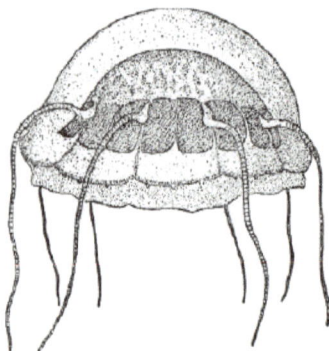

Fig. (3). *Aeginura grimaldii.*

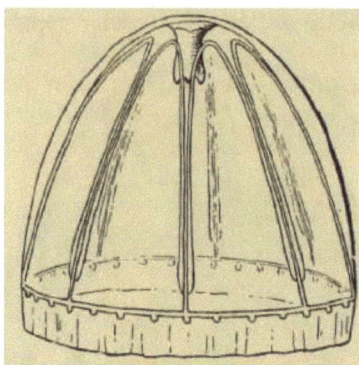

Fig. (4). *Colobonema sericeum.*

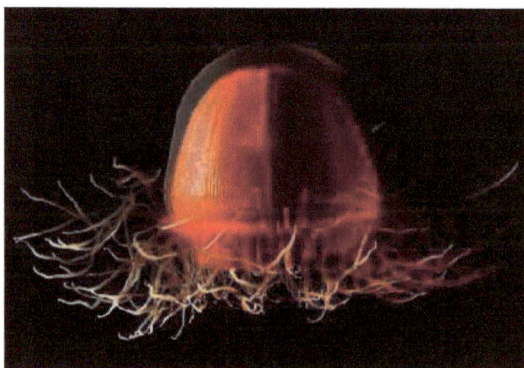

Fig. (5). .*Crossota* sp.

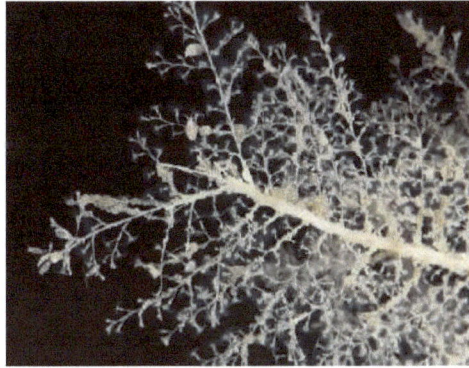

Fig. (6). *Halecium muricatum.*

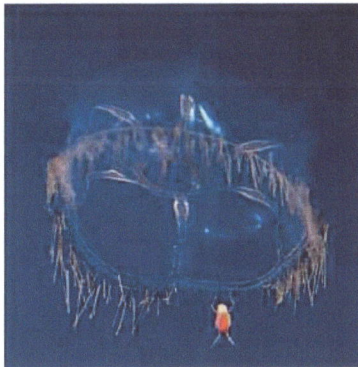

Fig. (7). *Halicreas minimum.*

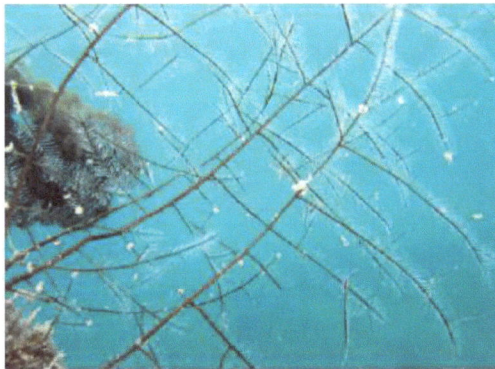

Fig. (8). *Macrorhynchia philippina.*

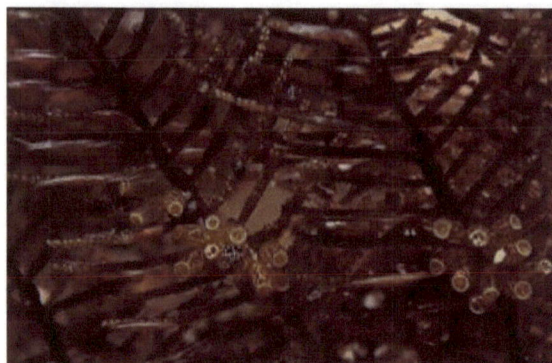

Fig. (9). *Thuiaria* sp.

Image credit: *Abylopsis* sp.: *Copepedia* (applied for permission); *Aegina citrea, Aeginura grimaldii, Colobonema sericeum, Crossota* sp., *Halecium muricatum,* and *Halicreas minimum,* Wikipedia; *Macrorhynchia philippina,* Wikipedia commons; *Thuiaria* sp., Wikipedia.

Anticancer Marine Hydrozoans

Investigations of the bioactive compounds of marine hydrozoans are very much limited and most of the findings relate to only anticancer compounds. The hydrozoan species possessing anticancer properties are given below (Table **1**).

Table 1. Anticancer activities of marine hydrozoans.

Species	Extract/Compound/Chemistry	Mechanism	Refs.
Abylopsis eschscholtzii	GFP-like proteins	Bioluminescence in cancer therapy	[70]
Aegina citrea	Extract-polypeptides (proteins).	Cytotoxic; IC_{50}, 100mg/ml	[71]
Aeginura grimaldii	Extract-polypeptides (proteins)	Cytotoxic; IC_{50}, 170mg/ml	[71]
Arctapodema sp.	Extract-polypeptides (proteins)	Cytotoxic: IC_{50}, 190mg/ml; hemolytic: IC_{50}, 110 mg/ml	[71]
Colobonema sericeum	Extract-polypeptides (proteins)	Cytotoxic: IC_{50}, 420mg/ml; hemolytic: IC_{50}, 190 mg/ml	[71]
Crossota rufobrunnea	Extract-polypeptides (proteins)	Hemolytic ; IC_{50}, 100mg/ml	[71]
Halecium muricatum and *Halecium beanie*	1- Tetradecylglycero-3-phosphocholine (1) and 1- Hexadecylglycero3-phosphocholine (2) ; SwissLipids	Anticancer; 1. against lung fibroblast cell line and 2 against human breast carcinoma at 100 µg/ mL	[7]
Halicreas minimum	Extract-polypeptides (proteins)	Cytotoxic-; IC_{50}, 750mg/ml;	[71]

(Table 1) cont.....

Species	Extract/Compound/Chemistry	Mechanism	Refs.
Macrorhynchia philippina	Macrophilone A,A1,B-G ; Quinones	Cytotoxic	[11]
Pantachogon haeckeli	Extract-polypeptides (proteins)	Cytotoxic; IC_{50}, 160mg/ml	[71]
Thuiaria breitfussi	Breitfussin C-D; Alkaloids	Cytotoxic	[11]

Class: Scyphozoa

The scyphozoan jellyfish are of two types *viz.* free-swimming medusae and sessile medusae (*i.e.*, stem animals that are attached to seaweed and other objects by a stalk). These sessile polyp-like forms constitute the order Stauromedusae. The free-swimming (planktonic) scyphozoan jellyfish which are disk-shaped organisms living in all oceans and are often found drifting along the shoreline. This class is composed of about 200 described species. While most of these jelly fishes live for only a few weeks, some species are known to survive a year or more. Bodies of the most jelly fishes range in size from about 2 to 40 cm in dia. and some species are fairly larger with dia. of up to 2 m. *Scyphozoan medusae* consist of almost 99 percent water. Several species of these jelly fishes are bioluminescent and are transparent with bright colours, such as yellow, blue, and pink. The calcium binding protein of jelly fish has been reported to be helpful to maintain healthy cells and is also considered good for human brain. The edible species of these jelly fishes contain low calories with carbohydrates and are therefore very good for weight loss. Further, they are also helpful for lowering high blood pressure. Many jellyfish species have been found to possess anticoagulant, antihypertensive and immune-stimulative effects.

Pharmaceutically Important Marine Scyphozoan medusae

Atolla vanhoeffeni, Atolla sp. (Fig. **10**), *Aurelia aurita* (Fig. **11**) and *Nemopilema nomurai* (Fig. **12**)

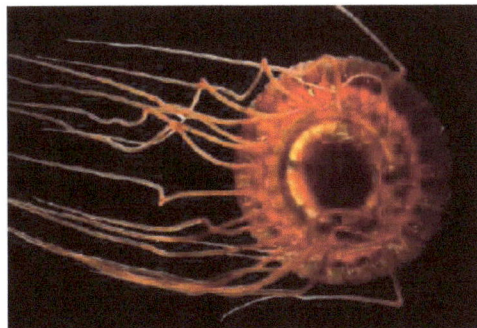

Fig. (10). *Atolla* sp.

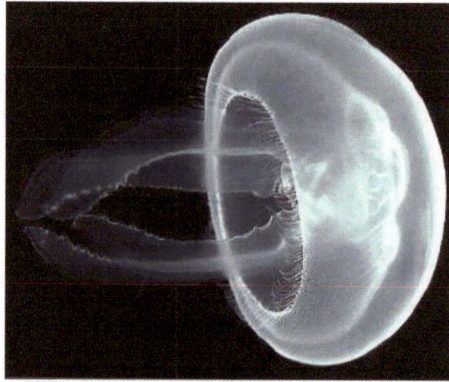

Fig. (11). *Aurelia aurita.*

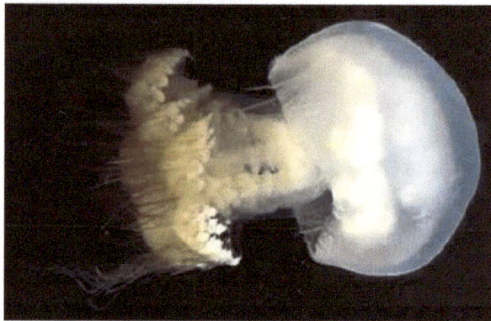

Fig. (12). *Nemopilema nomurai.*

Image credit: *Atolla* sp., Wikipedia; *Aurelia aurita* and *Nemopilema nomurai*, Wikipedia commons.

Therapeutic Activities of Marine *Scyphozoan medusae*

Atolla vanhoeffeni

The extracts of this species have been reported to contain polypeptides (proteins) which have cytotoxic properties with an IC_{50} value of 740mg/ml [71].

Aurelia aurita

The venom of this species has been reported to possess anticoagulant effects, which act through strong fibrinogrnolytic activity [72].

Aurelia coerulea

The extracts from the oral arms of this species showed significant antioxidant activity and lysozyme-like activity. The soluble and insoluble fractions of its oral arm samples had most of the antioxidant capacity (762.3 nmol of TE/mg of proteins and 518.8 nmol of TE/mg of proteins respectively). On the other hand, the soluble and insoluble fractions of the umbrella and whole jellyfish showed very low antioxidant activity (soluble fraction: 172.3 nmol of TE/mg of proteins and 147.4 nmol of TE/mg of proteins, respectively; and insoluble fraction: 55.6 nmol of TE/mg of proteins and 80.3 nmol of TE/mg of proteins respectively) [73].

Nemopilema nomurai

The nematocyst-derived venom of this species displayed cardiovascular effects in anesthetized rats. At concentrations of 0.1-2.4 mg protein/kg, a dose-dependent hypotension (65%) and bradycardia (80%) were recorded [74].

This jellyfish venom displayed a significant cytotoxic activity in H9C2 heart myoblast than in C2C12 skeletal myoblast (LC(50)=2 microg/mL *vs.* 12 microg/mL, respectively). Further, this venom showed concentration-dependent hemolysis in the dog erythrocyte (EC(50)=151 microg/mL) [75].

Its collagen extract displayed the regulatory effects on the immune system by stimulating the production of immunoglobulin as well as cytokines but without causing the allergic issues. Further, its glycoprotein, called qniunucin had the ability to inhibit the degeneration of articular cartilage. Furthermore, as it contains antioxidant property, it could be a potential food for human [72].

Class: Anthozoa

Among the different classes of Cnidaria, the class, Anthozoa with its order Octocorallia (formerly Orders, Alcyonacea and Gorgonacea) has been reported to yield the maximum number of most promising bioactive compounds. The coral reefs which are known as "jewels of the sea" are not only a nursery to several marine species but are also known for their excellent medicinal properties. The secondary metabolites of corals are an important source to treat diseases like arthritis, Alzheimer's, cancer, viral disease, bacterial diseases, heart disease, *etc.* Owing to their health benefits, several compounds of the class Anthozoa are presently used in the development of novel drugs and new commercial products including nutritional supplements [11]. A total of 5761 bioactive compounds have been described from these cnidarians during the period 2010–2019 and terpenoid compounds ranked first (67%) followed by steroids (21%), alkaloids (5%) and other compounds (6%). With regard to the bioactivities of these compounds, cytotoxicity against cancer cell lines is the most represented bioactivity (42%) followed by anti-inflammatory activity (29%), antimicrobial activity(8%), antifouling activity (7%), and antiviral activity (4%) [11, 68, 69].

Scleractinian Corals and Sea Anemones (Subclass: Hexacorallia)

Pharmaceutically Important Marine Scleractinian Corals and Sea Anemones

Antipathozoanthus hickmani (Fig. **13**), *Anthopleura* sp. (Fig. **14**), *Palythoa caribaeorum* (Fig. **15**), *Palythoa tuberculosa* (Fig. **16**) and *Zoanthus kuroshio* (Fig. **17**).

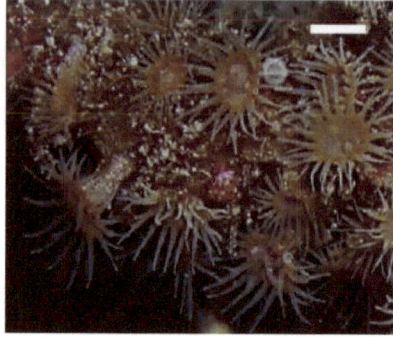

Fig. (13). *Antipathozoanthus hickmani.*

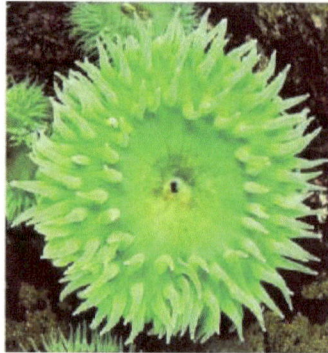

Fig. (14). *Anthopleura* sp.

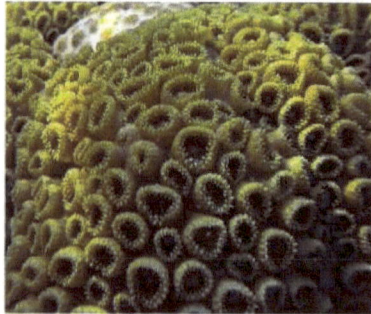

Fig. (15). *Palythoa caribaeoru.*

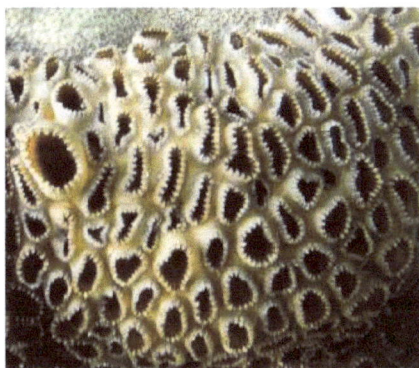

Fig. (16). *Palythoa tuberculosa.*

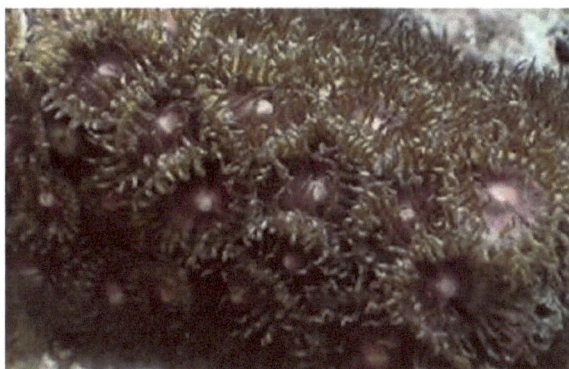

Fig. (17). *Zoanthus kuroshio.*

Image credit: *Antipathozoanthus hickmani*: Wikipedia commons; *Anthopleura* sp.: Wikipedia; *Palythoa caribaeor* and *Palythoa tuberculosa.* Wikipedia commons.

Promising Secondary Metabolites of Sea Anemones and Scleractinian Corals and their Bioactivities

Sea anemones (Class: Anthozoa; Order: Actiniaria) are fairly a good source of bioactive proteins and polypeptides. Further, many several cytolytic neuropeptides, toxins, and protease inhibitors have been reported from these organisms. Among the different species of these corals, the sea anemone Actinia equina is known to possess equinatoxins, cytolytic proteins and equistatin, an inhibitor of papain-like cysteine proteinase and aspartic proteinase cathepsin D. While the aspartic proteinase cathepsin D activates the pathogenesis of breast cancer and Alzheimer's disease, papain-like cysteine proteases are found involved in brain tumors, Alzheimer's disease, epilepsy and neurological autoimmune diseases. Among the scleractinian corals (Class: Anthozoa; Order: Scleractinia), species of Tubastrea and Cladocora are known to possess promising bioactive compounds. For example, a bis(indole) alkaloid, Cycloaplysinopsin C derived from an unidentified species of Tubastrea displayed antimalarial activity of two strains of Pasmodium falciparum *viz.* a chloroquine-sensitive (F32/Tanzania) and a chloroquine-resistant (FcB1/Colombia) with IC_{50} values of 1.5 and 1.2 µg/mL, respectively. Further, the sesterterpenoids, cladocorans A, B derived from Cladocora caespitosa displayed potent anti-inflammatory activity by inhibiting secretory phospholipase A2 and IC_{50} values recorded for these compounds were ranging from 0.8 to 1.9 µM [11].

Soft corals (Subclass: Octocorallia; Order: Octocorallia (Formerly Orders, Alcyonacea and Gorgonacea)

Pharmaceutically Important Marine Soft Corals

Antillogorgia acerosa (Fig. **18**), *Antillogorgia americana* (Fig. **19**), *Asterospicularia laurae* (Fig. **20**), *Astrogorgia dumbea* (Fig. **21**), *Briareum* sp. (Fig. **22**) *Carijoa riisei* (Fig. **23**), *Cladiella hirsuta* (Fig. **24**), *Clavulariaviridi* (Fig. **25**), *Conglomeratusclera coerulea* (Fig. **26**), *Convexella magelhaenica* (Fig. **27**), *Dichotella gemmacea* (Fig. **28**), *Eunicea* sp. (Fig. **29**), *Euplexaura robusta* (Fig. **30**), *Heteroxenia* sp. (Fig. **31**), *Isis hippuris* (Fig. **32**), *Junceella fragilis*, (Fig. **33**), *Klyxum simplex* (Fig. **34**), *Leptogorgia punicea* (Fig. **35**), *Litophyton* sp. (Fig. **36**), *Lobophytum* sp. (Fig. **37**), *Muricella* sp. (Fig. **38**), *Muriceopsis flavida* (Fig. **39**), *Pacifigorgia* sp. (Fig. **40**), *Paralemnalia thyrsoides* (Fig. **41**), *Paraminabea* sp.(Fig. **42**),. *Pinnigorgia* sp. (Fig. **43**), *Plumigorgia* sp., (Fig. **44**), *Pseudoplexaura* sp. (Fig. **45**), *Sarcophyton* sp. (Fig. **46**), *Scleronephthya* sp. (Fig. **47**), *Sclerophytum* sp. (Fig. **48**), *Sinularia brassica* (Fig. **49**), *Subergorgia* sp. (Fig. **50**), *Unomia stolonifera* (Fig. **51**), *Verrucella* sp. (Fig. **52**) and *Xenia umbellata* (Fig. **53**).

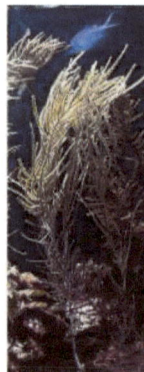

Fig. (18). *Antillogorgia acerosa.*

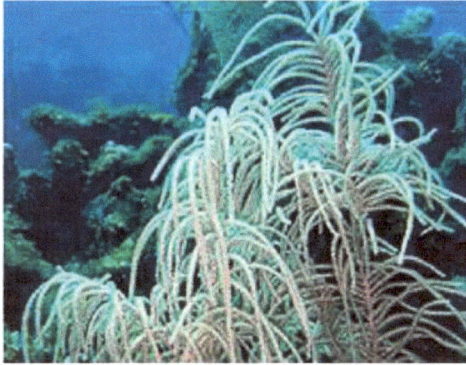

Fig. (19). *Antillogorgia americana.*

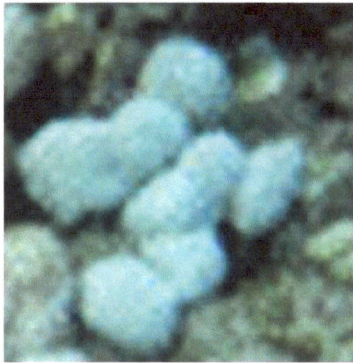

Fig. (20). *Asterospicularia laurae.*

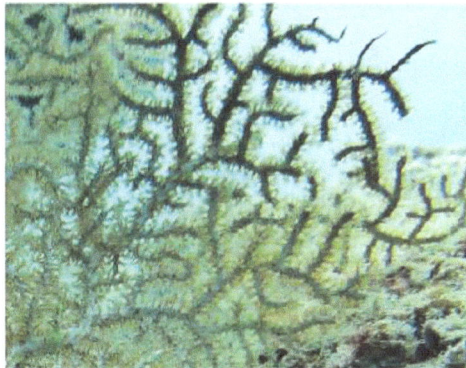

Fig. (21). *Astrogorgia dumbe.*

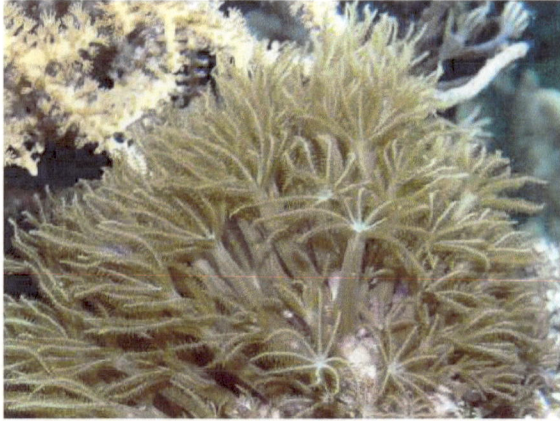

Fig. (22). *Briareum* sp.

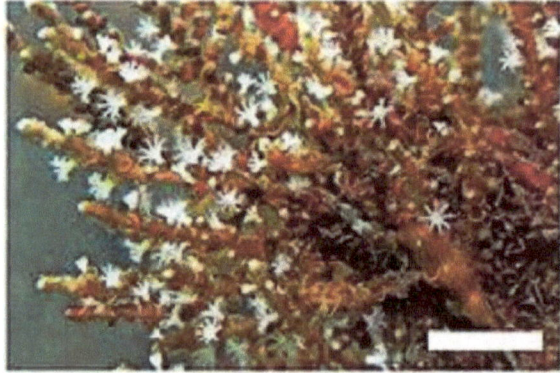

Fig. (23). *Carijoa riisei.*

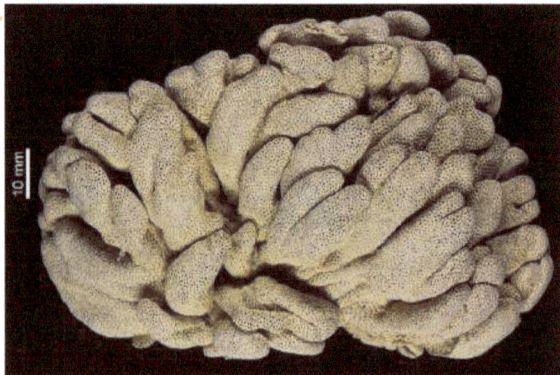

Fig. (24). *Cladiella hirsuta.*

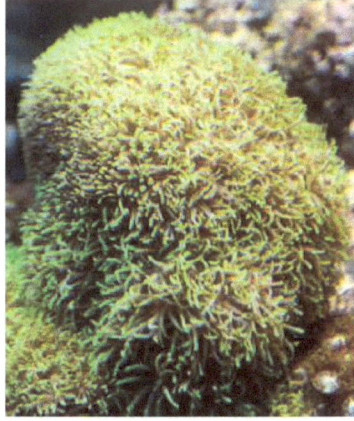

Fig. (25). *Clavularia viridis.*

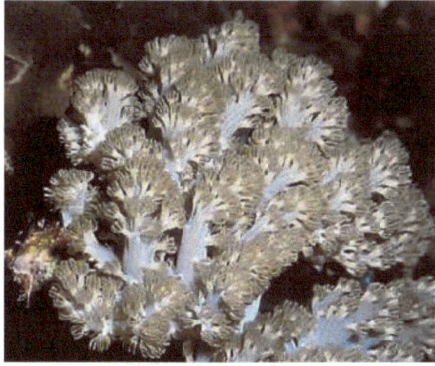

Fig. (26). *Conglomeratusclera coerulea.*

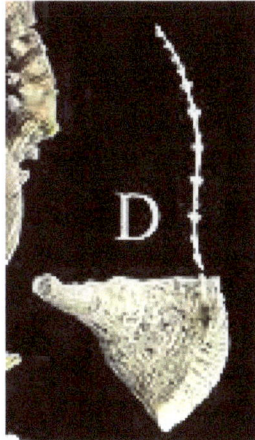

Fig. (27). *Convexella magelhaenica.*

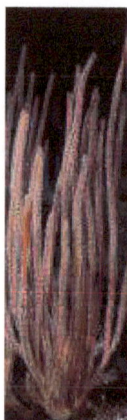

Fig. (28). *Dichotella gemmacea.*

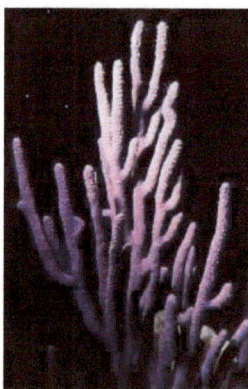

Fig. (29). *Eunicea* sp.

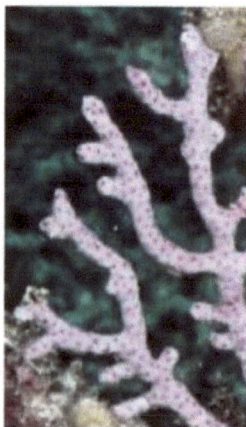

Fig. (30). *Euplexaura robusta.*

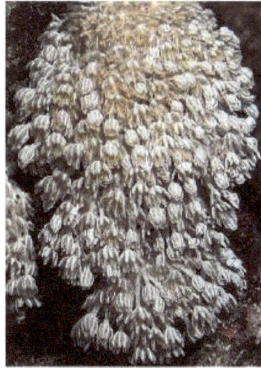

Fig. (31). *Heteroxenia* sp.

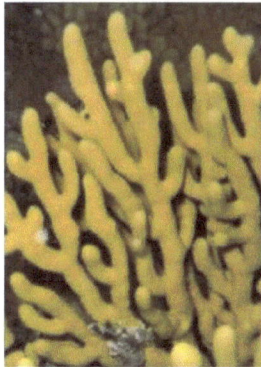

Fig. (32). *Isis hippuris.*

Image credit: *Antillogorgia acerosa*: Wikimedia commons; *Antillogorgia americana*: Wikidata; *Astrogorgia dumbea*: Wikimedia commons; *Briareum* sp. and *Carijoa riisei*: Wikipedia; *Cladiella hirsuta:* Wikidata; *Clavulari aviridi*s Wikimedia commons; *Conglomeratusclera coerulea*: Wikidata; *Convexella magelhaenica*: Wikimedia commons; *Eunicea* sp.: Wikiwand; *Heteroxenia* sp.: Wikipedia.

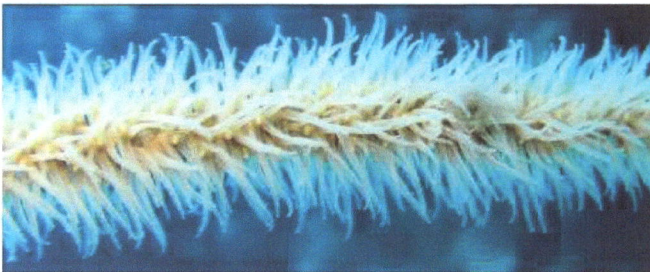

Fig. (33). *Junceella fragilis.*

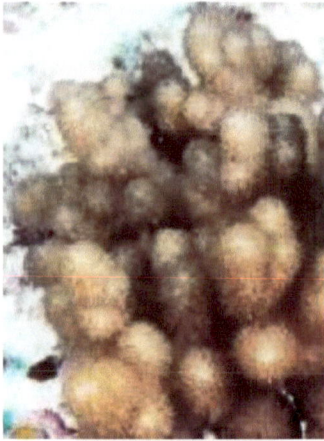

Fig. (34). *Klyxum simplex.*

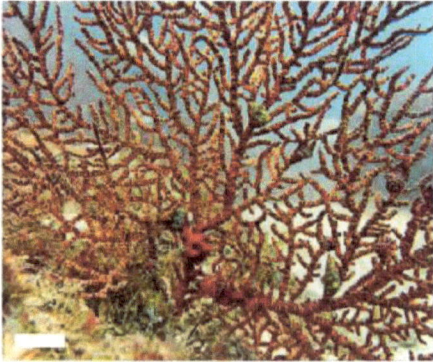

Fig. (35). *Leptogorgia punicea.*

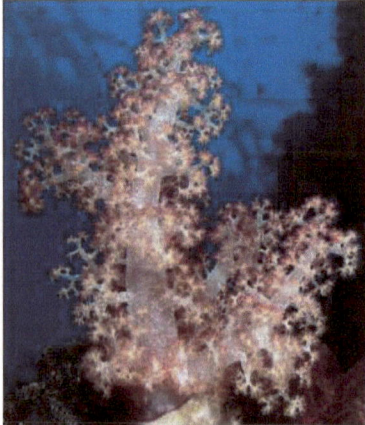

Fig. (36). *Litophyton* sp.

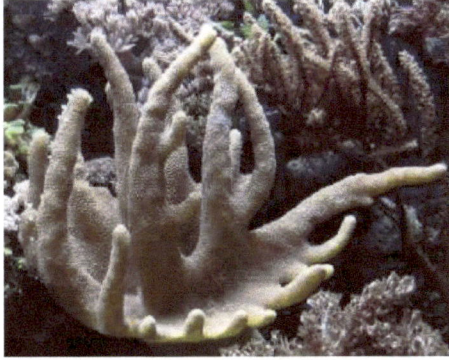

Fig. (37). *Lobophytum* sp.

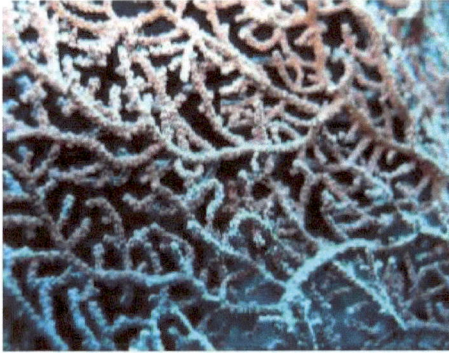

Fig. (38). *Muricella* sp.

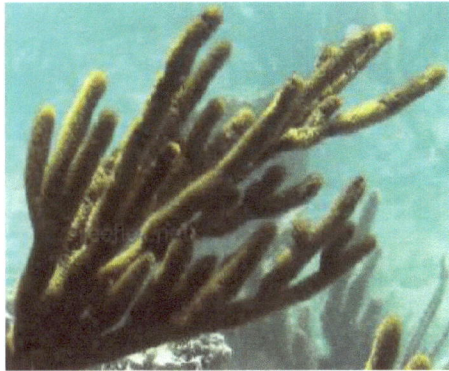

Fig. (39). *Muriceopsis flavida.*

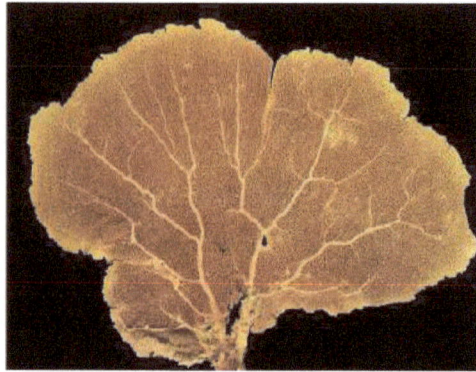

Fig. (40). *Pacifigorgia* sp.

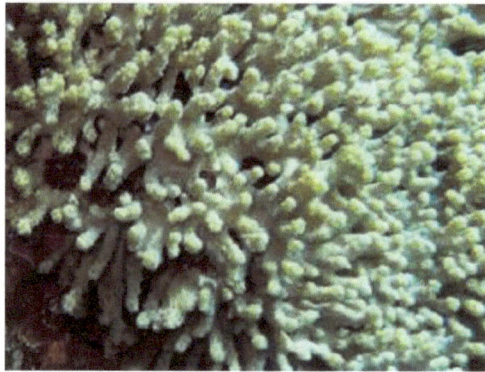

Fig. (41). *Paralemnalia thyrsoides.*

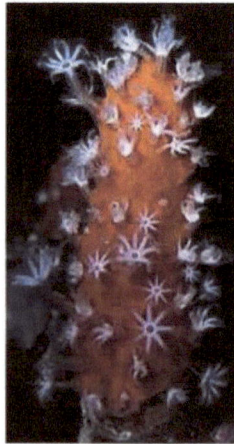

Fig. (42). *Paraminabea* sp.

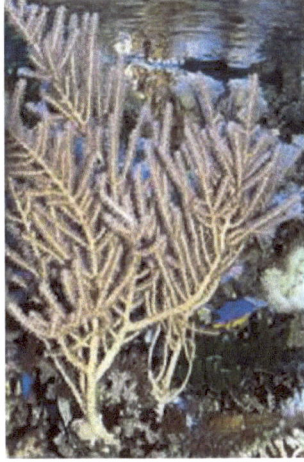

Fig. (43). *Pinnigorgia* sp.

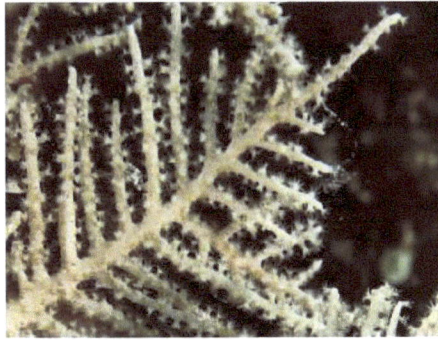

Fig. (44). *Plumigorgia* sp.

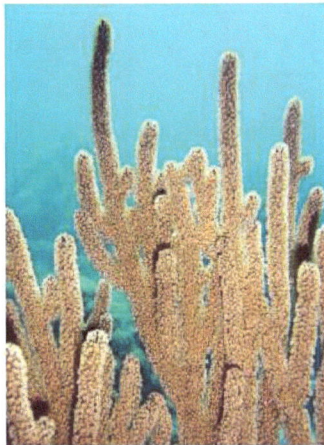

Fig. (45). *Pseudoplexaura* sp.

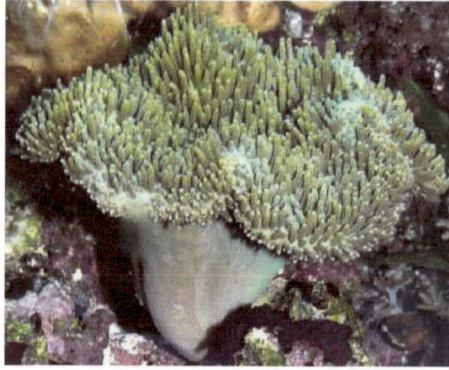

Fig. (46). *Sarcophyton* sp.

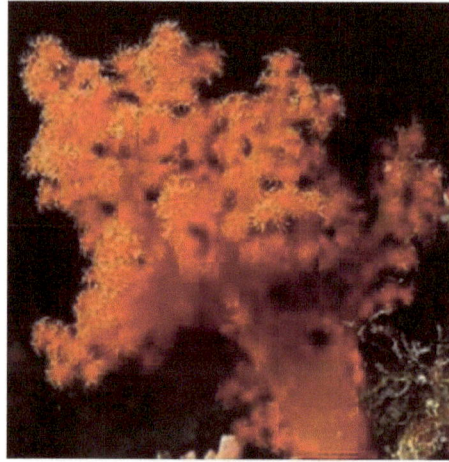

Fig. (47). *Scleronephthya* sp.

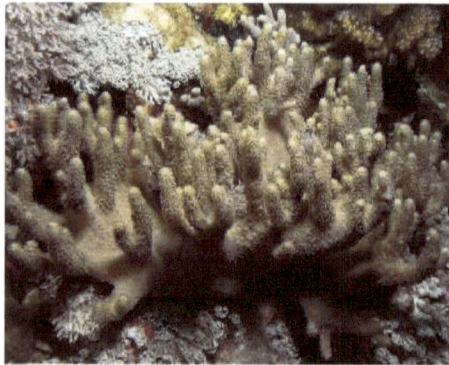

Fig. (48). *Sclerophytum* sp.

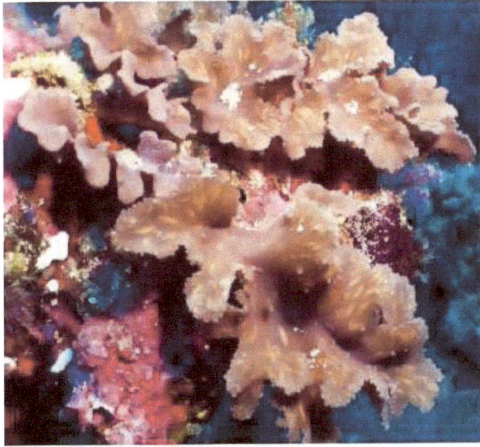

Fig. (49). *Sinularia brassica.*

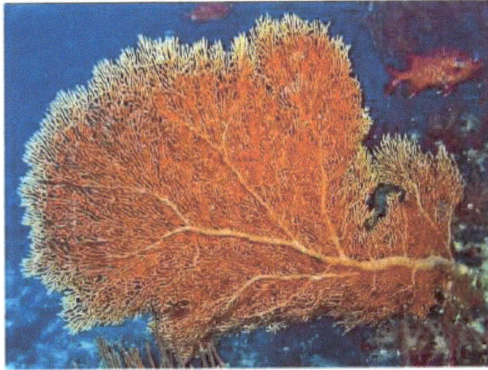

Fig. (50). *Subergorgia* sp.

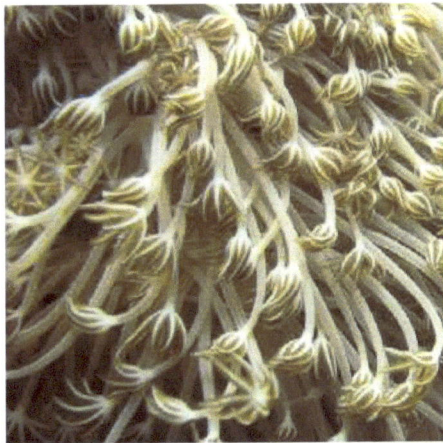

Fig. (51). *Unomia stolonifera.*

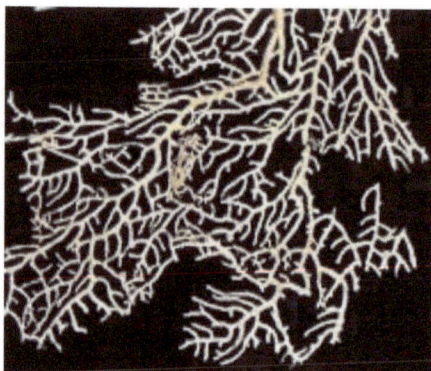

Fig. (52). *Verrucella* sp.

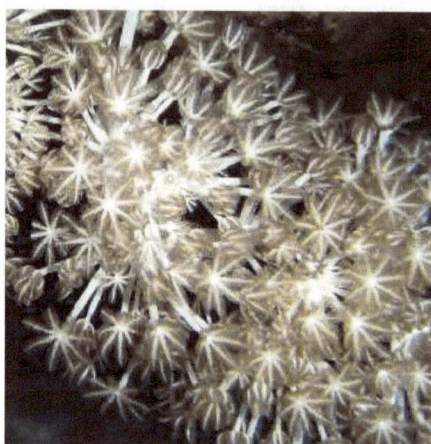

Fig. (53). *Xenia umbellata.*

Image credit: *Junceella fragilis* and *Leptogorgia punicea*: Wikipedia commons; *Litophyton* sp. and *Lobophytum* sp.: Wikipedia; *Muricella* sp.: Wikipedia commons; *Pacifigorgia* sp.: Marine Species org. (CC);*Paraminabea* sp.: Wikipedia commons; *Pinnigorgia* sp. and *Pseudoplexaura* sp.: Wikipedia; *Scleronephthya* sp*., Sclerophytum* sp.., *Sinularia brassica*: Wikipedia commons; *Subergorgia* sp. and *Xenia umbellata*: Wikipedia.

Promising Secondary Metabolites of Soft Corals and their Bioactivities

The secondary metabolites derived from the species of soft corals have shown promising bioactivities [11, 68], which are listed below.

Capnella imbricata

The sesquiterpenes *viz.* capnellenes isolated from this species displayed anti-inflammatory activity.

Dendronephthya rubeola

The sesquiterpene *viz.* dihydroxycapnellene (capnell-9(12)-ene-8β,10α-diol) of this species displayed potential antiproliferative activity against murine fibroblasts cell line (L-929) with a GI_{50} value of 6.8 μM/L). Further, this compound has been reported to display a significant cytotoxicity against human leukemia (K-562) and human cervix carcinoma (HeLa) cell lines with IC_{50} values of 0.7 μM and 7.6 μM, respectively. Capnell-9(12)-ene-8β,10α-diol has also been reported to strongly inhibit the interaction of the oncogenic transcription factor Myc with its partner protein Max, thereby making this compound a potential therapeutic in oncology.

Nephthea chabroli

A nor-sisquiterpene compound, chabranol produced by this species has shown moderate cytotoxicity against mouse lymphocytic leukemia cells (P-388 cell line) with an ED_{50} value of 1.8 μg/mL.

Nephthea erecta

At a concentration of 10 μM, the protein compounds *viz.* ergostanoid 1,3 derived from this species were found to significantly reduce the levels of inducible nitric oxide synthase (iNOS) and cyclooxygenase-2 protein (COX-2) with percentage values of 45.8 and 33.6 respectively; and 68.1 and 10.3% respectively.

Xenia novaebrittanniae

The diterpenoid, xeniolide I derived from this species displayed antibacterial activity against *Escherichia coli* ATCC and *Bacillus subtilis* at a concentration of 1.25 mg/mL.

Xenia plicata (= Xenia blumi)

The diterpenoid, Blumiolide C of this species displayed significant cytotoxicity against mouse lymphocytic leukemia (P-388) and human colon adenocarcinoma (HT-29) with ED_{50} values of 0.2 and 0.5 μg/mL, respectively.

Sarcophyton crassocaule

The cembranoids, crassocolide I,M derived from this species displayed significant cytotoxicity against human medulloblastoma (Daoy cells) cell line IC_{50} values of 0.8 and 1.1 μg/mL, respectively. Further, its crassocolide H was found to inhibit the growth of human oral epidermoid carcinoma (KB) cell line with an IC_{50} value of 5.3 μg/mL; and its crassocolide L was active against human cervical epitheloid carcinoma (HeLa) cell line with an IC_{50} value of 8.0 μg/mL.

Lobophytum cristagalli

A cembranolide diterpene of this species showed potent anticancer activity with an IC_{50} value of 0.15 μM.

Lobophytum durum and Lobophytum crassum

Produce durumolides A–C [60], durumhemiketalolide A–C [61] and crassumolides A and C [58], with anti-inflammatory effects. They have been shown to inhibit up-regulation of the pro-inflammatory iNOS and COX-2 proteins in LPS-stimulated murine macrophage cells at $IC_{50} < 10$ μM.

Lobophytum spp.

Other species of this genus also showed cembranolide diterpenes (lobophytene) with significant cytotoxic activity against human lung adenocarcinoma (A549) and human colon adenocarcinoma (HT-29) cell lines

The diterpenoids, lobohedleolide, (7Z)-lobohe dleolide, and 17-di-methyl-amino lobohed leolide, were isolated from the aqueous extract of *Lobophytum* species and exhibited moderate HIV-inhibitory activity (IC_{50} approximately 7–10 μg/mL) in a cell-based *in vitro* anti-HIV assay.

Klyxum simplex

This species produces diterpene compounds, such as simplexin E, which at a concentration of 10 μM, was found to considerably reduce the levels of iNOS and COX-2 proteins to 4.8 ± 1.8% and 37.7 ± 4.7%, respectively. These results have shown that this compound significantly inhibits the accumulation of the pro-inflammatory iNOS and COX-2 proteins in LPS-stimulated RAW264.7 macrophage cells.

This species also produces two diterpene compounds, klysimplexins B and H, exhibiting moderate cytotoxicity towards human carcinoma cell lines. Klysimplexin B exhibits cytotoxicity toward human hepatocellular carcinoma (Hep G2 and Hep 3B), human breast carcinoma (MDA-MB-231 and MCF-7), human lung carcinoma (A549) and human gingival carcinoma (Ca9-22) cell lines with IC_{50}s of 3.0, 3.6, 6.9, 3.0, 2.0, and 1.8 μg/mL, respectively. Metabolite klysimplexin H demonstrated cytotoxicity (IC_{50}'s 5.6, 6.9, 4.4, 5.6, 2.8 and 6.1 μg/mL) toward human hepatocellular carcinoma (Hep G2 and Hep 3B), human breast carcinoma (MDA-MB-231 and MCF-7), human lung carcinoma (A549) and human gingival carcinoma (Ca9-22) cell lines, respectively.

Sinularia sp.

In *Sinularia* sp. a tetraprenylated spermine derivative has been isolated — sinulamide — which revealed an H, K-ATPase inhibitory activity. H, K-ATPase is a gastric proton pump of stomach and is the enzyme primarily responsible for the acidification of the stomach contents. Its inhibition is a very common clinical intervention used in diseases including dyspepsia, peptic ulcer, and gastroesophageal reflux (GORD/GERD). Sinulide is a potential antiulcer drug, as it inhibits production of gastric acid by H,K-ATPase (IC_{50} 5.5 μM). Although it has been synthesized, no clinical trials seem to have been reported.

Sinularia gibberosa and Sinularia querciformis

The steroid gibberoketosterol, isolated from *Sinularia gibberosa*, and the diterpenoid querciformolide C from *Sinularia querciformis*, showed significant inhibition of the up-regulation of the pro-inflammatory iNOS and COX-2 proteins in LPS-stimulated murine macrophages at concentration <10 μM.

Sinularia spp.

Sinularia species produce significant molecules: lipids from *Sinularia grandilobata* and another unspecified species of *Sinularia* possesses antibacterial and antifungal activity [64]. The diterpene 11-episinulariolide from *Sinularia flexibilis* is an interesting antifoulant exhibiting strong algacidal properties. This species also produces cembrenoids, named flexilarins, which evidence cytotoxic activity in cancer cell lines. Flexilarin D exhibited potent cytotoxicity in human hepatocarcinoma (Hep2) cells with an IC_{50} value of 0.07 μg/mL, and moderate cytotoxic activity against human cervical epitheloid carcinoma (HeLa, IC_{50} 0.41 μg/mL), human medulloblastoma (Daoy, 1.24 μg/mL) and human breast carcinoma (MCF-7, 1.24 μg/mL) cell lines.

Paralemnalia thyrsoides

Paralemnalia thyrsoides showed significant inhibition of pro-inflammatory iNOS protein expression (70% at IC_{50} 10 μM).

Clavularia viridis

Prostanoids (claviridic acid) isolated from *Clavularia viridis* exhibited potent inhibitory effects on phytohemagglutinin-induced proliferation of peripheral blood mononuclear cells (PBMC, 5 μg/mL), as well as significant cytotoxic activity against human gastric cancer cells (AGS, IC_{50} 1.73–7.78 μg/mL) [71]. Claviridenone extracts also showed potent cytotoxicity against mouse lymphocytic leukemia (P-388) and human colon adenocarcinoma (HT-29), and exceptionally potent cytotoxic activity against human lung adenocarcinoma (A549) cells, with ED_{50} between 0.52 pg/mL and 1.22 µg/mL [45]. Halogenated Prostanoids also showed cytotoxic activity against human T lymphocyte leukemia cells (MOLT-4, IC_{50} 0.52 µg/mL), human colorectal adenocarcinoma (DLD-1, IC_{50} 0.6 µg/mL) and human diploid lung fibroblast (IMR-90, IC_{50} 4.5 µg/mL) cells [72]. The cyclopentenone prostanoid, bromovulone III-a promising marine natural compound for the treatment of prostate, colon and hepatocellular carcinoma-showed anti-tumor activity against human prostate (PC-3) and human colon (HT29) cancer cells at an IC_{50} of 0.5 µM [73], and induced apoptotic signaling in a sequential manner in Hep3B cells [74]. In case of prostate cancer cells, this compound displayed an anti-tumor activity 30 to 100 times more effective than cyclopentenone prostaglandins (known to suppress tumor cell growth and to induce apoptosis in prostate cancer cells), by causing a rapid redistribution and clustering of Fas (member of the tumor necrosis factor (TNF) receptor superfamily). Apoptotic stimulation of Fas by specific ligand or antibodies causes the formation of a membrane-associated complex comprising Fas clustering) in PC-3 cells. *C. viridis* also produces steroids that show cytotoxic activity against human colorectal adenocarcinoma (DLD-1, $0.02 < IC_{50} < 50$ µg/mL) and also against human T lymphocyte leukemia cells (MOLT-4, $0.01 < IC_{50} < 10$ µg/mL), in case of yonarasterols [75]. Stoloniferone additionally displayed potent cytotoxicity against mouse lymphocytic leukemia (P-388), human colon adenocarcinoma (HT-29) and human lung adenocarcinoma (A549) cells [45]. This species produces several compounds with anti-tumor activity in different types of human tumors, although more *in vitro* studies are needed to determine which compound are potential anticancer agents.

Clavularia koellikeri

Clavularia koellikeri produces diterpenoids as secondary metabolites, which display cytotoxic activity against human colorectal adenocarcinoma (DLD-1, IC_{50} 4.2 µg/mL) and strong growth inhibition against human T lymphocyte leukemia cells (MOLT-4, IC_{50} 0.9 µg/mL).

Clavularia spp.

The genus *Clavularia* contains secondary metabolites with unique structures and remarkable biological activities. Some of the species in this genus produce prostanoids (icosanoids) [45, 72, 73], steroids [75] and diterpenoids [70]. The bioactive marine diterpene, stolonidiol, isolated from an unidentified *Clavularia*, showed potent choline acetyltransferase (ChAT) inducible activity in primary cultured basal forebrain cells and clonal septal SN49 cells, suggesting that it may act as a potent neurotrophic factor-like agent on the cholinergic nervous system

[69]. Cholinergic neurons in the basal forebrain innervate the cortex and hippocampus, and their function may be closely related to cognitive function and memory. The degeneration of neuronal cells in this brain region is considered to be responsible for several types of dementia including Alzheimer's disease. One of the neurotransmitters, acetylcholine, is synthesized from acetyl coenzyme A and choline by the action of ChAT. Therefore, induction of ChAT activity in cholinergic neurons may improve the cognitive function in diseases exhibiting cholinergic deficits.

Cespitularia hypotentaculata

In the genus *Cespitularia*, several interesting diterpenes of cembrane and neodolabellane skeletons have been identified. In *Cespitularia hypotentaculata* (family Xeniidae) a significant production of diterpenoids was detected. Cespitularin C exhibited potent cytotoxicity against mouse lymphocytic leukemia (P-388, ED_{50} 0.01 μg/mL) and human lung adenocarcinoma (A549, ED_{50} 0.12 μg/mL) cells, while cespitularin E exhibited potent cytotoxicity against human lung adenocarcinoma (A549, ED_{50} 0.034 μg/mL) cell cultures.

Asterospicularia laurae

A less active diterpene, Asterolaurin A, from *Asterospicularia laurae* (a species from the same family) exhibited cytotoxicity against human hepatocellular carcinoma (HepG2) cells with an IC_{50} of 8.9 μM.

Telesto riisei

Telesto riisei produces punaglandins, highly functional cyclopentadienone and cyclopentenone prostaglandins. Cyclopentenone prostaglandins have unique antineoplastic activity and are potent growth inhibitors in a variety of cultured cells. These punaglandins have been shown to inhibit P53 accumulation (a tumor suppressor protein) and ubiquitin isopeptidase activity (IC_{50} between 0.04 and 0.37 μM) (enzyme involved in protein degradation system) *in vitro* and *in vivo* [76]. Since these proteasome inhibitors exhibit higher antiproliferative effects than other prostaglandins, they may represent a new class of potent cancer therapeutics.

Isis hippuris

Isis hippuris have resulted in the isolation of a series of novel metabolites such as sesquiterpenes, steroids, *A*-nor-hippuristanol and isishippuric acid B. These compounds exhibit potent cytotoxicity against cancer cell lines of human hepatocellular carcinoma (HepG2 and Hep3B, IC_{50} 0.08–4.64 μg/mL and

0.10–1.46 µg/mL, respectively), human breast carcinoma (MCF-7, IC_{50} 0.20–4.54 µg/mL and MDA-MB-231, IC_{50} 0.13–2.64 µg/mL), mouse lymphocytic leukemia (P-388), human lung adenocarcinoma (A549), and human colon adenocarcinoma (HT-29) with ED_{50} values less than 0.1 µg/mL and IC_{50} of 0.1 µg/mL.

Pseudopterogorgia bipinnata

Species from the genus *Pseudopterogorgia* are a rich source of unusual biologically active diterpenoids, sesquiterpenes, and polyhydroxylated steroids, which exhibit diverse structures. A sample of the organic extract of *Pseudopterogorgia bipinnata* was included in an initial screening carried out as part of an effort in the discovery of new antimalarial agents. This extract was found to be active in inhibiting the growth of *Plasmodium falciparum* (a protozoan parasite responsible for the most severe forms of malaria). Caucanolide A and D demonstrated significant *in vitro* antiplasmodial activity against chloroquine-resistant *P. falciparum* W2 (IC_{50} 17 µg/mL and IC_{50} 15 µg/mL, respectively).

Pseudopterogorgia spp.

Three secosterols isolated from an unidentified gorgonian from the genus *Pseudopterogorgia* inhibited human protein kinase C (PKC) α, βI, βII, γ, δ, ε, η, and ζ, with IC_{50} values in the range 12–50 µM. PKC is a key player in cellular signal transduction and has been implicated in cancer, cardiovascular and renal disorders, immunosuppression, and autoimmune diseases such as rheumatoid arthritis. Semisynthetic derivatives also showed a similar activity.

Promising antimicrobial substances were also reported from *Pseudopterogorgia rigida* (*e.g.*, curcuphenol and from *Pseudopterogorgia elisabethae* (*e.g.*, pseudopterosin X and Y). Ileabethoxazole, homopseudopteroxazole, caribenols A and B and elisapterosin B from *Pseudopterogorgia elisabethae* and bipinnapterolide B from *Pseudopterogorgia bipinnata* inhibit *Mycobacterium tuberculosis* $H_{37}Rv$ at a concentration of 12.5 µg/mL (for elisapterosin B and homopseudopteroxazole) and at a concentration range of 128–64 µg/mL (for others compounds). In fact, the inhibition of *Mycobacterium tuberculosis* $H_{37}Rv$ is within the ranges recorded for rifampin. *Pseudopterogorgia elisabethae* and *Pseudopterogorgia bipinnata* also produce antituberculosis compounds. Bielschowskysin, a naturally occurring diterpene isolated from *Pseudopterogorgia kallos* and aberrarone isolated from *Pseudopterogorgia elisabethae* exhibited antiplasmodial activity (IC_{50} 10 µg/mL) when tested against *Plasmodium falciparum*. The first compound was also found to display strong and specific *in vitro* cytotoxicity against the EKVX non-small cell lung cancer ($GI_{50} <$ 0.01 µM) and CAKI-1 renal cancer (GI_{50} 0.51 µM). Bis(pseudopterane) amine from *Pseudopterogorgia acerosa* was found to exhibit selective activity against HCT116 (IC_{50} 4 µM) cell lines.

Eunicea fusca

Fuscosides, originally isolated from *Eunicea fusca* selectively and irreversibly inhibited leukotriene synthesis. Leukotrienes are molecules of the immune system that contribute to inflammation in asthma and allergic rhinitis and their production is usually related to histamine release. Pharmacological studies indicated that fuscoside B inhibits the conversion of arachidonic acid (AA) to leukotriene B_4 and C_4 (LTB_4 and LTC_4) by inhibiting the 5-Lipoxygenase (5-LO), in the case of LTB_4 with an IC_{50} of 18 µM. These selective inhibitors of lipoxygenase isoforms can be useful as pharmacological agents, as nutraceuticals or as molecular tools. Sesquiterpenoid metabolites isolated from *Eunicea* sp. display antiplasmodial activity against the malaria parasite *Plasmodium falciparum* W2 (chloroquine-resistant) strain, with IC_{50} values ranging from 10 to 18 µg/mL.

Junceella fragilis

The gorgonian *Junceella fragilis* produces secondary metabolites, frajunolides B and C, with anti-inflammatory effects towards superoxide anion generation and elastase release by human neutrophils, with an IC_{50} > 10 µg/mL. When properly stimulated, activated neutrophils secrete a series of cytotoxins, such as the superoxide anion (O_2^{-}), a precursor of other reactive oxygen species (ROS), granule proteases, and bioactive lipids. The production of the superoxide anion is linked to the killing of invading microorganisms, but it can also directly or indirectly damage surrounding tissues. On the other hand, neutrophil elastase is a major secreted product of stimulated neutrophils and a major contributor to the destruction of tissue in chronic inflammatory disease. The anti-inflammatory butenolide lipide from the gorgonian *Euplexaura flava* can be currently synthesized, opening the possibility of advancing into a new level of anti-inflammatory pharmaceuticals.

Some of the most interesting compounds identified so far in the on-going search for new anti-fouling agents have been recorded in the order Gorgonacea. Good examples of such compounds are juncin ZII from *Junceella juncea*, homarine from *Leptogorgia virgulata* and *Leptogorgia setacea*, pukalide and epoxypukalide recorded so far only from *Leptogorgia virgulata*.

Briareum excavata

Species of the genus *Briareum* (family Briareidae) which commonly exhibit an incrusting appearance rather than the fan-like shape of many gorgonians) are widely abundant in Indo-Pacific and Caribbean coral reefs. These organisms have been recognized as a valuable source of bioactive compounds with novel structural features. Briarane-related natural products are a good example of such promising compounds due to their structural complexity and biological activity. Briaexcavatin E, from *Briareum excavata* (Nutting 1911), also occasionally referred to as *Briarium excavatum*, inhibited human neutrophil elastase (HNE) release with an IC_{50} between 5 and 10 µM. Briaexcavatolides L and P, diterpenoids from the same species exhibited significant cytotoxicity against mouse lymphocytic leukemia (P-388) tumor cells with ED_{50} of 0.5 and 0.9 µg/mL, respectively.

Briareum asbestinum (= Briareum polyanthes)

Diterpenoids produced from *Briareum polyanthes* (presently accepted as *Briareum asbestinum*), namely Briarellin D, K and L, exhibited antimalarial activity against *Plasmodium falciparum* with an IC_{50} between 9 and 15 µg/mL.

The promising secondary metabolites derived from the soft corals and their bioactivities are shown in Tables **2** to **7**.

Table 2. Anticancer/anti-tumor/cytotoxic compounds of soft corals.

Species	Compound (s)	Chemistry	Refs.
Alcyonium paessleri	Alcyopterosins A–O; Paesslerins A–B	Sesquiterpenoids	[76]
Anthomastus bathyproctus	Steroids 2–5	---	[76]
Anthoptilum grandiflorum	Bathyptilones A–C	Terpenoids	[76]
Anthopleura anjunae	AAP-H	Pentapeptide	[11]
Anthopleura midori	Epoxyergosterol 1,2	Steroids	[11]
Anthoptilum grandiflorus	Bathyptilone A	Terpenoid	[11]
Antipathozoanthus hickmani	Valdiviamide B	Dipeptide	[11]
Asterospicularia laurae	Asterolaurin A, K–M	Diterpenoids	[11, 68]
Astrogorgia dumbea	Astrogorgioside A-C	Steroidal saponins	[11]
Briareum excavata	Briaexcavatolide L,P	Diterpenoids	[68]
Briareum sp.	Brialalepolide A -D	Terpenoids	[11]
Carijoa riisei	15β-hydroxypregna-4,20-dien-3-one;	Pregnane steroid	[11]
Carijoa riisei	15β, 18, 20R -acetoxypregna-1,4,20-trien-3-one	Pregnane steroid	[11]

(Table 2) cont.....

Species	Compound (s)	Chemistry	Refs.
Carijoa sp.	Carijoside A	Steoid	[11]
Cespitularia hypotentaculata	Cespitularin C	Diterpenoid	[68]
Cespitularia stolonifera	2S, 3R-4E, 8E-2-(heptadecanoylamino)-heptadeca-4, 8-diene-1, 3-diol	Ceramide	[11]
Cespitularia taeniata	Cespitulone A, Cespitaenin A, Cespilamide E	Terpenoids	[11]
Cladiella hirsuta	Cladophenol glycoside A,B	Glycosides	[11]
Cladiella hirsuta	Hirsutosteroside A, B; Hirsutosterols A–G	Steroids	[11]
Cladiella krempfi	Krempfielins E–I ; Oxylitophynol, Litophynol A acetate, Litophynol C	Terpenoids	[11]
Cladiella pachyclados	Pachycladin A-E	Terpenoids	[11]
Cladiella tuberculosa	Cladieunicellin R, S	Diterpenoids	[11]
Cladiella spp.	Cladielloide A-D ; Cladieunicellin A-E, I- Q	Terpenoids	[11]
Clavularia koellikeri	Cembrane-type diterpenoid	------	[68]
Clavularia viridis	Claviridic acid, mor Clavulone, Claviridenone, Bromovulone III	Prostanoids	[68]
Clavularia viridis	Yonarasterol, Stoloniferone E	Steroids	[68]
Clavularia viridis	Dolabellane diterpenoids	------	[11]
Clavularia viridis	Clavuridin A,	Sesquiterpenes	[11]
Clavularia viridis	Claviridin A–D	Steroids	[11]
Clavularia sp.	Haebaruol	Steroid	[11]
Convexella magelhaenica	Dolabellane diterpenoids	------	[11]
Dasystenella acanthina	Polyoxygenated steroids	-------	[76]
Dendronephthya rubeola	Capnell-9(12)-ene-8β,10α-diol	Sesquiterpenoid	[68]
Dendronephthya sp.	Dendronephthol A, C	ylangene-type sesquiterpenoids	[11]
Dichotella gemmacea	Dichotellide A – E; Gemmacolide N–S, G-M, T-Y, AZ–BF, AA–AR	Terpenoids	[111]
Echinomuricea sp	Echinoclerodane A, Echinohalimane A, Echinolabdane A	Terpenoids	[11]
Eunicea pinta	Pintoxolanes A–C	Terpenoids	[11]
Euplexaura robusta	Malonganenones I–K	Alkaloids	[11]
Euplexaura sp.	Euplexaurenes A–C	Diterpenoids	[11]

Species	Compound (s)	Chemistry	Refs.
Heteroxenia ghardaqensis	2S,3R-4E,8E-2-(hexadecanoylamino)-docosa-4,8- diene-1,3-diol	Ceramide	[11]
Isis hippuris	Suberosenol B	Terpenoid	[68]
Isis hippuris	Isishippuric acid B	Steroid	[68]
Isis minorbrachyblasta	11-O-acetyl-22-epihippuristanol	Steroid	[11]
Junceella fragilis	Frajunolide H	Diterpenoid	[11]
Klyxum flaccidum	Klyflaccicembranols A–I ; Flaccidenol A, B	Terpenoids	[11]
Klyxum flaccidum	Klyflaccisteroids G–J; K-M.	Steroids	[11]
Klyxum molle	Klymollins T–Z; Klyxumollins A-D	Diterpenoids	[11]
Klyxum simplex	- Simplexin P–S; Klysimplexin B-H	Terpenoids	[11]
Lemnalia philippinensis	Philippinlin A, B	Terpenoids	[11]
Leptogorgia gilchristi	Malonganenone A–C	Alkaloids	[11]
Leptogorgia punicea	Punicinol A–E	Steroids	[11]
Litophyton mollis	4α-methylated steroids	Steroids	[11]
Lobophytum compactum	Lobocompactol A,B	Terpenoids	[11]
Lobophytum cristagalli	Cembranolide diterpene	Diterpenoid	[68]
Lobophytum crassum	24-methylenecholest-5-ene-1α,3β,11α-triol 1-acetate	Steroid	[11]
Lobophytum crassum	13-acetoxysarcophytoxide; Culobophylin A–C; Lobocrassin A–E	Terpenoids	[11]
Lobophytum cristatum	Lobophytumin C,D	Terpenoids	[11]
Lobophytum durum	Durumolide M–Q	Terpenoids	[11]
Lobophytum laevigatum	Lobophytosterol	Steroid	[11]
Lobophytum michaelae	Michaolides, Lobomichaolides, Michaolide L–Q	Terpenoids	[11]
Lobophytum michaelae	Michosterol A-C	Steroids	[11]
Lobophytum pauciflorum	Cyclolobatriene	Terpenoid	[11]
Lobophytum sp.	Lobophysterol D	Steroid	[11]
Lobophytum sp.	Lobophytene	Diterpenoid	[68]
Menella kanisa	Polyoxygenated steroids	--------	[11]

(Table 2) cont.....

Species	Compound (s)	Chemistry	Refs.
Menella sp	Menecubebane B	Sesquiterpene	[11]
Muriceides collaris	Muriceidine A–C	Alkaloids	[11]
Muriceides collaris	Muriceidone A	Bis-sesquiterpene	[11]
Muricella flexuosa	Muricellasteroid A– E	Steroids	[11]
Muricella sibogae	Sibogin A, B	Terpenoids	[11]
Muricella sibogae	Sibogol A–C	Steroids	[11]
Muriceopsis flavida	Muriflasteroid A–C	Steroids	[11]
Nephthea chabroli	Chabrolin A, Parathyrsoidin E-G; Chabranol	Terpenoids	[11, 68]
Nephthya chabrolii.	Nebrosteroids Q,R,S.	Steoids	[77]
Nephthea columnaris	Plumisclerin A	Terpenoid	[11]
Nephthea columnaris	Columnaristerol A	Steroid	[11]
Nephthea erecta	Kelsoenethiol	Terpenoid	[11]
Nephthea erecta	Nephtheasteroid A, B	Steroids	[11]
Nephthea sp.	Nephthoacetal	Steroid	[11]
Nephthea sp	10-hydroxy-nephthenol acetate, 7,8-epoxy-10-hydr-xy-nephthenol acetate, 6-acetoxy- 7,8-epoxy--0-hydroxy-nephthenol acetate	Diterpenes	[11]
Pacifigorgia senta	Cholesta-5,24-diene-3β,7β,19-triol	Steroid	[11]
Palythoa caribaeorum	6β-carboxyl-24(R)-(8→6)-abeo-ergostan-3β,5β-diol	Steroid	[11]
Palythoa tuberculosa	Palysterol F	Steroid	[11]
Palythoa variabilis	6β-carboxyl-24(R)-(8→6)-abeo-ergostan-3β,5β-diol	Steroid	[11]
Paralemnalia thyrsoides	Parathyrsoidin A-G; Paralemnolin J—O ; Chabrolin A	Terpenoids	[11]
Paraminabea acronocephala	Paraminabic acid A-C ; Paraminabeolide A-F	Steroids	[11]
Paraminabea sp.	Methyl-3-oxochola-1,4-dien-24-oate ; ((1a,3b,7a,11a,12b)-gorgost-5-ene-1,3,7,11,12-pentol 12-acetate	Steroids	[11]
Pinnigorgia sp.	Pinnisterol A–J	Steroids	[11]
Plumigorgia terminosclera	Plumisclerin A	Terpenoid	[11]
Protodendron repens	Protoxenicin A,-B	Terpenoids	[11]
Pseudoplexaura flagellosa	Asperdiol stereoisomer	Terpenoids	[11]

Species	Compound (s)	Chemistry	Refs.
Pseudopterogorgia acerosa	Bis(pseudopterane) amine	Dialkylamine	[68]
Pseudopterogorgia acerosa	15-chlorodeoxypseudopterolide	Diterpene	[11]
Pseudopterogorgia americana	Ameristerenol A, B	Steroids	[11]
Pseudopterogorgia kallos	Bielschowskysin	Diterpene	[68]
Pseudopterogorgia sp	Secosterol	Steroid	[68]
Sarcophyton auritum	2-epi-sarcophine ; (1R,2E,4S,6E,8R,11R,12R)- 2, 6-cembradiene-4,8,11,12-tetrol ;	Terpenoids	[11]
Sarcophyton crassocaule	Crassocolide H–M; Sarcocrassocolide M–O ; 13-acetoxysarcocrassolide; Crassocolide N-P; Sarcocrassocolide A–E	Terpenoids	[11]
Sarcophyton ehrenbergi	2-methyloctyl 4-(3- methoxyphenyl) propenoate	Polyhydroxylated steroid	[11]
Sarcophyton ehrenbergi	(+)-12-ethoxycarbonyl-11Z-sarcophine; Ehrenbergol A,B; 7-keto-8α-hydroxy-deepoxysarcophine; 7β-chloro-8α-hydroxy-12-acetoxy-deepoxysarcophine; (E)-methyl-3-(5-butyl-1-hydroxy-2,3-dimethyl-4-oxocyclopent-2-enyl) acrylate; 3,4-epoxyehrenberoxide A; Ehrenbergol D,E	Terpenoids	[11]
Sarcophyton elegans	Sarcophyolide B–E	Diterpenoids	[11]
Sarcophyton glaucum	Sarcophytolol, Sarcophytolide B,C; Glaucumolide A, B; Sarglaucol; (1S,2E,4R,6E,8S,11R,12S)-8,11-epoxy-4,12-epoxy-2,6-cembradiene ; (1S,2E,4R,6E,8R,11S,12R)-8,12-epoxy-2,6-cembradiene-4,11-diol ; (1S,4R,13S)-cembra-2E,7E,11E-trien-4,13-diol; 6-oxo-germacra-4(15),8-11-triene; 10(14)-aromadendrene, sarcophinediol, ent-deoxysarcophine and sarcotrocheliol acetate; 3,4,8,16-tetra-epi-lobocrasol, 1,15 -epoxy- deoxysarcophine, 3,4-dihydro-4 ,7 ,8 -trihydroxy- D2-sarcophine; Ent-sarcophyolide E; and 16- deacetylhalicrasterol B	Terpenoids	[11]
Sarcophyton pauciplicatum	Sarcophytolide M	Terpenoids	[11]
Sarcophyton trocheliophorum	Yalongene A,B	Terpenoids	[11]
Sarcophyton trocheliophorum	7α-hydroxy- crassarosterol A	Steroid	[11]
Sarcophyton sp.	Dihydrofuranocembranoids 1 and 2; Sarchophine-like - tepenoids	Terpenoids	[11]

(Table 2) cont.....

Species	Compound (s)	Chemistry	Refs.
Sarcophyton sp.	(24S)- ergostan-3β,5α,6β,18,25-pentaol 18,25-diacetate	Steroid	[11]
Scleronephthya flexilis	3β-methoxy-5,20-pregnadiene	Steroid	[11]
Scleronephthya gracillimum	Sclerosteroid J–N; Clerosteroids aei (1, 5, 6, 8e13)	Steroids	[11]
Sinularia capillosa	Capilloquinol	Quinone	[11]
Sinularia capillosa	Capilloquinone, capillobenzopyranol, capillobenzofuranol and apillofuranocarboxylate	Diterpenes	[11]
Sinularia crassa	Crassarosterol A,	Steroid	[11]
Sinularia crassa	Crassalone A	Diterpene	[77]
Sinularia depressa	Depressin	Diterpene	[11]
Sinularia erecta	3β,5α-dihydroxyeudesma-4(15),11-diene	Terpenoid	[11]
Sinularia flexibilis	Flexilarin D, Flexibilide, Flexibilisolides C–G ; 11-acetylsinuflexolide	Terpenoids	[11]
Sinularia gaweli	5a,8a-Etidioxysterol	Steroid	[77]
Sinularia gyrosa	Sinugyrosanolide A, Gyrosanol A-C	Terpenoids	[11]
Sinularia inelegans	Pambanolide A-C; 4,5-secosinulochmodin C	Terpenoids	[11]
Sinularia leptoclados	Leptoclalin A	Terpenoid	[11]
Sinularia microspiculata	7-oxogorgosterol -ster-cyto; 16α-hydroxysarcosterol	Steroid	[11]
Sinularia mollis	Mollisolactone A, B	Diterpenes	[11]
Sinularia nanolobata	24(S),28-epoxyergost-5-ene-3β,4α-diol	Steroid	[11]
Sinularia pavida	Pavidolide B,C	Terpenoids	[11]
Sinularia rigida	Sinulariol A - S	Terpenoids	[11]
Sinularia sandensis	Sandensone A	Sesquiterpenoid	[11]
Sinularia scabra	Scabralin A, B.	Terpenoids	[11]
Sinularia triangula	Sinutriangulin A.	Terpenoid	[11]
Sinularia acuta	Cyclopentenone 9	Steroid	[11]
Sinularia brassica	Sinubrasolide A–G; Sinubrassione	Steroids	[11]
Sinularia conferta	Ergosta-24(28)-ene-3β,5α,6β-triol-6-acetate ; 5,6β-epoxygorgosterol	Steroids	[11]
Sinularia flexibilis	7α-hydroxy- crassarosterol A	Steroid	[11]
Sinularia gibberosa	Flaccidoxide-13-acetate	Terpenoid	[11]
Sinularia leptoclados	5,6β-epoxygorgosterol	Steroid	[11]
Sinularia molesta	Molestin E	Diterpene	[11]

Species	Compound (s)	Chemistry	Refs.
Sinularia sp.	Ximaosteroid E, F; (22E)-24-methylenecholestane-22-ene-3β,5α,6β-triol	Steroids	[11]
Sinularia sp.	5-episinuleptolide acetate; Sinulariaoid A -D	Terpenoids	[11]
Subergorgia suberosa	(3b,12b,16b,23E)-cholesta-5,23-diene-3,12,16,20,25-pentaol ; (3b,12b,16b)-cholesta-5,25(26)-diene-3,12,16,20,24-pentaol; Subergorgol A–J	Steroids	[11]
Subergorgia suberosa	Suberosoid	Sesquiterpene	[11]
Stragulum bicolor	Amphidinolide P, T1, C4, B8, B9; Stragulin	Macrolides	[11]
Telesto riisei	Punaglandin.	Prostaglandin	[68]
Umbellulifera petasites	Petasitosterone A,B	Steroids	
Verrucella corona	Verrucorosterone	Steroids	[11]
Verrucella umbraculum	Verumbsteroid A, B	Steroids	[11]
Xenia plicata	Blumiolide C	Diterpene	[68]
Xenia umbellata	Xeniumbellal	Diterpene	[11]
Xenia sp.	Xenimanadins A–D	Diterpenes	[78]
Xenia sp.	12-epi-9-deacetoxyxenicin	Terpenoid	[11]
Zoanthus kuroshio	Kuroshine A, C–G	Alkaloids	[11]

Table 3. Anti-inflammatory compounds of soft corals.

Species	Compound (s)	Chemistry	Refs.
Briareum asbestinum,	Seco-briarellinone, briarellin S	Terpenoids	[11]
Briareum excavatum	Briaexcavatin E ; Excavatoids L—N	Terpenoids	[68]
Briareum violaceum	Briaviolides K-N,V; Briaviodiols B, D, E ; Briaviotriols A-B; Fragilide S	Terpenoids	[11]
Briareum sp.	Briarenolide K,L, U-Y	Terpenoids	[11]
Capnella sp.	Capgermacrene A, B	Sesquiterpenoids	[11]
Cladiella hirsuta	Hirsutalin A- M	Terpenoids	[11]
Cladiella hirsuta	Hirsutosterol A-G	Steroids	[11]
Cladiella krempfi	8-n-butyryl-litophynol A, 6-keto-litophynol B; 6- epi-litophynol B; Krempfielin A-D, J–M	Diterpenes	[11]
Cladiella sp.	Cladielloide C, D; Cladieunicellin A- F, X ; solenopodin C	Terpenoids	[11]

(Table 3) cont.....

Species	Compound (s)	Chemistry	Refs.
Dendronephthya mucronata	5-α-pregn-20-en-3,6-dione	Steroid	[11]
Dendronephthya sp.	Dendronesterone D, E	Steroids	[11]
Echinogorgia sassapo	Sassapol A	Steroid	[11]
Eunicea fusca	Fuscoside E	Diterpene	[11]
Eunicea succinea	Uprolide N, O, P	Terpenoids	[11]
Euplexaura flava	Butenolides	Lactones	[68]
Heteractis crispa	Rhcgs1.19, rhcgs1.36	Peptides	[11]
Junceella fragilis	Frajunolide B,C, L–S; Fragilide K,L, W ; Cladieunicellin U; Klyflaccicembranols A–I	Terpenoids	[11]
Junceella juncea	Juncenolides M–O	Terpenoids	[11]
Klyxum flaccidum	23,24-dimethylated steroids; 9,11-secogorgosteroids; Klyflaccisteroids G–J.	Steroids	[11]
Klyxum flaccidum	Gyrosanolides A–F; Klyflaccilide A;	Terpenoids	[11]
Klyxum molle	Klymollins A–H, I-S, Y,Z	Terpenoids	[11]
Klyxum simplex	Klysimplexin sulfoxides A–C; Simplexin E; Klysimplexins I–T; Simplexins J–O	Terpenoids	[11]
Lemnalia flava	Flavalins A-D	Terpenoids	[11]
Lobophytum crassum	Crassumolide A, C; Lobophyolide A; Locrassumins A–G; Menelloide E; Lobocrasol A,B; Lobocrassin A–F ; 13-acetoxysarcophytoxide; (–)-laevigatol B; (–)-isosarcophine; (–)-7R,8S-dihydroxydeepoxysarcophytoxide;	Terpenoids	[11, 68]
Lobophytum durum	Durumolide A–C; Durumhemiketalolide A–C;	Terpenoids	[68]
Lobophytum laevigatum	Laevigatol A–D	Terpenoids	[11]
Lobophytum michaelae	Michosterol A-C	Steroids	[11]
Lobophytum pauciflorum	Lobophytone A-S, U–Z1	Terpenoids	[11]
Lobophytum sarcophytoides	Sarcophytosterol	Steroid	[11]
Lobophytum sarcophytoides	Lobophytin A, B	Terpenoids	[11]
Lobophytum varium	Lobovarols A–E.	Terpenoids	[11]
Menella sp.	Menellsteroid C	Steroid	[11]
Menella sp.	Menelloide A- D; (-)-Hydroxylindestrenolide; Menellin A; Menelloide E, Lobocrassin F	Terpenoids	[11]

Species	Compound (s)	Chemistry	Refs.
Nephthea columnaris	Columnaristerol B, C	Steroids	[11]
Nephthea erecta	Ergostanoid 1, 3	Polyhydroxyoctane	[68]
Paraminabea acronocephala	Paraminabic acid A-C	Steroids	
Pennatula aculeata	2-acetoxyverecynarmin C	Terpenoid	[11]
Pinnigorgia sp.	Pinnigorgiols A-C; Pinnigorgiols D and E ; 11-acetox--9,11-secosterols, pinnisterols D–J (1–7) ; 5 ,6 -epox--(22E,24R)-3 ,11-dihydroxy-9,11- secoergosta-7-e--9-one ; (22R)-acetoxy-(24x)-ergosta-5-en-3 ,25-diol	Steroids	[11]
Rumphella antipathies	Rumphellol A, B; Rumphellaoic acid A; Rumphellaone B,C ; Rumphellclovane B; 2β-acetoxyclovan-9α-ol (1), 9α-acetoxyclovan-2β-ol	Terpenoids	[11]
Sarcophyton cherbonnieri	Cherbonolide A-E	Terpenoids	[11]
Sarcophyton crassocaule	Sarcocrassocolide A-E, M	Terpenoids	[11]
Sarcophyton ehrenbergi	Sarcoehrenolide A,B,D	Terpenoids	[11]
Sarcophyton glaucum	Glaucumolide A,B	Terpenoids	[11]
Sarcophyton pauciplicatum	Sarcopanol A	Terpenoid	[11]
Sarcophyton tortuosum	Tortuosene. A,B	Terpenoid	[11]
Scleronephthya gracillimum	Sclerosteroid J–N	Steroids	[11]
Sinularia arborea	Sinularbol A,B.	Diterpenoids	[11]
Sinularia brassica	Sinubrasone A–D; Sinubrasolide H–L	Terpenoids	[11]
Sinularia crassa	Crassarine A–H	Terpenoids	[11]
Sinularia erecta	Sinulerectol A,B.	Terpenoids	[11]
Sinularia flexibilis	Thioflexibilolide A; Flexibilin D; Xidaosinularide A; Flexibilisin C-E; Secoflexibilisolide A,B; Flexibilisolide C- H; 11,12-secoflexibillin	Terpenoids	[11]
Sinularia flexibilis	Flexibilisquinone	Quinone	[11]
Sinularia gaweli	Flexibilin D, Sinulacembranolide A	Terpenoids	[11]
Sinularia gibberosa	Gibberoketosterol	Steroid	[68]
Sinularia granosa	8ah-3b,11-dihydroxy-5a,6a- expoxy-24-methylene-9-11-secocholestan-9-one	Steroid	[11]

(Table 3) cont.....

Species	Compound (s)	Chemistry	Refs.
Sinularia gyrosa	Gyrosanin A	Terpenoid	[11]
Sinularia leptoclados	Leptocladolin A,B	Terpenoids	
Sinularia lochmodes.	Lochmolin A–G	Terpenoids	[11]
Sinularia maxima	12-hydroxy-scabrolide A ; 13-epi-scabrolide	Terpenoid	[11]
Sinularia numerosa	Sinumerolide A ; 7E-sinumerolide A	Terpenoids	[11]
Sinularia querciformis	Querciformolide C	Terpenoid	[11]
Sinularia scabra	Scabralin A, B	Sesquiterpenes	[11]
Sinularia sp.	Chloroscabrolide A,B; Prescabrolide R; Sinularcasbane A, B; Sinularianin C-F; Sinularolide	Terpenoids	[11]
Sinularia sp.	Sinulasulfoxide, Sinulasulfone	Alkaloids	[11]
Sinularia sp.	Sinularioside	Glycerolipid	[11]
Umbellulifera petasites	Petasitosterone C	Steroid	[11]
Zoanthus kuroshio	5α-iodozoanthenamine; 11β-chloro-11- deoxykuroshine A	Alkaloids	-

Table 4. Antiviral compounds of soft corals.

Species	Compound (s)	Chemistry	Refs.
Briareum excavatum	Briacavatolides A–C	Terpenoids	[11]
Briareum violacea	Briaviolides A–J	Terpenoids	[11]
Briareum sp	Briarenolide J	Terpenoid	[11]
Cladiella hirsuta	Eunicellin-type hirsutalins N–R	Terpenoids	[11]
Cladiella krempfi	Krempfielin N-R	Terpenoids	[11]
Echinogorgia pseudossapo	Pseudozoanthoxanthin III	Alaklaoid	[11]
Echinogorgia rebekka	Echrebsteroids A–D	Steroids	[11]
Isis hippuris	Hipposterone M–O	Steroids	[11]
Junceella fragilis	Fragilolides B-Q	Diterpenoids	[11]
Klyxum molle	Klymollin I-X	Terpenoids	[11]
Lobophytum crassum	Secocrassumol	Terpenoid	[11]
Lobophytum durum	Durumolide M–Q	Terpenoids	[11]

(Table 4) cont.....

Species	Compound (s)	Chemistry	Refs.
Lobophytum sp.	Lobohedleolide, (7Z)-lobohedleolide, 17-dimethylamino lobohedleolide	Diterpenoids	[68]
Palythoa mutuki	Palythone A	Ecdysteroid	[11]
Sarcophyton ehrenbergi	Ehrenbergol C, Acetyl ehrenberoxide B, Cembranoid, Lobophynin C, Ehrenberoxide A-C; (+)-12-ethoxycarbonyl--1Z-sarcophine; Ehrenbergol A,B	Terpenoids	[11]
Sinularia candidula	3β-25-dihydroxy-4-methyl-5α,8α-epidioxy-2- ketoergost-9-ene (1) along with three new ceramides, N-[(2S,3R,E)-1-3-dihydroxyhexacos-4- en-2-yl]icosanamide (2), N-[(2S,3S,4R--1,3,4- trihydroxyhexacosan-2-yl]icosanamide (3), and (R)- 2'-hydroxy-N-[(2S,3S,4R)-1,3,4- trihydroxypentacosan-2-yl] nonadecanamide (4)	Steroids	[11]
Sinularia candidula	N-[(2S,3R,E)-1,3-dihydroxyhexacos-4-en-2- yl]icosanamide (2), N-[(2S,3S,4R)-1,3,4- trihydroxyhexacosan-2-yl]icosanamide (3), and (R)- 2'-hydroxy-N-[(2S,3S,4R)-1,3,4- trihydroxypentacosan-2-yl] nonadecanamide (4)	Terpenoids	[11]
Sinularia mollis	Mollisolactone A,B	Terpenoids	[11]
Sinularia nanolobata	9,11-secosteroids, 22α-acetoxy-24-methylene- 3β,6α,11-trihydroxy-9, 11-seco-cholest-7-en-9-one (1) and 11-acetoxy--4-methylene-1β,3β,6α- trihydroxy-9, 11-seco-cholest-7-en-9-one (2)	Steroids	[11]
Subergorgia suberosa	Subergorgol T–X	Steroids	[11]
Zoanthus sp.	Zoanthone A	Steroid	[11]

Table 5. Antimalarial compounds of soft corals.

Species	Compound (s)	Chemistry	Refs.
Briareum asbestinum	Briarellin D, K,L	Diterpenoids	[68]
Eunicea sp.	Sesquiterpenoid	------	[68]
Pseudopterogorgia bipinnata	Caucanolide A,D	Diterpenoids	[68]
Pseudopterogorgia elisabethae	Aberrarone	Diterpenoid	[68]
Pseudopterogorgia kallos	Bielschowskysin	Diterpenoid	[68]
Sinularia sp	Sinuketal, Sinulin A, B	Terpenoids	[11]

Table 6. Anti-tubercular compounds of soft corals.

Species	Compound (s)	Chemistry	Refs.
Nepthea sp.	Linosterol, nephalsterol C	Steroids	[79]
Pseudopterogorgia bipinnata	Bipinnapterolide B	Terpenoid	[68]
Pseudopterogorgia elisabethae	Ileabethoxazole, Homopseudopteroxazole, Caribenol A,B; Elisapterosin B	Terpenoids	[68]
Pseudopterogorgia elisabethae	Cumbiasin A,B	Diterpenoids	[79]
Pseudopterogorgia elisabethae	Pseudopteroxazole,homopseudopteroxaz ole, Seco-pseudopteroxazole - benzoxazole diterpene	Benzoxazole diterpene alkaloids	[79]

Table 7. Miscellaneous bioactive compounds of soft corals.

Species	Drug class	Compound (s)	Chemistry	Refs.
Acanthoprimnoa cristata	Antiprotozoal	Cristaxenicin A	Terpenoid	[11]
Briareum asbestinum	Antiparasitic	Briarellin 1-9; Polyanthellin A	Terpenoids	[11]
Capnella fungiformis	Antiparasitic	Ethyl 5-[(1E,5Z)-2,6-dimethylocta-1,5,7-trienyl]furan-3-carboxylate	Terpenoid	[11]
Capnella fungiformis	Antiparasitic	Oxyfungiformin	Sesquiterpenoid	[11]
Clavularia sp.	Neuroprotective	Stolonidiol	Diterpenoid	[11]
Eunicea sp.	Antiplasmodial	Cembradiene diterpenoid	-	-
Gorgonia sp.	Anti-leishmanial	Oxysterol	Steroid	[11]
Leptogorgia sp.	Antidiabetic	Chloro-furanocembranolides; 1,4-diketo cembranolides; seco- furanocembranolide	-	[11]
Plumarella delicatissima	Anti-leishmanial	Keikipukalides B–E; Pukalide aldehyde	Terpenoids	[76]
Sarcophyton stellatum	Antiparasitic	(1E,3E,11E)-7,8-epoxycembra-1,3,11,15-tetraene	Terpenoid	[11]
Sinularia sp.	Antiulcer	Sinularamide derived spermine	Terpenoid	[68]
Soft coral	Anti-leishmanial	Shagene A,B	Terpenoids	[76]

CONCLUSION

Although the phylum Cnidaria is not the most significantly bioprospected at present, this review shows that some cnidarian species are promising sources of marine bioactive compounds of medical, economic and scientific interest. Green fluorescent protein (GFP), GPF-like proteins, red fluorescent and orange fluorescent protein (OPF) are good examples of biotechnological metabolites currently employed as molecular biomarkers. They were first purified from a fluorescent hydrozoan medusa [68] and since then have been recorded in other cnidarian species.

Even though most pharmaceutical industries abandoned their natural product-based discovery programs over a decade ago, the lack of new compounds in their pipelines in some strategic areas (*e.g.*, antibiotics) suggests that renewed interest in this field is imminent. The establishment of small biotech companies can play a decisive role in the initial discovery of promising marine bioactive compounds, as these enterprises will work closely together with academics and governmental agencies performing the initial steps in the discovery of new MNPs. Collaboration between private companies and public institutions can be of paramount importance for financial support in the discovery process. On the other side, crude extracts and pure compounds produced by academic laboratories may be screened by diverse bioassays as a part of broader collaboration programs, nationally and internationally, with private biotech companies. One challenge for universities is to devise mechanisms that protect intellectual property and simultaneously encourage partnerships with the private sector, by recognizing that the chances of a major commercial pay-off are small if drug discovery is pursued by a single institution [3].

The commercial use of some promising marine bioactive compounds isolated from cnidarians may be several years away. New compounds other than toxins and venoms produced by members of this highly diverse group of marine invertebrates may be discovered in the quest for new marine products.

CHAPTER 6

Promising Pharmaceutical Compounds of Marine Bryozoans: Their Chemistry and Therapeutic Applications

Abstract: This chapter deals with the pharmaceutically important marine bryozoans, their promising secondary metabolites, and bioactivities. All the bioactive compounds of this marine invertebrate group are dealt with as per their chemical classes.

Keywords: Bryostatins, *Bugula neritina*, Cheilostomatida, Gymnolaemata, Marine bryozoans.

INTRODUCTION

The phylum Bryozoa is one of the excellent marine invertebrate sources of pharmacologically interesting substances. The bryozoans are found distributed from tropical to polar regions particularly in New Zealand, Antarctica, the North Pacific around Japan, the northern Mediterranean and the Adriatic and North Sea. While many marine bryozoans are colonial, they are also benthic or epibiotic on algae, seagrass, and marine animals. There are more than 6000 species of marine bryozoans and the species of the class Gymnolaemata are considered to be important sources of marine drug leads. Bryostatins of Bugula neritina with remarkable antineoplastic activity have attracted researchers' interests worldwide. However, this phylum has so far received little attention and most studied species belong to the order Cheilostomatida, the species of which possess erect, foliose, and large colonies. The major reason for these scarce studies is believed to be the insufficient biomass of bryozoan samples for the use of the isolation of bioactive compounds. Further, many species of bryozoans are heavily calcified with encrusting growth and difficulty in taxonomical identifications. The origin of the bioactive compounds in marine invertebrates is said to be either from de novo biosynthesis, from the diet, or from symbiotic microorganisms. In bryozoans, the origin of the most important bioactive compounds *viz.* bryostatins has been traced to bacterial symbiont *Endobugula sertula* but it is still unknown for many such compounds. Intensive and coordinated research is therefore required to isolate and

Santhanam Ramesh, Ramasamy Santhanam & Veintramuthu Sankar

characterize the secondary metabolites of bryozoans with pharmaceutical applications [79].

MARINE BRYOZOANS WITH PROMISING BIOACTIVE COMPOUNDS

Amathia convoluta, Amathia tortusa, Amathia verticillata (= Zoobotryon verticillatum) Amathia wilsoni, Biflustra grandicella, Aspidostoma giganteum, Bidenkapia spitzbergensis (= Tegella spitzbergensis), Biflustra perfragilis (= Membranipora perfragilis), Bugula longissima, Bugula neritina, Caulibugula intermis, Chartella papyracea, Cryptosula pallasiana, Dendrobeania murrayana, Euthyroides episcopalis, Flustra foliacea, Hincksinoflustra denticulate, Myriapora truncata, Paracribricellina cribraria (= Cribricellina cribraria), Pentapora fascialis, Pterocella vesiculosa, Securiflustra securifrons, Sessibugula translucens, Terminoflustra membranaceotruncata Virididentula dentata (= Bugula dentata), Wateripora subtorquata, and Watersipora cucullaa (Figs. **1 - 15**).

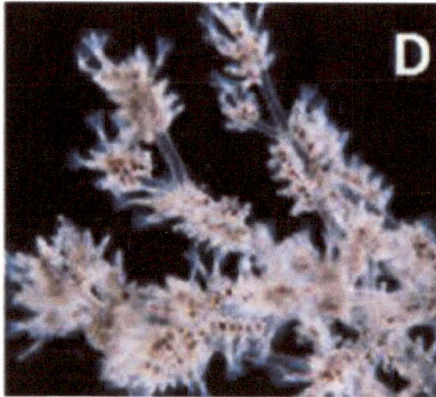

Fig. (1). *Amathia verticillata.*

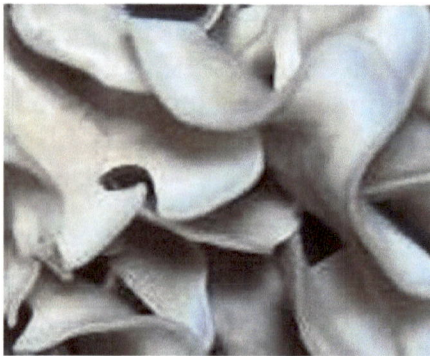

Fig. (2). *Biflustra* sp.

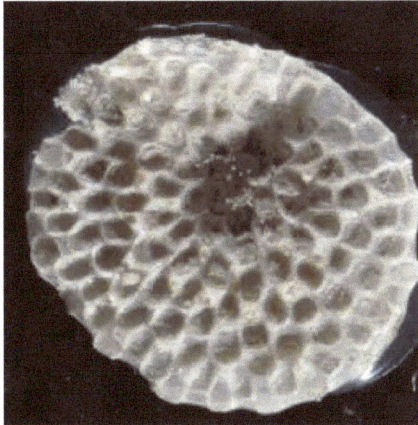

Fig. (3). *Bidenkapia spitzbergensis.*

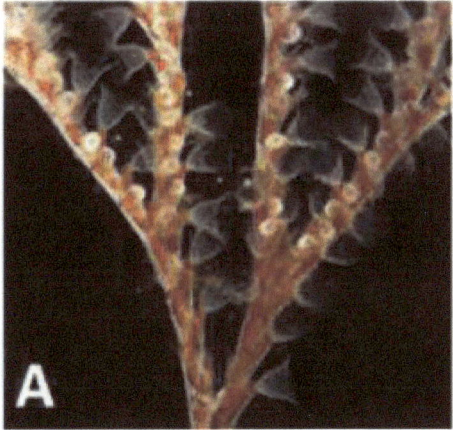

Fig. (4). *Bugula neritina.*

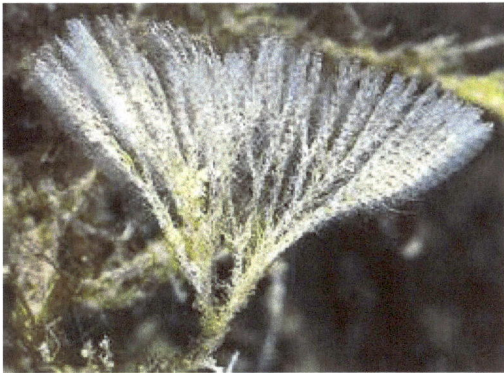

Fig. (5). *Caulibugula* sp.

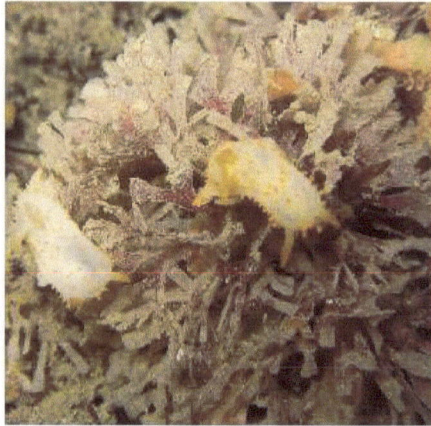

Fig. (6). *Chartella papyracea.*

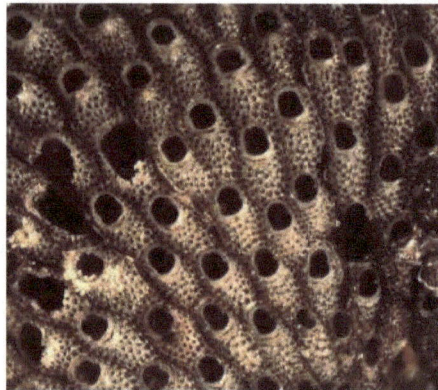

Fig. (7). *Cryptosula pallasiana.*

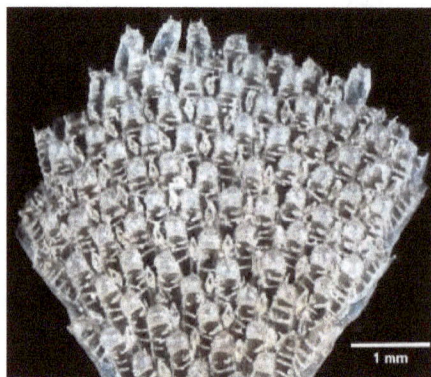

Fig. (8). *Dendrobeania murrayana.*

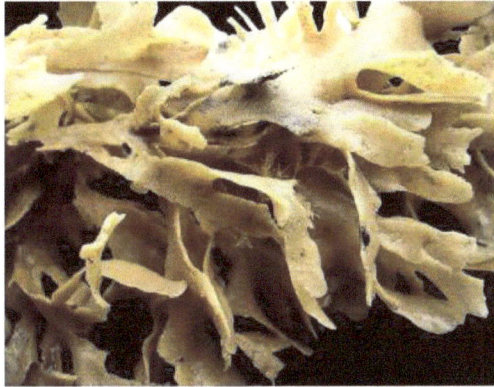

Fig. (9). *Flustra foliacea.*

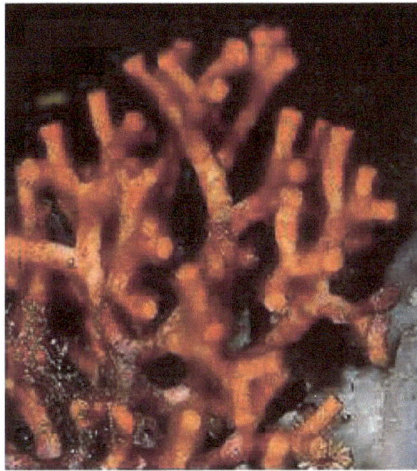

Fig. (10). *Myriapora truncata.*

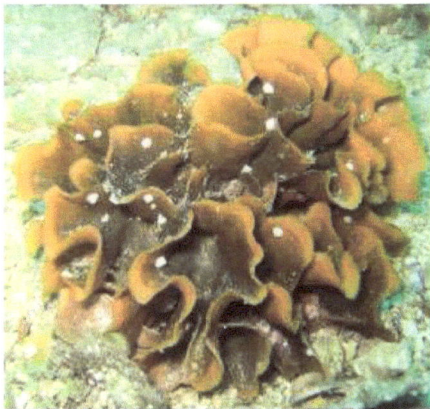

Fig. (11). *Pentapora fascialis.*

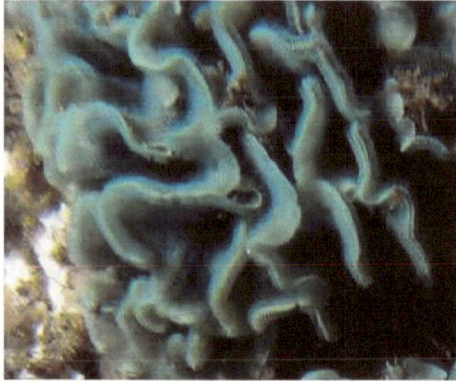

Fig. (12). *Sessibugula translucens.*

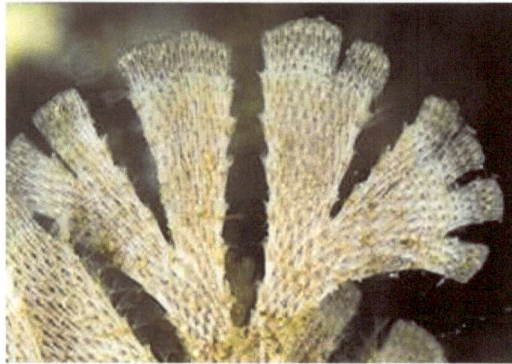

Fig. (13). *Securiflustra securifrons.*

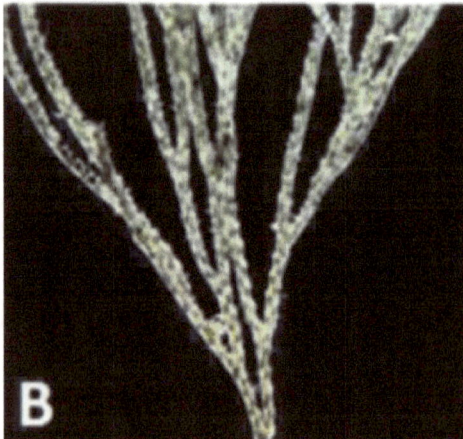

Fig. (14). *Virididentula dentata.*

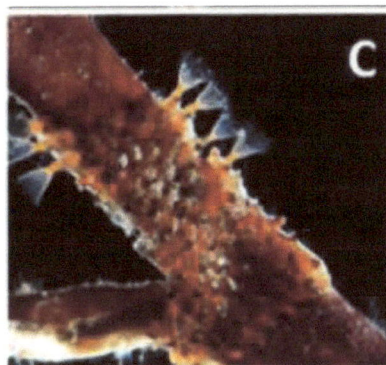

Fig. (15). *Wateripora subtorquata.*

Image credit: *Amathia verticillata, Bugula neritina, Virididentula dentata, Wateripora subtorquata*: Ciavatta, *et al.*, CC; *Amathia wilsoni, Bidenkapia spitzbergensi*: Wikipedia; *Biflustra* sp.: *Chartella papyracea, Cryptosula pallasiana, Dendrobeania murrayana*: Wikimedia commons; *Flustra foliacea*: Wikipedia.

The promising biopharmaceutical compounds of marine bryozoans and their bioactivities are detailed below.

ANTICANCER AND CYTOTOXIC ACTIVITIES OF MARINE BRYOZOANS

Alkaloids

Marine bryozoans possess the most common class of natural products *viz.* alkaloids which have been reported to have a huge potential as new anticancer drugs. The cytotoxic and anticancer activities of the different alkaloid compounds as reported by Figuerola, and Avila [79] are given below.

Dibrominated alkaloids

Thee dibrominated alkaloids, *viz.* amathaspiramides A–F, a series of six dibrominated alkaloids, were isolated from Amathia wilsoni. These compounds, with four analogues were tested for antiproliferative activity against human cancer cell lines such as HCT-116 (colon cancer), PC-3 (prostate cancer), MV4-11 (acute myeloid leukemia), and MiaPaCa-2 (pancreas cancer). Among the different compounds, amathaspiramide C only displayed significant antiproliferative activity (5.8 µM) against MiaPaCa-2 cell line and with other cell lines, the IC_{50} values recorded were 63, 80, and 64 µM, respectively. Amathaspiramide A recorded IC_{50} values of 46, 67, 48, and 14 µM against the HCT-116, PC-3, MV4-

11, and MiaPaCa-2 cell lines, respectively; and for amathaspiramide E, the IC_{50} values were 29, 81, 55, and 15 µM, respectively.

Bromopyrrole alkaloids

A series of bromopyrrole alkaloids *viz.* Aspidostomides A–H were isolated from the Patagonian bryozoan *Aspidostoma giganteum*. Among these compounds, aspidostomide E displayed moderate inhibitory activity towards the 768-O renal carcinoma cell line with an IC_{50} value of 7.8 µM.

Brominated alkaloids

A bromated alkaloid, 7-bromo-2,4(1H,3H)-quinazolinedione isolated from the cheilostome bryozoan, *Cryptosula pallasiana* did not show significant cytotoxicity against human myeloid leukemia HL-60 cells and the IC_{50} value recorded in this case was 11.87 µg/mL.

β-Carboline alkaloids

The crude extracts of the cheilostomes *Paracribricellina cribraria* containing the β-carboline alkaloids compound, 1-vinyl-8-hydroxy-β-carboline displayed potent cytotoxicity against an NCI-60 cell tumor. This compound also showed cytotoxicity against P-388 cell line with an IC_{50} value of 0.1 µg/mL. While the other β-carboline alkaloids of this species viz 1-vinyl-8-acetoxy-β-carboline displayed cytotoxicity against P-388 cell line with an IC_{50} value of 0.67 µg/mL, the other related compounds *viz.* 1-ethyl-4-methylsulfone-β-carboline, 1-ethyl-8-hydroxy-β-carboline, 1-ethyl-8-methoxy-β-carboline and 8-hydroxyharman showed cytotoxicity against P-388 cell line with IC_{50} values greater than 12.5 µg/mL. Moreover, another β-carboline alkaloid, 5-bromo-8-methoxy-1-me-hyl-β-carboline derived from the cheilostome *Pterocella vesiculosa* showed relatively moderate cytotoxicity against P-388 cells with an IC_{50} value of 5.089 µg/mL. It has also been demonstrated that the vinyl substituent at C-1 or bromine at C-5 is important for the cytotoxicity against the P-388 cell line.

Caulamidines

Among the heterocyclic alkaloids caulamidine A and B derived from the cheilostome *Caulibugula intermis*, caulamidine A did not exhibit cytotoxicity in an NCI-60 cell screen with a single dose of 40 µM.

Caulibugulones

The alkaloids, caulibugulones A–F isolated from *Caulibugula. intermis* exhibited cytotoxicity against the murine IC-2wt tumor cell line *in vitro* with IC_{50} values ranging from 0.03 to 1.67 µg/mL.

Convolutamides

The alkaloids, convolutamides A–F were isolated from the ctenostome *Amathia convoluta*. Among these compounds, the mixture of convolutamides A and B exhibited cytotoxicity against L-1210 murine leukemia cells and human epidermoid carcinoma (KB) cells with IC_{50} values of 4.8 and 2.8 µg/mL respectively).

Convolutamydines

The alkaloids, convolutamydines A–D have been isolated from *Amathia convoluta*. Among these compounds, convolutamydine A (1,4,6-dibromo-3-hydroxy-3-(2-oxopropyl)-2-indolinone) displayed potent activity in the differentiation of HL-60 human plomyelocytic leukemia cells at concentrations of 0.1–25 µg/mL. The biological evaluation of the dibromohydroxyoxindole derivatives *viz.* convolutamydines B–D. could not be achieved due to their small amounts.

Convolutamines

The brominated β-phenylethylamine alkaloids *viz.* convolutamines A–G and lutamides A and C (2,4,6-tribromo-3-methoxyphenethylamine alkaloids) were isolated from *Amathia convoluta*. Among these compounds, convolutamines A, C, and F have been reported to show inhibition against adriamycin (ADM)-resistant P-388/ADM (IC_{50} values 7.0, 3.0, and 9.5 µg/mL, respectively) and vincristine (VCR)-resistant P-388/VCR (IC_{50} values 3.0, 1.4, and 8.0 µg/mL, respectively). Further, the convolutamines B and D also displayed cell growth inhibitory activity against P-388 with IC_{50} values of 4.8 and 8.6 µg/mL, respectively; and convolutamine F against its vincristine-resistant KB/VJ-300 cells with an IC_{50} value of 9.6 µg/mL. Lutamides A and C of *Amathia convoluta* displayed inhibition against KB/VJ300 cells (IC_{50} values 7.5 and 6.5 µg/mL, respectively) and lutamide C against P-388/VCR (IC_{50} value 4.8 µg/mL). Furthermore, the convolutamines I–J, derived from *Amathia tortuosa* have been reported to serve as potential ATP competitive inhibitors.

Eusynstyelamides

The alkaloids, brominated tryptophan-derived ent-eusynstyelamide B and three derivatives, eusynstyelamides D, E, and F, have been isolated from *Tegella* cf. *spitzbergensis*. Among these compounds, eusynstyelamide D and E, did not display activity against the human melanoma A-2058 cell line (IC_{50} values 57 and 114.3 µg/mL, respectively). Eusynstyelamide B, together with its two isomers *viz.* eusynstyelamide A and C, have been reported to be nontoxic toward the three human tumor cell lines MCF-7 (breast), SF-268 (central nervous system), and H460 (lung) at concentrations of up to 32 mM. Further, Eusynstyelamide D, was also nontoxic towards human colon cancer cell line HCT-116.

Perfragilins

The isoquinoline quinones *viz.* perfragilins A and B were derived from *Biflustra perfragilis*. These perfragilins exhibited cytotoxic activity towards murine leukemia cell (P-388) lines with ED_{50} values of 0.8 and 0.07 µg/mL, respectively.

Polycyclic indole alkaloids

The chief source of these alkaloids are *Chartella papyracea, Securiflustra securifrons, Hincksinoflustra denticulata* and *Flustra foliacea*. The polycyclic indole alkaloids *viz.* chartellines A–C and chartellamides A–B were derived from *Chartella papyracea*. Among these compounds, chartelline A, was found to be inactive against leukemia cells in the NCI test. Three halogenated, hexacyclic indole-imidazole alkaloids,viz. securamines H–J, and securamines C and E, were derived from *Securiflustra securifrons* Among these compounds, securamines C, E, and H–J were evaluated for their cytotoxic activity against human cancer cell lines A-2058 (skin), HT-29 (colon), and MCF-7 (breast), as well as against non-malignant human MRC-5 lung fibroblasts. However, securamines C, E, H, and I have been reported to affect cell viability, with H, I, and E being the most potent and with IC_{50} values ranging from 1.4 to 10 µM. On the other hand, the crude extract of Flustra. foliacea displayed activity against human colon cancer cell line HCT-116. Further, its deformylflustrabromine compound showed the strongest cytotoxicity (IC_{50} value 5.8 µM) and flustramines A and D and dihydroflustramine C did not display cytotoxicity (IC_{50} value 26 µM).

Pterocellins

The alkaloids, pterocellins A–F have been derived from *Pterocella vesiculosa*. Among these compounds, pterocellins A and B displayed relatively potent antitumor activity against the murine leukemia cell line P-388 *in vitro* with IC_{50} values of 0.477 and 0.323 µg/mL, respectively. Further, pterocellins A and B were evaluated against a variety of human tumor cell types (leukemia, non-small cell lung, colon, central nervous system, melanoma, ovarian, renal, prostate, and breast cancers), and these compounds showed potent cytotoxicity overall (panel average values of GI50 (growth inhibition of 50%) 1.4 µM, TGI (tumor growth inhibition) 4.8 µM, and LC_{50} 17.0 µM for pterocellin A and GI50 0.7 µM, TGI 2.1 µM, and LC_{50} 6.9 µM for pterocellin B). The most sensitive cell lines to pterocellins A and B were leukemia (CCRF-CEM: GI50 0.05 µM, TGI 0.8 µM) and melanoma (MALME-3M: GI50 0.03 µM, TGI 0.1 µM), respectively. Non-small cell lung (NCI-H23: GI50 0.3 and 0.1 µM, TGI 1.0 and 0.3 µM, and LC_{50} 6.1 and 0.7 µM, respectively), melanoma (MALME-3M: GI50 0.1 and 0.03, TGI 0.3 and 0.1 µM, and LC_{50} 0.8 and 0.3 µM, respectively; M-14: GI50 0.2 and 0.1 µM, TGI 0.8 and 0.2 µM, and LC_{50} 4.6 and 0.5 µM, respectively; SK-MEL-5: GI50 0.2 and 0.1 µM, TGI 0.3 µM, and LC_{50} 0.6 and 0.5 µM, respectively) and breast (MDA-MB-435: GI50 0.2 µM, TGI 0.3 µM, and LC_{50} 0.6 µM, respectively, and MDA-N: GI50 0.2 µM, TGI 0.4 and 0.3 µM, and LC_{50} 0.6 µM, respectively). Further, only pterocellin A was found to be cytotoxic to Hela human cervical cancer cells, with an IC_{50} of 0.886 µg/mL. Furthermore, among the four new pterocellins (C–F) isolated from *Pterocella vesiculosa,* only pterocellin D displayed moderate activity against the P-388 cell line with an IC_{50} value of 4.773 µg/mL.

Tambjamines

The 2-2′-bipyrrolic class of cytotoxic alkaloids *viz.* tambjamines A–K are a 2-2--bipyrrolic class of cytotoxic alkaloids derived from marine bryozoans. *Virididentula (Bugula) dentata* yielded tambjamines A, B and K (isopentenyl derivative of tambjamine A). Among these compounds, tambjamine K displayed antiproliferative and cytotoxicity against tumor and non-tumor cell lines with an IC_{50} value against the human epithelial colorectal adenocarcinoma CaCo-2 cells within the nano-molar range (CaCo-2 cells: IC_{50} 3.5 × 10−3 µM; H9c2 cells: IC_{50} 2.7 µM). However, tambjamine K was found to be not active (IC_{50} 13.7 µM and IC_{50} 15.3 µM, respectively) against human colon cancer HCT-116 and breast carcinoma MB-231 cell lines.

Terminoflustrindoles

The brominated akaloids *viz.* terminoflustrindoles A–C were isolated from *Terminoflustra (Chartella) membranaceotruncata.* Among these compounds, terminoflustrindole A displayed cytotoxic activity against human neuroblastome SK-N-SH, and histiotypic leukemia U-937 cells) at concentrations of 10 µM,.

Lactones

Bryostatins

The macrocyclic lactones, bryostatins 1-18 are the oxygenated macrolides are complex polyketides derived from the marine bryozoan, *Bugula neritina*. These compounds are the most promising compound candidates as anticancer and antitumor agents due to their antineoplastic activity and low toxicity. Further, these compoundsare able to selectively modulate the function of several protein kinase C (PKC) enzymes, which possess an important role in the regulation of cell growth and death.Among *in vitro* and *in vivo* anticancer effects against a range of tumor lines, these bryostatins have been shown to exhibit activity against several cancer cell lines such as histiocytic lymphoma cell U-937, human leukemia HL-60, lymphocytic leukemia P-388, melanoma B-16, murine melanoma K1735-M2, prostate cancer cells LNcaP and M-5076 reticulum cell sarcoma. The important bryostatins and their anticancer activities as reported by Ciavatta, *et al.* [80] are given below.

Bryostatin-1

It is the first macrocyclic lactone identified from *Bugula neritina* and is the most studied compound among all bryostatins Apart from being a PKC inhibitor, this compound has been reported to induce differentiation and promote apoptosis in various tumor cell lines, immunomodulatory properties (*e.g.*, stimulation of cytokine production and activation of cytotoxic T lymphocytes) and antitumor activity in preclinical models. Therefore, his compound is a promising compound against several tumor cell types, although this drug candidate is still under Phase II clinical trials for cancer.

Bryostatin-5

It showed a strong differentiation-inducing ability in human myeloid blast cells at a concentrations of 10 nM and inhibited the growth of murine melanoma K1735-M and HL-60 leukemic cells at an optimal concentration of 5–10 nM. Further, this compond has been reported to promote the activation of PKC.

Bryostatin-8

This compound has been reported to promote the activation of PKC for a short period followed by its deregulation, leading to growth inhibition, cell differentiation, and programmed cell death.

Bryostatin-19

This compound displayed strong cytotoxic activity against the U-937 cell line with an *in vitro* ED_{50} value of 3.2 nmol/L.

Bryostatin Analogues (Bryostatins (1, 2, 3, 7, 9, and 16))

Among these compounds, the bryostatin-7 was the first member of the synthesized bryostatins, It showed the most potent binding affinity to PKC and therefore this compound is considered as an effective substitute for the bryostatin-1. All other analogues have also shown PKC inhibition activity with strong *in vitro* antitumor effects. For example, the simplified bryostatin analogue 1, picolog, has been reported to show potent growth inhibition of MYC-induced lymphoma *in vitro* compared with bryostatin-1 at concentrations from 1 nM to 10 μM.

Neristatin 1

A macrocyclic lactone, neristatin 1 derived from *Bugula neritina* displayed weak cytotoxic activity (ED_{50} = 10 μg/mL) against the P-388 leukemia cell line [80].

Myriaporones

The polyketide-derived metabolites *viz.* myriaporones 1–4 were isolated from the bryozoan, *Myriapora trunca*. Among these compounds, myriaporones 3 (hemiketal, myriaporone 3) and 4 (hydroxy ketone) have been reported to show 88% inhibition against murine leukemia L-1210 cells at a concentration of 0.2 μg/mL [80].

Other Lactones

A lactone isolated from *Cryptosula pallasiana* displayed stronger cytotoxicity against HL-60, human hepatocellular carcinoma Hep-G2, and human gastric carcinoma SGC-7901, with IC_{50} values ranging from 4.12 to 7.32 μM [80].

Ceramides

Two sulfates of ceramides isolated from *Watersipora cucullata* have been reported to act as inhibitors of the principal target of anticancer drugs DNA topoisomerase I enzyme, with IC_{50} values of 0.4 and 0.2 μM, respectively. Further, five ceramides *viz.* neritinaceramides A–E (2S, 3R, 3'S, 4E, 8E, 10 E)- 2-(hexa decanoy lamino) -4, 8,10-octa decatri ene-1,3,3'-triol, (2S,3R,2'R,4E,8E,10E)-2-(hexadecanoylamino)-4,8,10-octadecatriene-1,3,2'-triol, (2S,3R,2'R,4E,8E,10E)-2-(octadecanoylamino)-4,8,10-octadecatriene-1,3,2'-triol,

(2S,3R,3'S,4E,8E)-2-(hexa decano ylamino)-4,8-octade cadiene-l,3,3'-triol, and (2S,3R,3'S,4E)-2-(hexadecanoylamino)-4-octadecene-l,3,3'-triol derived from Bugula. neritina were found to be inactive against HepG2, human gastric carcinoma SGC-7901, and NCI-H460 cells (IC$_{50}$ > 47.3 µM). Furthermore, two ceramides *viz.* (2S,3R,4E,8E)-2-(tetradecanoylamino)-4,8-octadecadien-l,3-diol and (2S,3R,20R,4E,8E)-2-(tetradecanoylamino)-4,8-octadecadien-l,3,20-triol derived from *Cryptosula pallasiana* did not display cytotoxicity against HL-60, Hep-G2, and SGC-7901 (IC$_{50}$ values from 21.13 to 58.15 µM) [80].

Sterols

Two oxygenated sterols, *viz.* 3β,24(S)-dihydroxycholesta-5,25-dien-7-one and 3β,25-dihydroxycholesta-5,23-dien-7-one, were isolated from cheilostome Bugula. neritina and these compounds have not been reported to display cytotoxicity towards three human cancer cell lines, namely, HepG2, HT-29, and NCI-H460. In these compounds, the IC$_{50}$ values ranged between 22.58 and 53.41 µg/mL). Further, this bryozoan species also yielded three new sterols (22E)-cholest-4,22-diene-3β,6β-diol, (23S,24R)-dimethylcholest-7-ene-3β, 5α,6β-triol) and (22E,24S)-24-methylcholest-4,22-diene-3β,6β-diol); a steroid glycoside, and six other sterols and these compounds were found to be inactive against human tumor cell lines Hep-G2, NCI-H460, and SGC-7901 (IC$_{50}$ > 36.6 µM). Thirteen sterols were isolated from the cheilostome *Cryptosula pallasiana*. Among these sterols, seven compounds *viz.* (23E)-25-methoxycholesta-5,23-dien-3β-ol, (22E)-7β-methoxy-cholesta-5,22-dien-3β-ol, 7β-methoxy-cholest-5-en-3β-ol, (23E)- 3β-hydroxy-27- norcholesta-5, 23-dien- 25-one, (23Z)- cholesta- 5,23 -diene- 3β,25-diol, (22E)- 3β- hydroxycholesta-5, 22 -dien-7-one, and (22E) -3β -hydroxy -2--norcholesta -5,22- dien-7 -one) did not display cytotoxic effects against human myeloid leukemia HL-60 cells and the IC$_{50}$ values reported in these experiments were found to range from 14.73 to 22.11 µg/mL). Furthermore, *Cryptosula pallasiana* collected from another region yielded a sterol, (23R)-methoxycholes--5,24-dien-3β-ol, together with three other sterols and all these compounds did not show cytotoxicity against human tumor cell lines HL-60, Hep-G2, and SGC-7901, and the IC$_{50}$ values in this regard ranged from 12.34 µM to 18.37 µM [80].

Other Anticancer and Cytotoxic Compounds

The bryoanthrathiophene, 5,7-dihydroxy-1-methyl-6-oxo-6H-anthra[1,9-bc] thiophene isolated from the bryozoan *Watersipora subtorquata* has been reported to serve as inhibitor of the proliferation of endothelial cells and was found to be the most active anticancer compound with an IC$_{50}$ value of 0.005 µM. Further, three aromatic compounds *viz.* p-methylsulfonylmethyl-phenol, p-hydroxyben-zaldehyde, and methylparaben, isolated from the bryozoan species *Cryptosula pallasiana*, were evaluated for cytotoxicity against HL-60 cells and p-methylsulfonylmethyl-phenol which appeared to be inactive [80].

Antiviral Activity

The pyridine paralleled indolizine alkaloid pterocellin A derived from *Pterocella vesiculosa* displayed strong antiviral activity. The macrocyclic lactone, bryostatin-1 derived from *Bugula neritina* displayed activity against Human Immunodeficiency Virus-1 (HIV-1) and it is suggested that this compound may be used for anti-retroviral treatment (HAART)-treated patients. Further, the bryostatin-1 analogues have been reported as potent protective agents against Chikungunya Virus (CHIKV) -mediated cell death. Furthermore, the alkaloid, amathaspiramide E has shown activity against polio virus type 1 at a concentration of 40 µg/well [80].

Antiparasitic Activity

Antiprotozoal (Antitrypanosomal) Activity

Trypanosomiasis which is caused by the protozoan parasite *Trypanosoma brucei* is mostly transmitted through the bite of infected tsetse flies and, if it is left untreated, this parasite is known to cause debilitating symptoms as it infects the central nervous system including confusion, sensory disturbances, personality changes, disturbance of the sleep cycle, and death [80]. Further, the β-phenylethylamine alkaloids, convolutamine I, J and H derived from *Amathia tortusa* displayed antitrypanosomal activity against the parasite *Trypanosoma brucei*. While the compounds, I and H recorded an IC_{50} value of 1.1 compound J had an IC_{50} value of 3.7 µM [81].

Anthelmintic (Nematocidal) Activity

The β-phenylethylamine alkaloid convolutamine H derived from *Amathia tortusa* exhibited anthelmintic activity against the potent nematocide parasite, *Haemonchus contortus* with an LD99 value of 0.2 µg/ml. It is worth-mentioning here that the commercial anthelmintic, levamisole as a reference compound showed an LD99 value of 1.6 µg/ml. Further, the disulfides, pentaporins A–C derived from the bryozoan *Pentapora fascialis* displayed anthelmintic activity against the nematode parasite, *Trichinella spiralis*, otherwise known as the pork worm [81]. The compounds, convolutamine H and convolutindole A derived from *Amathia convoluta* were found to be active against the free-living larval stages of the blood-feeding nematode *Haemonchus contortus*, which is known to cause excessive anemia, oedema, and sudden death especially in infected sheep and other ruminants [80].

Antimalarial (Anti-plasmodial) Activity

The brominated alkaloid compound *viz.* wilsoniamine A derived from *Amathia wilsoni* has shown anti-plasmodial activities. Further, the trihalogenated (heterocyclic) alkaloid, caulamidine A isolated from *Caulibugula intermis* has shown inhibitory effect against drug-resistant strains of *Plasmodium falciparum* with IC_{50} values ranging from 8.3 to 12.9 μM [80]. Further, its compounds caulamidine A and B showed antimalarial activity towards *Plasmodium falciparum* with IC_{50} values from 8.3 to 12.9 μM [79].

Antiangiogenic Activity

The sulfur-containing aromatic compound, bryoabthrathiophene (5,7-dihydroxy-1-methyl-6-oxo-6H-anthra[1,9-bc]thiophene) isolated from the bryozoan *Wateripora subtorquata* displayed potent antiangiogenic activity against basic fibroblast growth factor (bFGF) -induced proliferation of BAEC (Bovine aorta endothelial cell) with an IC_{50} value of 0.005 μM. It is also suggested that this compound may be useful for the development of novel antiangiogenic agent [80].

Topoisomerase Inhibitory Activity

The sphingolipids such as two sulfates of ceramides derived from the bryozoan *Watersipora cucullata* have been reported to demonstrate significant inhibition against human topoisomerase I (TRP1) with IC_{50} values of 0.4 and 0.2 μM, respectively. This topoisomerase enzyme has been reported be associated with essential genome functions, including DNA replication and transcription [80].

Metalloprotease Collagenase IV Inhibitory Activity

The tetracyclic terpenoid lactone, murrayanolide derived from the bryozoan *Dendrobeania murrayana* has been reported to show 54% inhibition against metalloprotease collagenase IV at a dose of 25 $\mu g/ml$. The type IV collagenase is often closely linked with malignant ascites and overexpression of this enzyme has been demonstrated in a variety of cancers [80].

Anti-Alzheimer's Activity

Alzheimer's disease (AD) is a multifactorial neurodegenerative disorder and the presently approved drugs may only ameliorate symptoms in a restricted number of patients for a restricted period of time. The macrolide lactone, bryostatin-1 derived from *Bugula neritina* has been reported to mediate the activation of protein kinase C (PKC) isozyme which possesses cognitive restorative and antidepressant effects. Bryostatin-1 represents a novel, potent and long-acting memory enhancer with future clinical applications in the treatment of AD patients. Further, the tribrominated indolic derivatives- *viz.* Kororamides A and B isolated from *Amathia tortuosa* have been reported as novel DYRK1A (dual specificity tyrosine phosphorylation-regulated kinase 1A) inhibitors for the treatment of Alzheimer's disease [80].

Antiparkinson Activity

The tribrominated indolic derivative, kororamide B isolated from *Amathia tortuosa* has been reported to display significant effects on early endosomes when profiled on human olfactory neurosphere-derived cells (hONS) from a Parkinson's disease patient [80].

Anti-Post-stroke Activity

THC ischemia and ischemic stroke are caused by the restriction of blood flow to the brain; these symptoms can cause death as well as life-changing physical and mental damage. The macrolide lactone, bryostatin-1 derived from *Bugula neritina* has shown anti- post-stroke activity. When administered within a time window of 24 hours post global cerebral ischemia/hypoxia, this compound has been reported to reduce neuronal and synaptic damage and help in the recovery of spatial learning and memory abilities through the activation of particular l protein kinase C (PKC) isozymes. Further, bryostatin-1 treatment was found to improve survival rate, inhibit lesion volume, salvage tissue in infarcted hemisphere by reducing necrosis and peri-infarct astrogliosis besides improving the functional outcome [80].

CONCLUSION

Although several pharmaceutical drug candidates have been discovered from the marine bryozoans, no new drugs from this source have been approved and marketed. The most promising compound *viz.* bryostatin 1 still finds it difficult to pass through the phase III clinical trial as an antitumor drug. Intensive investigations are the need of the hour to make use of this prominent invertebrate group pharmaceutically.

CHAPTER 7

Promising Pharmaceutical Compounds of Marine Worms: Their Chemistry and Therapeutic Applications

Abstract: This chapter deals with the promising bioactive compounds of marine worms such as nemertines, sipunculids, and annelids. Further, the chemical classes and the bioactivities of these secondary metabolites are dealtwith.

Keywords: Marine polychaete annelids, Nemertine worms, Peanut worm, Sipunculid worm, Spatial learning and memory, Wound healing.

INTRODUCTION

Recent investigations have demonstrated that the bioactive compounds of marine worms nemertines, sipunculids and polychaete annelids) such as peptides and polysaccharides have several health promoting functions, namely, anti-cancer, anti-inflammatory, anti-oxidant, anti-hypertensive, immunomodulatory, wound healing, and anti-hypoxia activities. While the bioactive potential of marine nemertines has been fairly studied, sipunculids and marine polychaete annelids are not at all explored for this aspect even though marine environment is rich in polychaete fauna compared to nemertines and sipunculids.

Marine Nemertine Worms

The phylum Nemertini (Nemertina, Rhyncocoeles or Nemertea) includes "ribbon worms" which are found closely related to flatworms comprising about 1300 species. While most species are found in marine environments, 22 species have been reported to occur in freshwater. These ribbon worms are poorly known to the general public and only little information is available on the biology and ecology of this group. Recent research conducted on these worms has reported that certain nemertean species are known to possess potent toxins including pyridine alkaloids, tetrodotoxin, and cytolytic or neurotoxic peptides. A few of these compounds have been found to be pharmacologically important and are of potential medicinal use or for application in biotechnology.

Santhanam Ramesh, Ramasamy Santhanam & Veintramuthu Sankar

Pharmaceutically Important Species of Marine Nemertine Worms: *Amphiporus lactifloreus* and *Notospermus geniculatus*

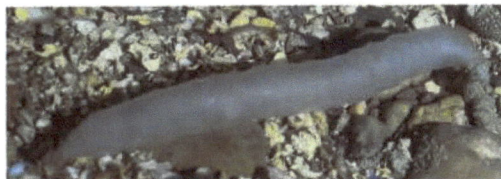

Fig. (1). *Amphiporus lactifloreus*. Image credit: Wikipedia.

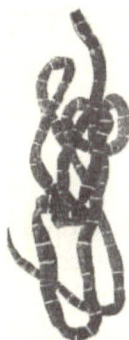

Fig. (2). *Notospermus geniculatus*. Image credit: Wikipedia.

Bioactivities of Marine Nemertine Worms

Amphiporus lactifloreus

Anti-Alzheimer's Activity

The toxin of this species *viz.* GTS21 (DMXB), 3- (2, 4- dimethoxy benzylidene)-anabaseine, has been reported to be a selective α7 nAChR partial agonist. This compound showed improvement in learning performance and memory retention in passive avoidance models in nucleus basalis magnocellularis (NbM)-lesioned rats. It has also been found to reduce neo- cortical cell loss in NbM lesioned rats and cell death induced by β-amyloid or glutamate in cultures of neuronal cells. This compound is currently in clinical trials for possible treatment of Alzheimer's dementia [82].

Notospermus geniculatus

Bioactivities

The toxins Q7T3S7, P0C929 and Q38L02 of this nemertine species inhibited platelet aggregation. Further, its toxins P0DN10 and C1 IC_{50} served as serine protease inhibitors which possess therapeutic benefits in treating cancer, blood coagulation disorders and viral infections [83].

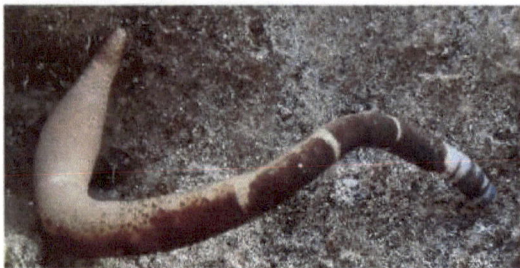

Fig. (3). *Phascolosoma sp.*. Image credit: Wikimedia commons.

Sipunculids

Sipunculid or peanut worm is a member of the invertebrate phylum Sipuncula, a group of unsegmented worms. Its common name is due to its general shape of shelled peanut. There are about 320 described species of sipunculids which are all marine and mostly from shallow waters. These worms have been reported to be a good source of several bioactive compounds which are of great use in food and pharmaceutical industries. For instance, the peptides and polysaccharides derived from these worms have been reported to possess anti-cancer, anti-hypertensive, anti-oxidant, immunomodulatory, anti-inflammatory, anti-hypoxia and wound healing activities by modulating various molecular mechanisms. However, studies of these compounds in humans have not been performed considerably. Therefore, it is important to undertake active research on this aspect.

Pharmaceutically Important Species of Sipunculids: *Phascolosoma esculenta, Phascolosoma* **sp. and** *Sipunculus (Sipunculus) nudus*

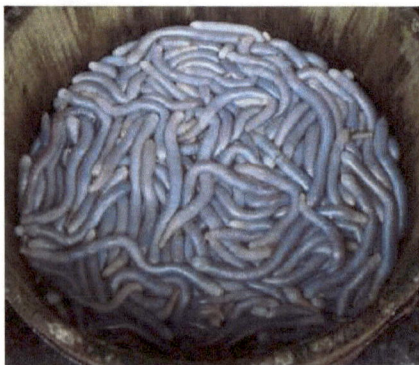

Fig. (4). *Sipunculus (Sipunculus) nudus (Mass)*. Image credit: Wikimedia commons.

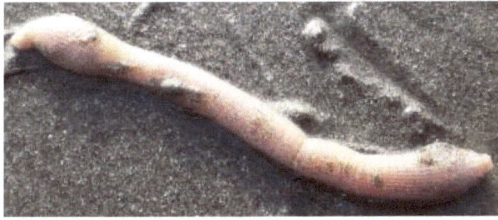

Fig. (5). *Sipunculus (Sipunculus) nudus.* Image credit: Wikimedia commons.

Bioactivities of Promising Polysaccharides and Peptides of Peanut Worms, *Phascolosoma esculenta* and *Sipunculus nudus*

Anti-cancer Activity of Polysaccharides

Sipunculus nudus

At concentrations of 0.13, 0.25, 0.5, and 1 mg/mL, the unidentified polysaccharides of this species exhibited anti-cancer activities by preventing the DNA synthesis of Hepg2.2.15 cells; increasing the expression of pro-apoptosis proteins, TNF-α, caspase-3, and Bax; and decreasing the expression of the anti-apoptosis proteins survivin, Bcl-2, and VEGF. Further, its polysaccharides displayed anti-tumor activity at concentrations of 50,100, and 200 mg/kg in hepatoma HepG2-bearing mice by inhibiting the growth of HepG2 cells through an increase of ATF4, DDIT3, and IkBα expression and a decrease of CYR61, HSP90, and VEGF expression.

Anti-oxidant Activity of Polysaccharides

Phascolosoma esculenta

At the concentrations of 1, 10 and 5 mg/mL, the unidentified oligosaccharides of this species displayed antioxidant activity by increasing the enzyme activities of GSH-Px and SOD and by regulating Nrf2 mRNA expression in sepsis mice model. Further, at concentrations of 0.2, 0.4 and 0.8 g/kg, the polysaccharides of this species displayed antioxidant activities in mice by increasing the superoxide dismutase and glutathione peroxidase activities in serum and liver. In another experiment, at concentrations of 1,5,10,15,20, and 25 mg/mL, the polysaccharide of this species displayed DPPH and hydroxyl radical scavenging and reducing power with IC_{50} of 0.57 and 0.61, 2.98 mg/mL, respectively.

Sipunculus nudus

At the concentrations of 0.25, 0.5, 1.0, 2.0, 5.0,10.0, and 20.0 mg/mL, the unidentified polysaccharide of this species displayed significant scavenging activity on hydroxyl radical in a dose-dependent manner. Further, the free radical scavenging rates increased significantly with the increase of concentration of polysaccharides. For example, at the concentration of 0.20 mg/mL, the scavenging activities of hydroxyl radical and DPPH radical were found to be-12.6%.

Anti-inflammatory Activity of Polysaccharides

Phascolosoma esculenta

At the concentrations of 1, 10 and 5 mg/mL, the unidentified oligosaccharides of this species displayed anti-inflammatory activity by considerably reducing the secretion of IL-1β and TNF-α and increasing the IL-10 in sepsis mice.

Sipunculus nudus

At the concentration of 50, 100 and 200 mg/k, the water extract from the body wall of this species containing unidentified polysaccharides displayed dose-dependent anti-inflammatory activity in the carrageenan-induced paw oedema, dextran-induced rat paw oedema, cotton pellet granuloma, carrageenan-induced peritonitis, xylene-induced ear oedema, and acetic acid-induced vascular permeability models in mouse and rat.

Anti-hypoxia Activity of Polysaccharides

Sipunculus nudus

At the concentration of 10, 30, 100 mg/kg, the extracted unidentified polysaccharide of this species displayed significant anti-hypoxic activity on normobaric hypoxia, chemical intoxicant hypoxia and acute cerebral ischemia hypoxia models in mice.

Immunomodulatory Activity of Polysaccharides

Phascolosoma esculenta

At the concentration of 3.0, 6.0, 9.0 mg/kg, the unidentified polysaccharides of this species displayed immunosuppressive activity by significantly enhancing the liver, spleen and thymus index of mice and Con A-stimulated mouse spleen cells.

Sipunculus nudus

At the concentration of 5–80 μg/mL, the water soluble and unidentified polysaccharide extracted from tis species displayed immune-stimulating activity by activating mice and human macrophages through the upregulation of expression of cytokines, IL-6 and TNF-α, and inducing the expression of iNOS and COX-2. It has also been reported that the polysaccharides from this species promoted cellular immunity and humoral immunity by enhancing the phagocytosis function and NK cell activity in mice. Further, at concentrations of 50,100, and 200 mg/kg, the polysaccharide extract from this species increased the immune response by increasing the thymus and spleen indexes and upregulating the IL-2, IFN-γ, and TNF-α cytokines in the serum of mice. Furthermore, at the concentration of 50,100, and 200 mg/kg, its polysaccharide increased the index of immune organs and enhanced the secretion of cytokines IL-2, IFN-γ and TNF- α.

Anti-oxidant Activity of Peptides

Phascolosoma esculenta

At the concentrations of 50, 100 and 150 mg/kg, the unidentified peptides of this species have been reported to dose-dependently improve oxidative stress status (GSH-Px, SOD, TAC and MDA) in mice. Similarly, its collagen peptides showed in-vitro total anti-oxidant capacity with a value of 3.8 U/mg.

Sipunculus nudus

The unidentified polypeptide of this species showed significant *in-vitro* hydroxyl radical scavenging activity with 95.42% inhibition.

Anti-inflammatory Activity of Peptides

Sipunculus nudus

At the concentrations of 30, 60, 120 mm, the unidentified peptides (LSPLLAAH and TVNLAYY) of this species displayed anti-inflammatory activity **by** inhibiting NO production and decreasing the expression of pro-inflammatory iNOS, IL-6, TNF-α, and COX-2, in LPS-stimulated RAW264.7 macrophages. Further, at a concentration of 2 g/mL, the peptides of this species displayed anti-inflammatory activity by reducing mRNA levels of TGF-β1, TNF-α, and IL-1β in the wound of mice skin.

ACE-inhibitory/Anti-hypertensive Activity of Peptides

Phascolosoma esculenta

The unidentified peptide of this species has been reported to inhibit ACE (IC_{50} value of 135 M) through competitive inhibition and display anti- hypertensive effects in experimental rats by significantly reducing the systolic blood pressure by about 30 mmHg. The unidentified peptides of this species also significantly reduced both diastolic blood pressure (DBP) and systolic blood pressure (SBP) and inhibited ACE *in vitro* in spontaneously hypertensive rats. The IC_{50} values recorded in this case were 0.67 and 0.24 mg/mL. In an another experiment, the peptides of this species displayed ACE inhibitory activity with IC_{50} values ranging from 3.4 to 4.2 U/mL. Further, its three peptides *viz.* RYDF, YASGR and GNGSGYVS have also been reported to inhibit ACE (IC_{50} values of 235, 184 and 29 µM, respectively) and reduce systolic blood pressure 31 mmHg at 2 h after oral administration in spontaneously hypertensive rats.

Sipunculus nudus

The peptides IND, VEPG, and LADEF displayed ACE inhibition activity with IC_{50} values of 34.72, 20.55, and 22.77 µmol/L, respectively.

Effects of Peptides on Wound Healing and Spatial Learning and Memory

Phascolosoma esculenta

At concentrations of 100 mg/kg, the unidentified peptides of this species have been reported to improve the spatial learning and memory ability significantly through the up-regulation of NR2A, NR2B, BDNF and CREB mRNA expressions in the hippocampus of mice.

Sipunculus nudus

At a concentration of 2 g/mL for 28 days and 500 µg/mL for 12, 24, 30, 36 h, the unidentified collagen peptides derived from this species displayed *a* significant capacity to induce human umbilical vein endothelial cells (HUVEC), human immortalized keratinocytes (HaCaT) and human skin fibroblasts (HSF) cells proliferation and migration *in vitro*. Further, these peptides amazingly improved the healing rate and inhibited scar formation in mice through the mechanisms of reducing inflammation, enhancing collagen deposition, and recombination and blockade of the TGF-β/Smads signal pathway.

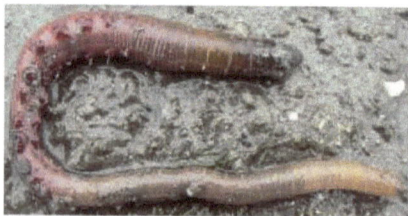

Fig. (6). *Arenicola marina.* Image credit: iNaturalist and Wikipedia.

Marine Annelids

The marine polychaete annelids are much less studied group as far as the bioactive compounds are concerned. Very recently two species have been reported with their bioactive compounds of therapeutic and biotechnological importance.

Pharmaceutically Important Species of Marine Annelids: *Arenicola marina* and *Hermodice carunculata*

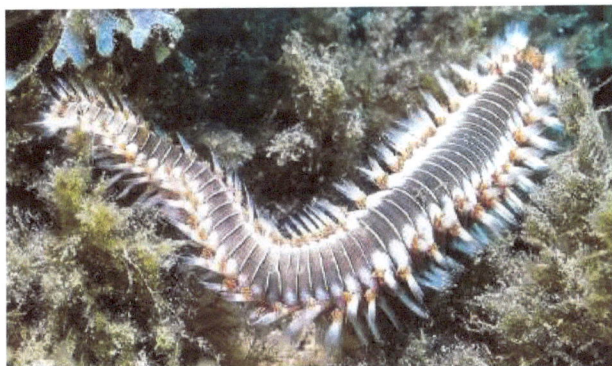

Fig. (7). *Hermodice carunculata.* Image credit: Wikipedia.

Bioactive Compounds of Marine Annelids

Arenicola marina

The identified bioactive compounds isolated from this species may be of great use in treating a variety of pathophysiological disorders including arthritis, osteoporosis, and bone cancer, among others [12].

Hermodice carunculata

This species has been reported to yield Eight betaine-derived unprecedented, quaternary ammonium compounds, named "carunculines" which are believed to possess biotechnological implications [85].

CONCLUSION

Among the marine invertebrates, the marine worms are not at all explored for their bioactive potential. This calls for intensive investigations on this aspect so as to discover their promising secondary metabolites and their molecular mechanisms of action.

CHAPTER 8

Promising Pharmaceutical Compounds of Marine Shellfish: Their Chemistry and Therapeutic Applications

Abstract: This chapter deals with the promising bioactive compounds of marine shellfish *viz.* crustaceans, molluscs, and echinoderms. Among the marine crustaceans, the extracts of shrimps and crabs containing astaxanthin showed major bioactivities. On the other hand, among molluscs, gastropods possessed the maximum number of secondary metabolites and associated bioactivities compared to the bivalves and cephalopods. Further, among echinoderms, the asteroids and holothurians showed maximum number of secondary metabolites compared to their counterparts *viz.* echinoids and crinoids.

Keywords: Bioactivities, Cephalopod ink, Echinoderms, Marine crustaceans, Marine molluscs, Secondary metabolites.

INTRODUCTION

The Marine crustaceans such as shrimps and crabs; marine molluscs and echinoderms are known for their biodiversity as they possess a considerable number of species. While the crustaceans are largely exploited as fisheries resources for edible purposes, the molluscs and echinoderms are only important biologically. In recent years, considerable research has been made on the potential bioactive compounds of gastropod molluscs and echinoderms. Among echinoderms, the sea cucumbers possess novel compounds with several bioactivities.

Marine Crustaceans

Marine crustaceans such as shrimps, prawns, lobsters and crabs are considered a healthy diet choice as they are a good source of various nutrients such as proteins, chitin, chitosan, lipids, carotenoids (pigments), and minerals. About 15 million tons of these organisms are captured annually around the world and Asian countries rank first in this regard. The structurally diverse bioactive nitrogenous components (10–23% (w/w)) of these organisms serve not only as functional food ingredients but they also possess several bioactivities including anti-cancer, anti-diabetic, antihypertensive, antioxidant, anti-microbial, anti-coagulant, immunostimulatory, calcium-binding, hypocholesterolemic and appetite suppression [86]. Among the compounds of these crustaceans, the carotenoid astaxanthin is of great interest to researchers and to the food, feed, pharmaceutical, and nutraceutical industries. Its potent antioxidant properties have been considered to be stronger than vitamin E, vitamin C, and β-carotene [87]. Further, its bioactivity has been found to be associated with beneficial health effects for humans, namely its anti-cardiovascular, anti-inflammatory, and antiaging potentials as well as other favorable cosmetic benefits, such as improvement of skin moisture and elasticity. In 2020, the global astaxanthin market size was estimated at USD 1371 million, and it is expected to grow. Although the production of astaxanthin by chemical synthesis is less expensive (about $1000 per kilo); this process does not yield a pure compound and the combination of different isoforms are believed to be 20 times lower antioxidant capacity than their natural counterpart. Further, this synthesized compound has not been approved for human consumption. Therefore, the demand for the naturally extracted astaxanthin products is expected to rise. At the industrial level, astaxanthin is presently extracted from krill and crustacean byproducts. As there is a continuous demand for natural astaxanthin, marine crustaceans and their byproducts present a great opportunity for the whole sector.

Pharmaceutically Important Shrimps, Prawns and Crabs

Shrimps and Prawns

Aristaeomorpha foliacea, Metapenaeus sp., *Mierspenaeopsis hardwickii (= Parapenaeopsis hardwickii), Mierspenaeopsis sculptilis (= Parapenaeopsis sculptilis), Pandalus borealis, Parapenaeus longirostris, Penaeus chinensis (= Fenneropenaeus chinensis), Penaeus japonicus, Penaeus merguiensis, Penaeus monodon, Penaeus subtilis (= Farfantepenaeus subtilis)* and *Penaeus vannamei (= Litopenaeus vannamei)* (Figs. **1-12**).

Crabs

Callinectes sapidus, Cancer pagurus., Portunus segnis, and *Scylla serrata* (Figs. **13-16**).

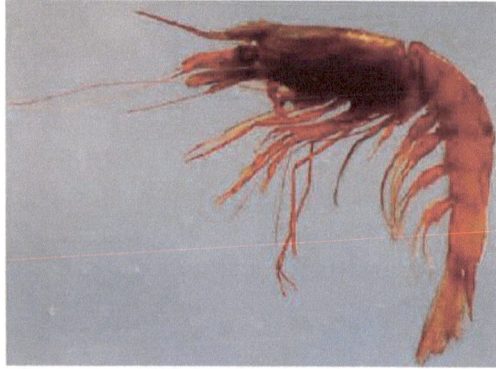

Fig. (1). *Aristaeomorpha foliacea.*

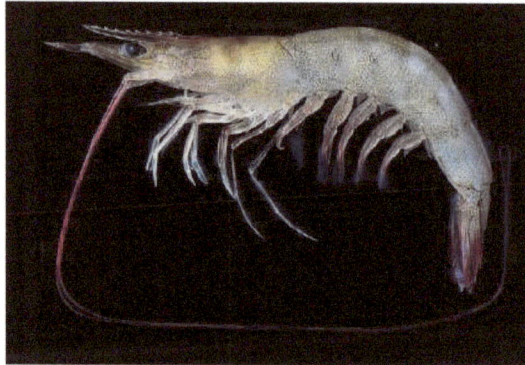

Fig. (2). *Metapenaeus* sp.

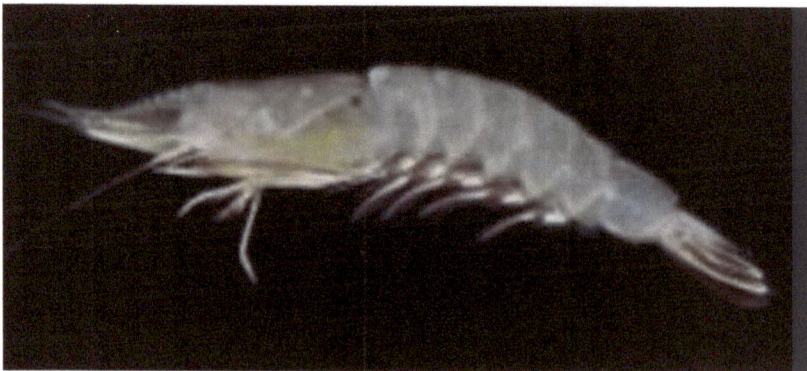

Fig. (3). *Mierspenaeopsis hardwickii.*

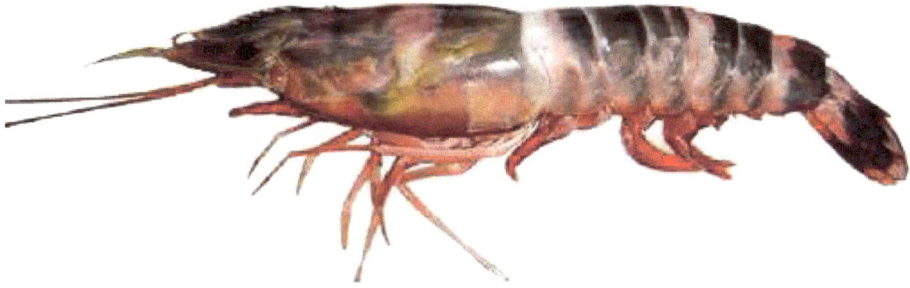

Fig. (4). *Mierspenaeopsis sculptilis.*

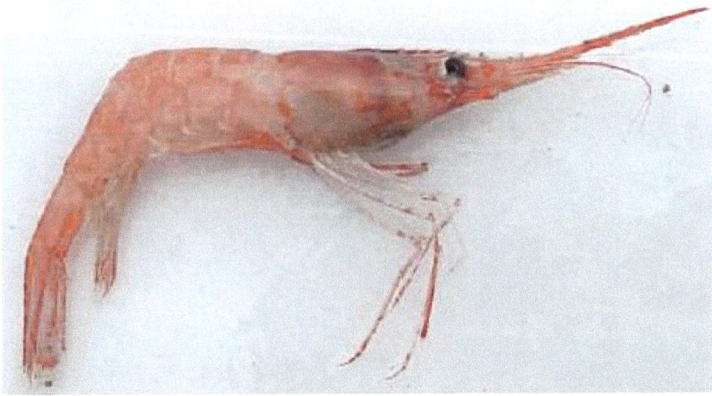

Fig. (5). *Pandalus borealis.*

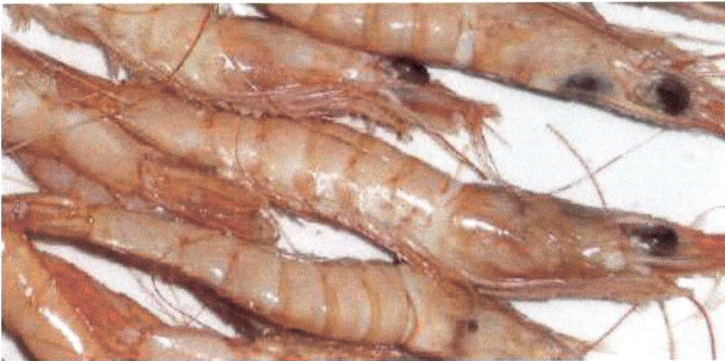

Fig. (6). *Parapenaeus longirostris.*

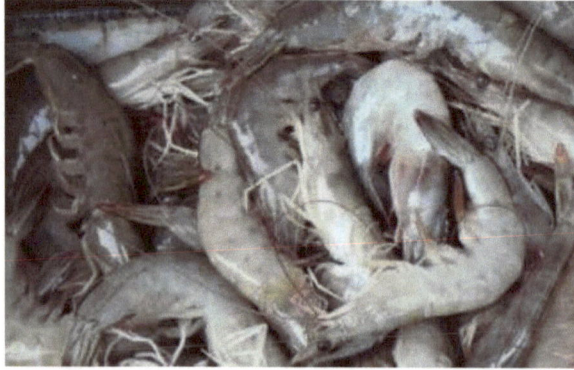

Fig. (7). *Penaeus chinensis.*

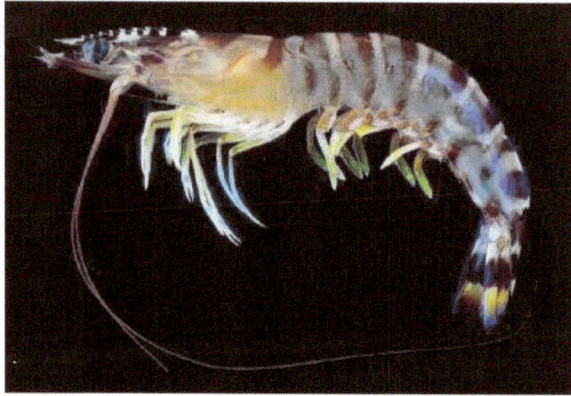

Fig. (8). *Penaeus japonicus.*

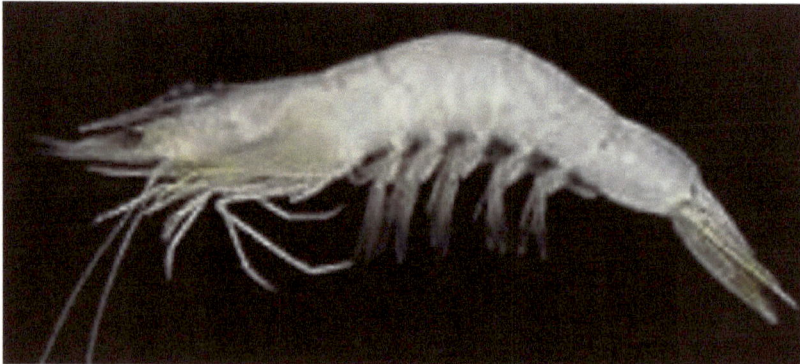

Fig. (9). *Penaeus merguiensis.*

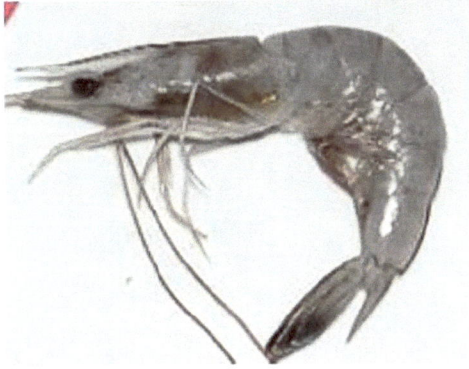

Fig. (10). *Penaeus monodon.*

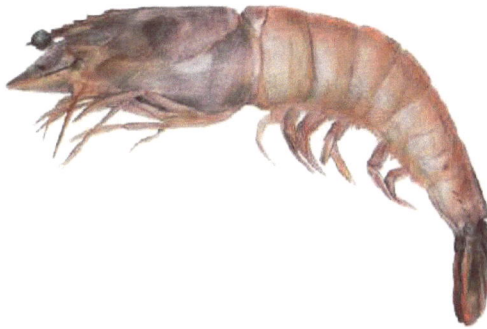

Fig. (11). *.Penaeus subtilis.*

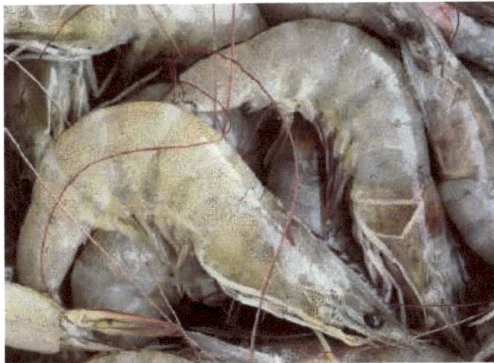

Fig. (12). *Penaeus vannamei.*

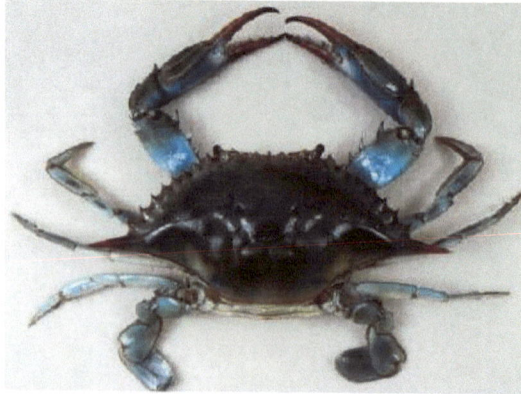

Fig. (13). *Callinectes sapidus.*

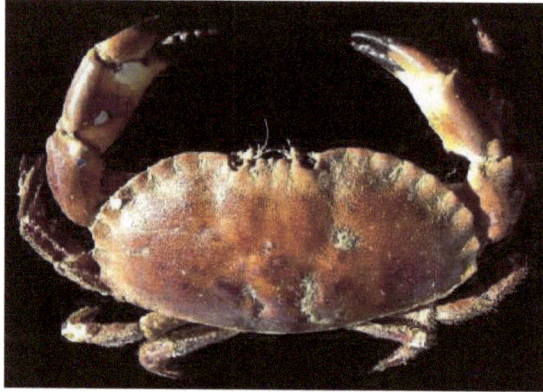

Fig. (14). *Cancer pagurus.*

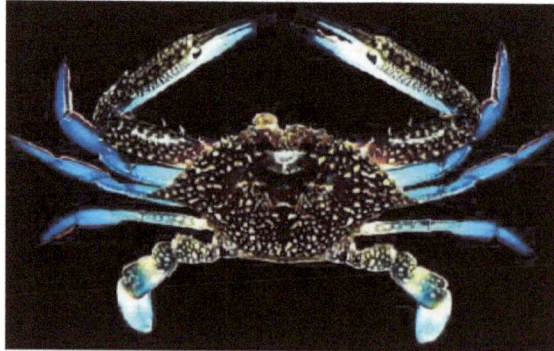

Fig. (15). *Portunus segnis.*

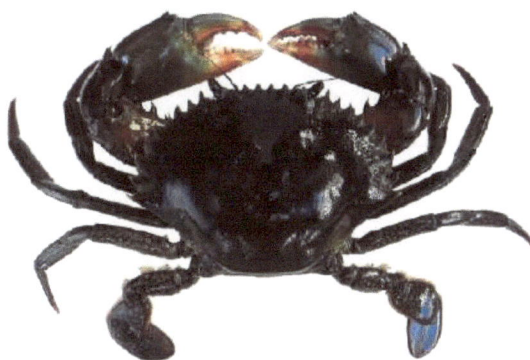

Fig. (16). *Scylla serrata.*

Image credit: *Aristaeomorpha foliacea:* Wikipedia; *Metapenaeus lysianassa:* Wikispecies; *Mierspenaeopsis sculptilis, Pandalus borealis, Parapenaeus longirostris*: Wikipedia; *Penaeus japonicus*: Wikimedia commons; *Penaeus monodon, Penaeus subtilis*: Wikipedia; *Callinectes sapidus, Cancer pagurus*: Wikipedia; *Scylla serrata*: Wiktionary.

Major Bioactive Compound of Marine Crustaceans

In the therapeutically important marine crustaceans, a reddish pigment *viz.* xanthophyll carotenoid astaxanthin (Fig. **17**) is invariably present in all the species of shrimps, prawns and crabs. This pigment has been reported to possess antioxidant, anti-inflammatory, and antineoplastic (cancer-treating) properties. Further, according to some research reports, this carotenoid belongs to a group of medicines called "antioxidants" which is mainly used to treat Alzheimer's, Parkinson's diseases, stroke, high cholesterol levels, liver diseases, age-related macular degeneration (vision loss) and prevent cancer. Further, it is also used to improve exercise performance and treat metabolic syndrome that leads to various conditions like heart disease, stroke, and diabetes [88].

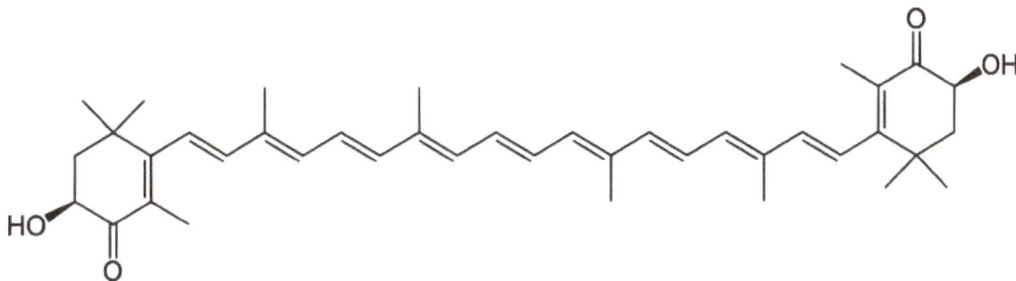

Fig. (17). Astaxanthin.

Bioactivities of Marine Crustaceans

Simat *et al.* [87] reported on the various bioactivities of astaxanthin of marine crustaceans as detailed below.

Anticancer, Antiproliferative and Cytotoxic Activity

i) Intragastrically administered astaxanthin in mice with PC-3 xenograft prostate tumor inhibited the tumor growth significantly.

ii) Astaxanthin has been reported to suppress the occurrence of N-nitrosomethylbenzylamine-induced esophageal cancer in experimental rats through the increase of antioxidant and anti-inflammation capacity.

iii) Astaxanthin-alpha tocopherol nanoemulsions displayed significant wound healing activity through scratch assay on CT26, HeLa, and T24 cell lines.

iv) Astaxanthin-alpha tocopherol nanoemulsions also exhibited cytotoxicity in cancer cell lines *viz.* CT26, HeLa, Panc1, and T24 along with significant decrease in *via*bility after 1 and 2 days of exposure.

v) In diethylnitrosamine-treated mice, astaxanthin displayed significant inhibition of the development of liver cell adenoma and hepatocellular carcinoma by reducing serum adiponectin level and improving oxidative stress.

vi) The effect of astaxanthin was tested on the subchronic testis injury induced by SnS2 nanoflowers in mice. The treatment has been reported to reduce testicular ultrastructure alterations and histopathological injury; and alleviate testicular inflammation, apoptosis, necroptosis, and oxidative stress.

vii) Gold nanoparticles synthesized using astaxanthin showed dose-dependent toxicity and antiproliferative effect against MDA-MB-231 (human breast cancer cells). Microencapsulated astaxanthin displayed significant cytostatic activity on adipose-derived stem cells by inhibiting lipid peroxidation.

viii) Oral treatment of astaxanthin nanoemulsion in mice with lung metastatic melanoma yielded a chemotherapy effect which is by triggering apoptosis.

Anti-inflammatory Activities

i) Astaxanthin of marine crustaceans has been found to be effective in a number of diseases (such as diabetes mellitus, Alzheimer's and Parkinson's diseases, neuropathic pain, kidney-related diseases, hepatitis, dry eye disease, atopic dermatitis, and inflammatory bowel disease) by suppressing proinflammatory cytokines and inflammatory mediator production in rats with monosodium urate crystal-induced arthritis.

ii) In rats with epilepticus-induced hippocampal injury, the astaxanthin has been reported to reduce the injury and improve cognitive dysfunction.

iii) In mice with ovalbumin-induced asthma, orally administered astaxanthin showed significant anti-inflammatory effect.

Antioxidant Activity

i) Astaxanthin derived from crabs has been reported to possess significant scavenging activity against hydrogen peroxide and 2,2-diphenyl-1-picryl hydrazyl (DPPH) radicals.

ii) The water-dispersible, astaxanthin-rich nanopowder of marine crustaceans has been reported to possess *in vivo* antioxidant efficiency on the alcohol-induced oxidative damage in mice.

iii) Astaxanthin biopolymer nanoparticles have shown improved antioxidant properties *in vitro* scavenging activity against 2, 2' -azino- bis(3-ethyl benzo thiazo line- 6-sulfo nic acid) (ABTS).

iv) Encapsulated astaxanthin in ethyl cellulose derived from applied supercritical emulsions extraction technology displayed good antioxidant activity

v) Astaxanthin in the form of nanohydrogels has shown profound effects in the neutralization of ROS *in vitro*.

Antidiabetic Activity

i) Treated rats with astaxanthin has shown significant reduction of total cholesterol and blood glucose levels and increase of high-density lipoprotein cholesterol levels.

ii) Oral administration of astaxanthin in rat pups has been reported to reduce lung damage with bronchopulmonary dysplasia induced by hyperoxia and lipopolysaccharide.

Hepatoprotective Activity

i) Astaxanthin-rich nanopowder produced by nanoencapsulation and freeze-drying technology displayed *in vivo* antioxidant effect on the alcohol-induced oxidative damage in mice, thereby hepatic injury was made less severe.

ii) Astaxanthin-loaded liposomes have shown therapeutic and reparative effects on experimental mice affected by alcoholic liver fibrosis.

iii) Astaxanthin encapsulated within liposomes yielded a significant reduction of lipopolysaccharide-induced acute hepatotoxicity in rats.

iv) Astaxanthin pretreatment in mice has been reported to reduce the effect of acetaminophen-induced liver injury through reduction of ROS generation, inhibition of oxidative stress, and reduction of apoptosis.

v) In rats affected by acute pancreatitis, astaxanthin treatment showed protection from pancreatic damage and a decrease in oxidative stress in rats with acute pancreatitis.

Anti-aging Activity

i) Astaxanthin treatment has shown protective effects on age-related skin deterioration and environmentally induced damages.

ii) In mice with phthalic anhydride-induced atopic dermatitis, liposomal astaxanthin treatment has shown antidermatotic effects.

Eye Health and Vision

i) Astaxanthin treatment has displayed protective effects against dry eye disease *in vitro* on human corneal epithelial cells cultures.

Marine Molluscs

The phylum Mollusca with its enormous diversity of species (about 80,000) constitutes about 7% of living animals on Earth and is distributed from tropical seas and temperate waters to polar regions [11]. Several species of marine gastropods and bivalves have been reported to yield a diversity of chemical classes and several drug leads currently in clinical trials. Cephalopods, which is a small and exclusively marine group of highly advanced and organized molluscs include octopus, squid, cuttlefish and nautilus. Among these animals, the octopus and squid possess human health benefits. The cephalopod ink which is a mixture of the co-secretions from the ink sac and funnel organ has several applications in the food industry. Processed ink is utilized as a food coloring and due to its antimicrobial properties, cuttlefish ink is also used to cure and, thus, extend the shelf life of cuttlefish meat. Many health benefits have been attributed to the cephalopod ink as a traditional medicine, both in Western culture (ancient Greece and Rome) and Eastern culture (China). More recently, this ink has been used in an attempt to develop new drugs. Further, the cephalopod ink is also being used in the development of eye cosmetic products such as mascara and eyeshadow [89, 90]. However, a tiny proportion (<1%) of molluscan species has been studied for its secondary metabolites. In the last decade, the number of new bioactive compounds from these marine molluscs substantially increased, and 255 new compounds have been reported between 2010 and 2019. Of these compounds, only 26% of these compounds %) were found to be bioactive. Among these bioactive compounds, cytotoxic and anti-proliferative compounds account for 36% and 12%, respectively. Further, the conotoxin of marine molluscs with inhibitory activity on voltage gated ion channels accounted for 22% [11]. Furthermore, among the reported bioactive compounds in the selected period, the peptides, terpenes, polyketides and sterols accounted for 31, 24, 15 and 8%, respectively; and polyphenols and other compounds combined accounted for 22% of the compounds [11].

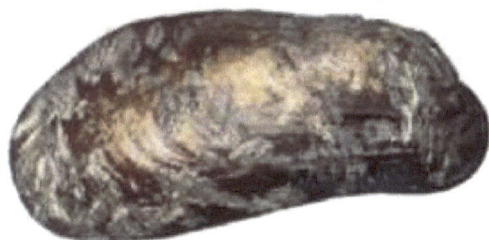

Fig. (18). *Bathymodiolus thermophilus.*

Pharmaceutically Important Marine Bivalves

Bathymodiolus thermophilus, Mactromeris polynyma (= Spisula polynyma), Mytilus edulis, Perna viridis, Protapes gallus (= Paphia malabarica), and *Villorita cyprinoides* (Figs. **18-23**).

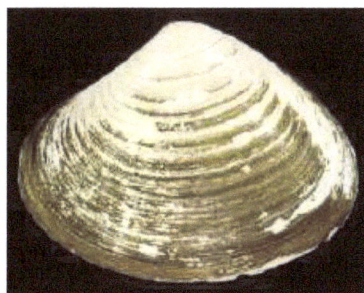

Fig. (19). *Mactromeris polynyma.*

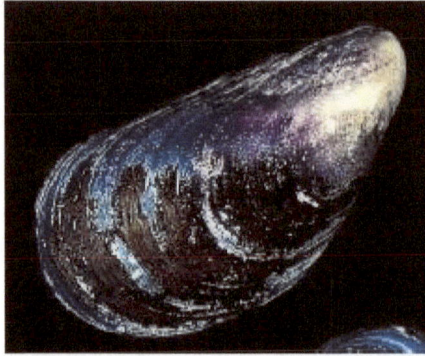

Fig. (20). *Mytilus edulis.*

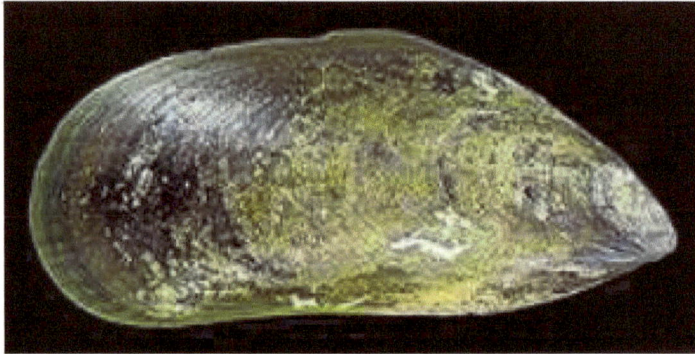

Fig. (21). *Perna viridis.*

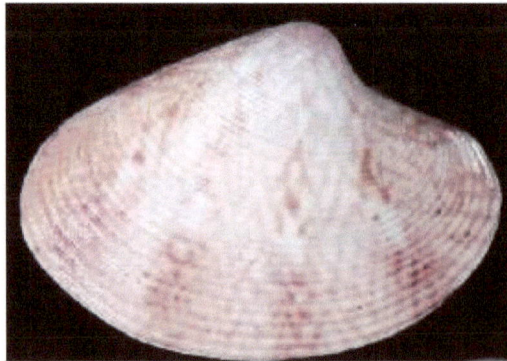

Fig. (22). *Protapes gallus.*

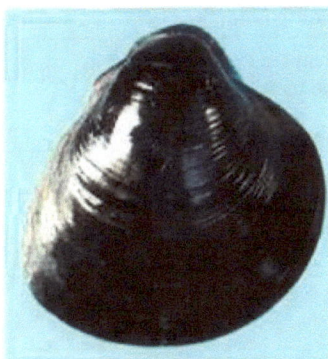

Fig. (23). *Villorita cyprinoides.*

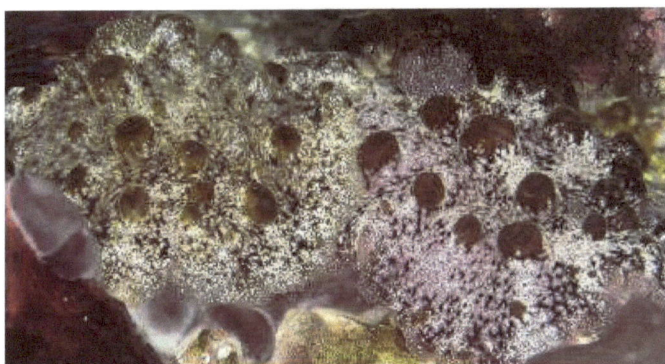

Fig. (24). *Actinocyclus papillatus.*

Therapeutic Activities in Marine Bivalves

The secondary metabolites and associated bioactivities are given in Table **1**.

Table 1. The bioactive compounds and associated therapeutic activities in marine bivalves.

Species	Compound(s)	Chemistry	Activity	Refs.
Bathymodiolus thermophilus	Bathymodiolamide A	Sphingolipid	Antiproliferative	[11]
Mytilus edulis	Azaspiracid 7-10	Polyketides	Cytotoxic	[11]
Paphia malabarica	18 (4 → 14), 19 (4 → 8)-bis-abeo C19 norditerpenoid	Terpenoid	Cytotoxic	[11]
-do-	Aryl polyketide	Polyketide	Anti-inflammatory	[91]
Perna viridis	Brassicasterol; 24-Methylenecholesterol	Sterols	-do-	[91]
Spisula polynyma	Spisulosine ES-285	Alkyl amino alcohol	Anticancer	[91]

(Table 1) cont.....

Species	Compound(s)	Chemistry	Activity	Refs.
Villorita cyprinoides	Isochromenyl meroterpenoids; furano meroterpenoid	Terpenoids	-do-	[11]
-do-	Several sterols	-	Anti-inflammatory	[91]

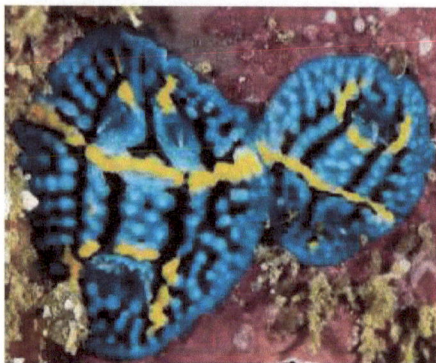

Fig. (25). *Aldisa andersoni.*

Pharmaceutically Important Marine Gastropods

Actinocyclus papillatus, Aldisa andersoni, Aplysia dactylomela, Aplysia kurodai, Aplysia oculifer, Cellana grata, Cellana toreuma, Dicathais orbita, Dolabrifera dolabrifera, Dollabellaaa uricularia, Doris kerguelenensis (= Austrodoris kerguelenensis), Drupella margariticola (= Drupa margariticola), Elysia ornaae, Elysia rufescens, Goniobranchus splendidus, Haliotis tuberculata coccinea, Haliotis tuberculata, Hexabranchus sanguineus, Monodonta labio, Onchidium sp., *Phyllidia coelestis, Phyllidia ocellata, Phyllidiella pustulosa, Pleurobranchus forskalii, Stylocheilus longicauda, Tambja ceutae, Trochus tentorium, Turbo stenogyrus* (Figs. **24-51**).

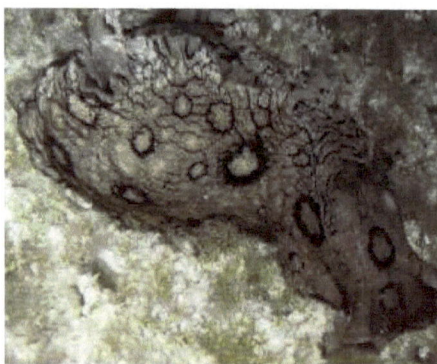

Fig. (26). *Aplysia dactylomela.*

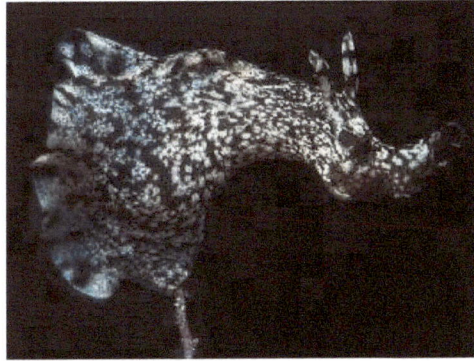

Fig. (27). *Aplysia kurodai.*

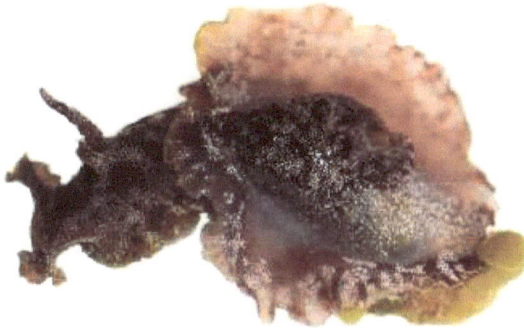

Fig. (28). *Aplysia oculifer.*

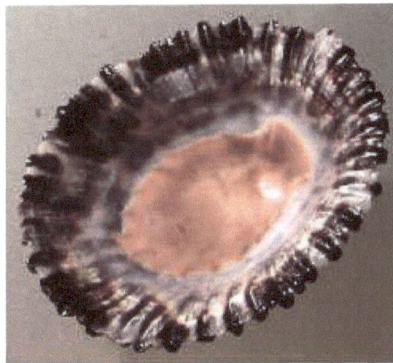

Fig. (29). *Cellana grata.*

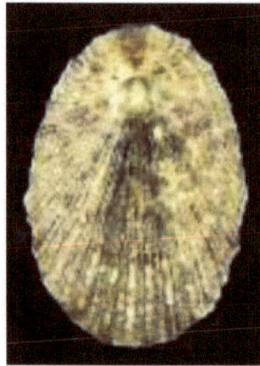

Fig. (30). *Cellana toreuma.*

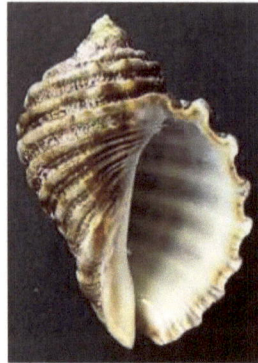

Fig. (31). *Dicathais orbita.*

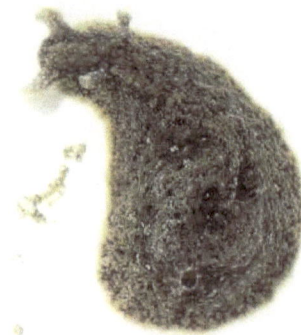

Fig. (32). *Dolabrifera dolabrifera.*

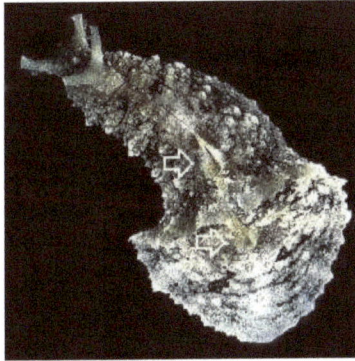

Fig. (33). *Dollabellaaa uricularia.*

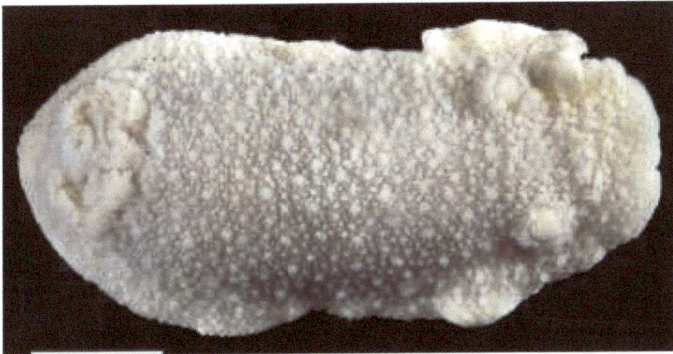

Fig. (34). *Doris kerguelenensis.*

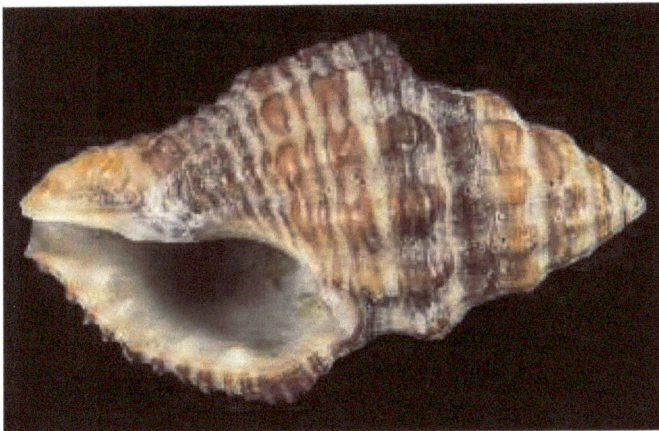

Fig. (35). *Drupella margariticola.*

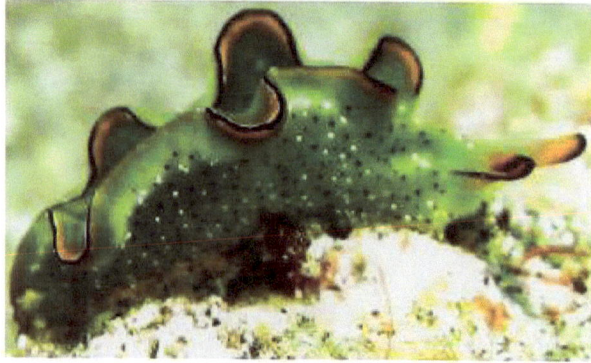

Fig. (36). *Elysia ornata.*

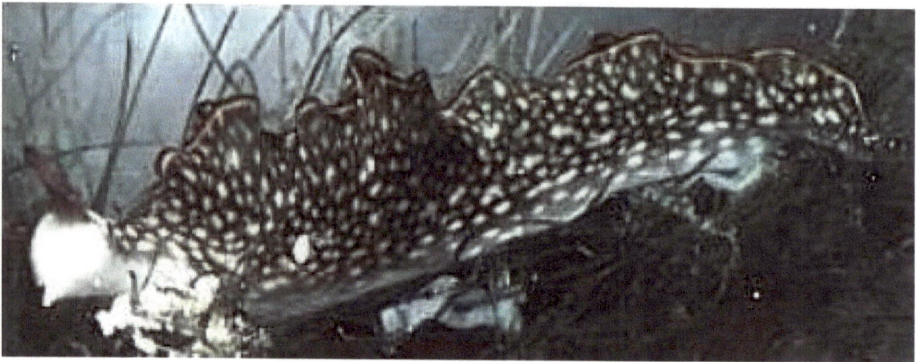

Fig. (37). *Elysia rufescens.*

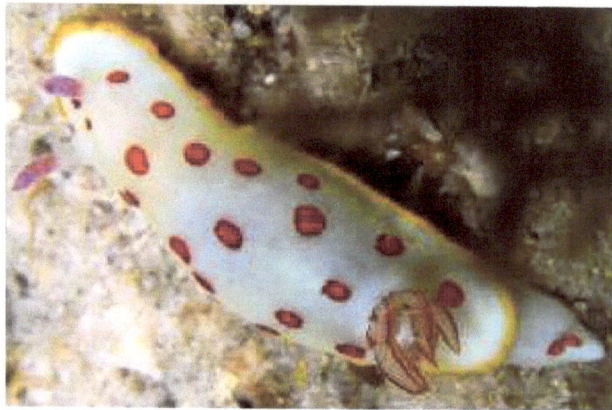

Fig. (38). *Goniobranchus splendidus.*

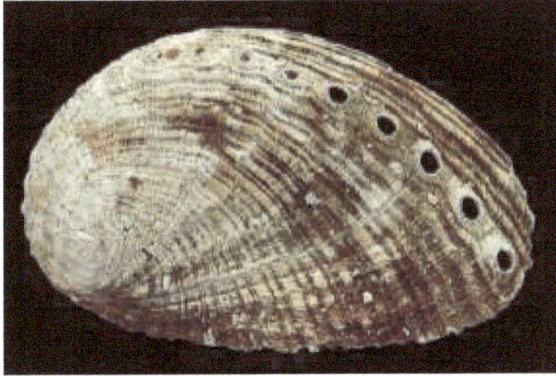

Fig. (39). *Haliotis tuberculata coccinea.*

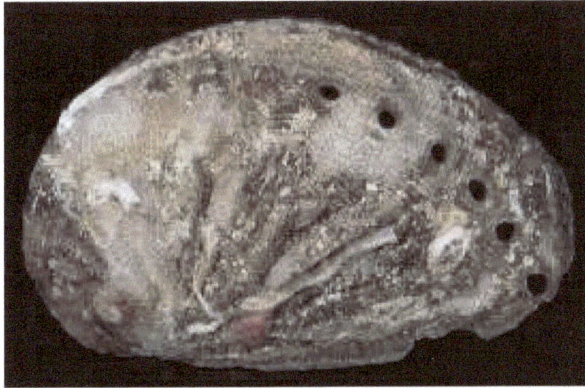

Fig. (40). *Haliotis tuberculata.*

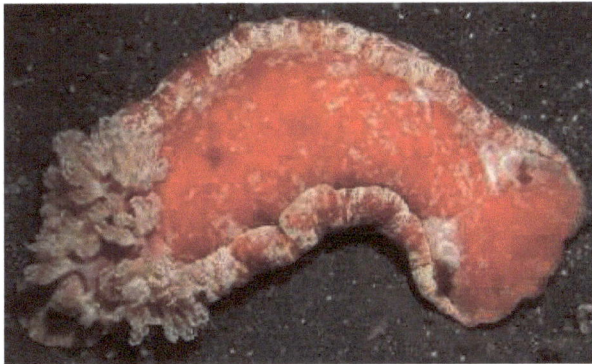

Fig. (41). *Hexabranchus sanguineus.*

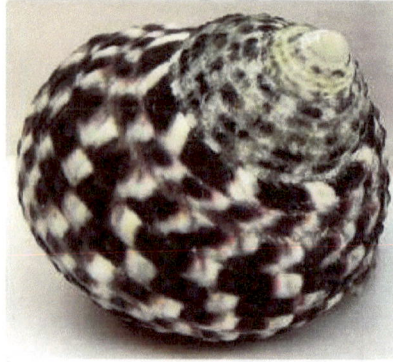

Fig. (42). *Monodonta labio.*

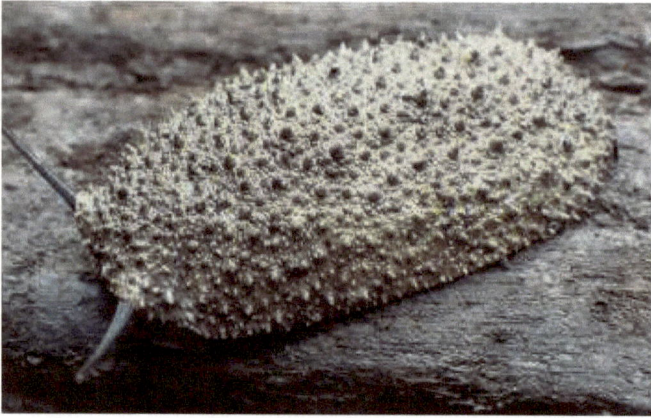

Fig. (43). *Onchidium* sp.

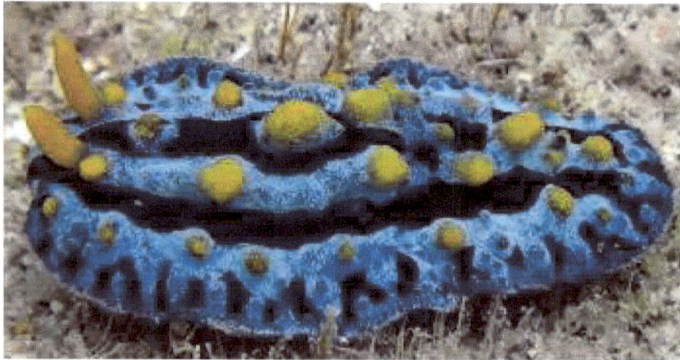

Fig. (44). *Phyllidia coelestis.*

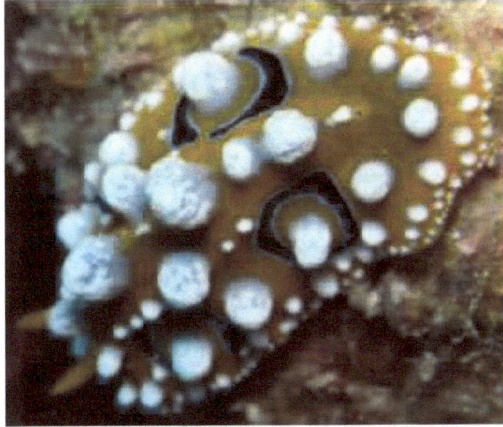

Fig. (45). *Phyllidia ocellata.*

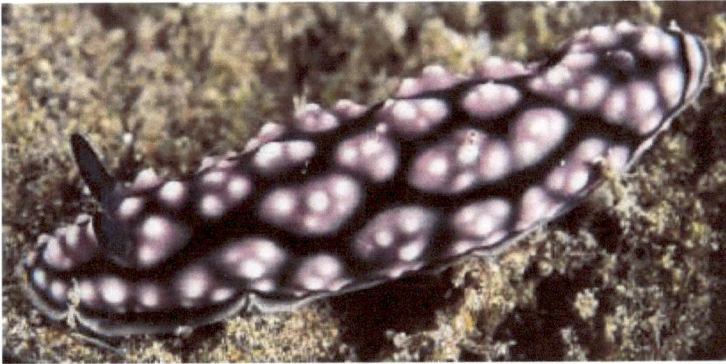

Fig. (46). *Phyllidiella pustulosa.*

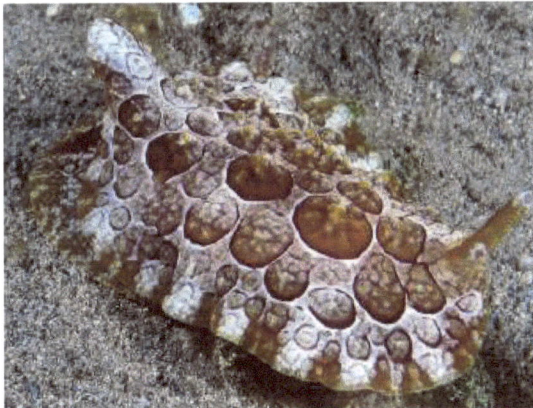

Fig. (47). *Pleurobranchus forskalii.*

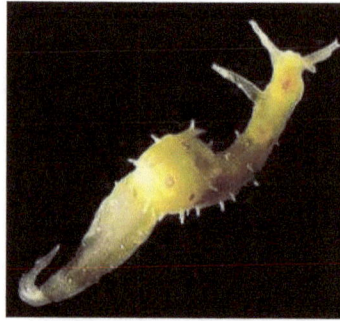

Fig. (48). *Stylocheilus longicauda.*

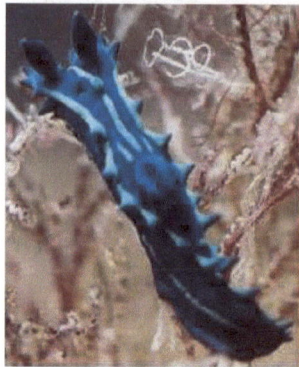

Fig. (49). *Stylocheilus longicauda.*

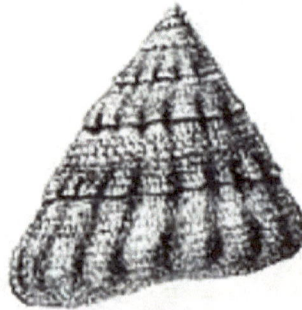

Fig. (50). *Trochus tentoriu.*

Image credit: *Actinocyclus papillatus, Aldisa andersoni,, Aplysia dactylomela, Cellana grata, Cellana toreuma, Dicathais orbita, Dolabrifera dolabrifera, Doris kerguelenensis (= Austrodoris kerguelenensis), Drupella margariticola (= Drupa margariticola), Elysia ornata, Elysia rufescens, Goniobranchus splendidus, Hexabranchus sanguineus, Monodonta labio, Onchidium* sp. *Phyllidia ocellata, Phyllidiella pustulosa,* and *Pleurobranchus forskalii,* Wikipedia;

Image credit: *Elysia ornaae, Haliotis tuberculata coccinea, Phyllidia coelestis* and *Trochus tentorium*, Wikimedia commons;

Image credit: *Aplysia kurodai Aplysia oculifer, Dollabellaaa uricularia, Elysia rufescens, Stylocheilus longicauda, Tambja ceutae,* Australian Museum (applied for permission).

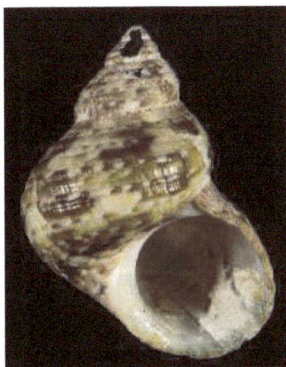

Fig. (51). *Turbo stenogyrus.*

Secondary Metabolites of Marine Gastropods and their Bioactivities

The secondary metabolites of marine gastropods and their bioactivities are given in Table **2**.

Table 2. Secondary metabolites of marine gastropods and their bioactivities.

Species	Compound(s)	Chemistry	Activity	Refs.
Actinocyclus papillatus	Actisonitrile	vinyl cyanide	Cytotoxic	[11]
-do-	Actinofide	Metal	Antiproliferative	[11]
Aldisa andersoni	Phorboxazole	Macrolide	-do-	[11]
Aplysia dactylomela	Aplysqualenol A	Bromotriterpene polyether	Cytotoxic	[11]
Aplysia kurodai	Aplyronine congeners D–H; Aplyronine A and C	Macrolides	-do-	[11]
Aplysia kurodai	Aplysiasecosterol A	Sterol	-do-	[11]
Aplysia oculifera	Palmadorins	Diterpene glycerides	Antiproliferative	[11]
Dicathais orbita	Extract	-	Necrosis in HT29; apoptosis in Jurkat	[91]
Dollabella auricularia	Dolastatin 10; Dolastatin 15-	Peptides	Anticancer	[91]
Elysia rufescens	Kahalalide F	Peptide	-do-	[91]

(Table 2) cont.....

Species	Compound(s)	Chemistry	Activity	Refs.
Elysia ornata	Kahalalide Z1,Z2	Depsipeptides	-do-	[11]
Goniobranchus splendidus	Gracilins O, P and Q	Norditerpenes	Cytotoxic	[11]
Haliotis tuberculata coccinea	Ethyl acetate extract	-	-do-	[92]
Hexabranchus sanguineus	Ulapualide-A	Macrolide	Cytotoxic	[91]
Monodonta labio	Monodontins A and B	Polyketides	Cytotoxic	[11]
Onchidium sp.	Onchidione	Ilikonapyrone	Cytotoxic	[11]
Phyllidia coelestis	1-formamido-10(1→2).	Abeopupukeanane	Antiproliferative	[11]
Pleurobranchus forskalii	Cycloforskamide	Synthetic alkylating agent	Cytotoxic	[11]
-do-	Keenamide A	Hexapeptide	-do-	[91]
Stylocheilus longicauda	Aplysiatoxin	Dermatoxin	Antiproliferative	[11]
Tambja ceutae	Tambjamine	Alkaloid	Anticancer	[11]
Turbo stenogyrus	Turbostatins 1-4	Depsipeptides	-do-	[91]

The anti-inflammatory and antiparasitic activities of the marine gastropods in relation to their bioactive compounds are given in Table **3**.

Table 3. Bioactive compounds and their Anti-inflammatory and Antiparasitic activities in marine gastropods.

Species	Compound(s)	Chemistry	Activity	Refs.
Cellana grata	4-methyl and 4,4- dimethyl sterols	Steroids	Anti-inflammatory	[91]
Cellana toreuma	-do-	-do-	-do-	[91]
Drupa margariticola	100% acetone extract	-	-do-	[91]
Scaphander lignarius	Lignarenone	Synthetic	Anti-inflammatory/ Immunomodulatory	[91]
Trochus tentorium	100% acetone extract	-	Anti-inflammatory	[91]
Dolabrifera dolabrifera	5α,8α-Epidioxycholest-6-en-3β-ol	Steroidal Endoperoxide	Anti-Leishmanial	[11]
Haliotis tuberculata coccinea	Ethyl acetate extract	-	Anthelmintic activity	[92]

(Table 3) cont.....

Species	Compound(s)	Chemistry	Activity	Refs.
Phyllidia ocellata	2-Isocyanoclovene; 2- Isocyanoclovane; 1- Isothiocyanatoepicaryolane; 4,5- Epi-10-isocyanoisodauc-6-ene;13-Isocyanocubebane	Sesquiterpene isonitriles	Antiplasmodial	[11]
Phyllidiella pustulosa	Pustulosaisonitrile-1	Terpenoid	antiparasitic	[11]

Pharmaceutically Important Cephalopods

Sepiella inermis, Loligo vulgaris, Uroteuthis (Photololigo) duvaucelii, Dosidicus gigas and *Octopus vulgaris* (Figs. **52 - 56**).

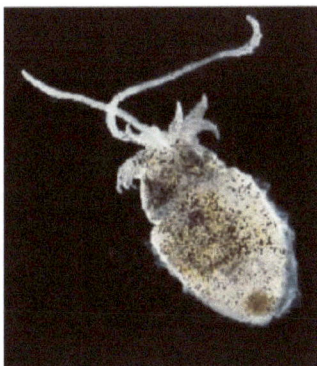

Fig. (52). *Sepiella inermis.*

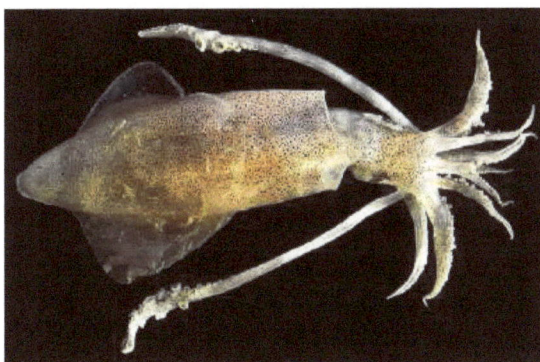

Fig. (53). *Loligo vulgaris.*

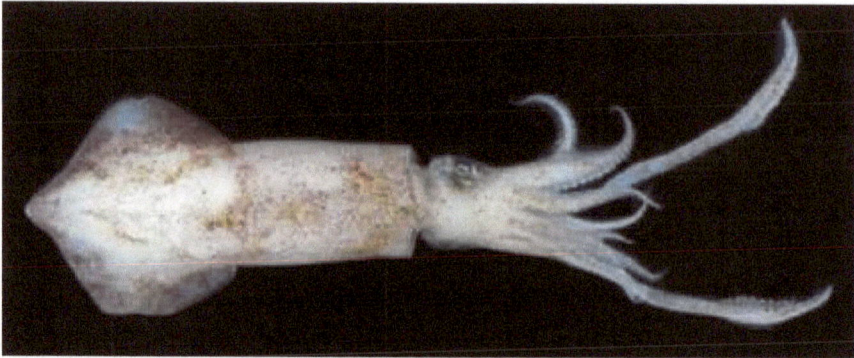

Fig. (54). *Uroteuthis (Photololigo) duvaucelii.*

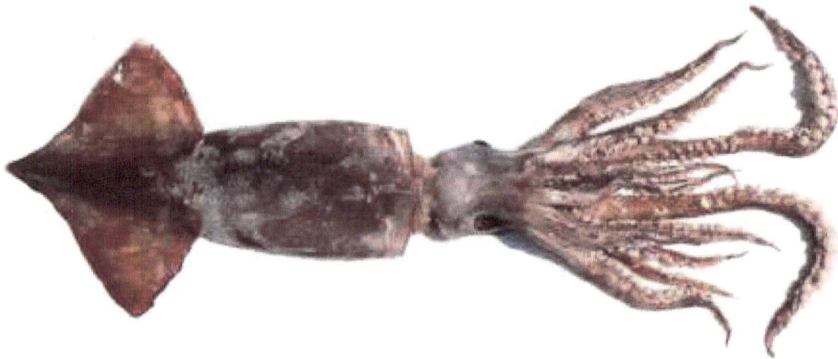

Fig. (55). *Dosidicus gigas.*

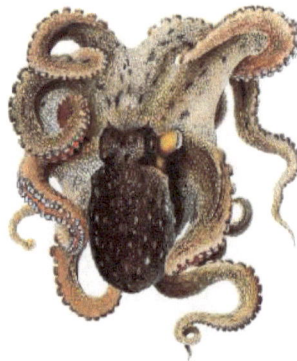

Fig. (56). *Octopus vulgaris.*

Image credit: 48, 49: Wikipedia; 50: Singapore Biodiversity (applied for permission); 51: Neptune Fisheries (applied for permission); 52: Wikispecies.

Therapeutic Values of Cephalopods

Dosidicus gigas

The Xanthommatin and dihydroxanthommatin, pigments and kynurenine compounds derived from the methanol-HCl and ethanol-HCl skin extracts of this species displayed antioxidant activity with IC_{50} DPPH values of 1.14 and 1.74 mg/mL, respectively. Among these extracts, the methanol-HCl yielded a higher recovery rate of pigments [93].

Uroteuthis (Photololigo) duvaucelii (= Loligo duvaucelii)

The ethyl acetate:methanol extract of this squid species yielded C19 furano-norditerpenoid, C15 sesquiterpenoid and C20 diterpenoid compounds. Among these compounds, the C19 furano-norditerpenoid showed antioxidant activity with significantly effective 2,2-diphenyl-1-picrylhydrazyl radical inhibition (IC_{50} 0.60 mg/mL). The 2,2'-azino-bis-3-ethylbenzothiozoline-6-sulfonic acid inhibition and ferrous ion chelating potentials were found to be higher for C19 furano-norditerpenoid C15 sesquiterpenoid compounds (IC_{50} 0.69 and 0.84 mg/mL, respectively). It is suggested that these compounds could be utilised as natural antioxidants and anti-inflammatory functional food ingredients [94].

The methanolic extract of the ink of this species possessed high +++ flavonoids and biologically and therapeutically active alkaloids such as morphine, atropine and quinine. Among these compounds, alkaloids have been reported to exhibit antioxidant activity through a scavenging or chelating process. Further, its saponins showed antiallergic, anti-inflammatory, antimicrobial and anticancer activities besides having the properties of precipitating and coagulating red blood cells; and cholesterol binding properties [95].

Xanthommatin and dihydroxanthommatin, pigments and kynurenine compounds derived from the methanol-HCl and ethanol-HCl skin extracts of this species displayed antioxidant activity with IC_{50} DPPH values of 1.14 and 1.74 mg/mL respectively. Among these extracts, the methanol-HCl yielded a higher recovery rate of pigments [93].

Loligo vulgaris

The ethanolic extracts of this squid ink showed the presence of functional groups such as 1° and 2° amines, amides, alkynes (terminal), alkenes, aldehydes, nitriles, alkanes, aliphatic amines, carboxylic acids, and alkyl halides, Owing to these compounds, this squid species exhibited an antioxidant activity of 83.5%. Further,

68.9% inhibition of protein denaturation by this squid ink extract indicated that it has very good *in vitro* anti-inflammatory properties [96].

Octopus vulgaris

The hexane, dichloromethane- (DM), and water ink extracts of this species exhibited anti-proliferative effects against human colorectal (HT-29/HCT116) and breast (MDA-MB-231) cancer cells. Among the DM fractions (F1/F2/F3), DM-F2 exhibited the highest anti-proliferative effect (LC$_{50}$ = 52.64 µg/mL), inducing pro-apoptotic morphological disruptions in HCT116 cells. Metabolomic analysis of DM-F2 showed the presence of hexadecanoic acid and 1-(15-methy--1-oxohexadecyl)-pyrrolidine as the most important metabolites [97].

The xanthommatin and dihydroxanthommatin, pigments and kynurenine compounds derived from the methanol-HCl and ethanol-HCl skin extracts of this species displayed antioxidant activity with IC$_{50}$ DPPH values of 0.48 and 1.24 mg/mL respectively. Among these extracts, the methanol-HCl yielded a higher recovery rate of pigments [93].

Therapeutic Values of the Ink of Cephalopods, *Sepiella inermis* and *Loligo duvauceli*

The chemistry of cephalopod ink can only be understood from studies of the ink sac as the chemical analyses of the contents of the funnel organ have not so far been reported. Melanin that provides the distinctive black color of cephalopod ink, is a major component of ink. Each ink sac of Sepia has about 1 g of melanin and melanin constitutes ~15% of the total wet weight of ink. Proteins make up another 5%–8% of the weight of Sepia ink [89]. The potential therapeutic properties of the cephalopod ink as reported by Derby [89] are given below.

Anticancer Activity

The anticancer activity of the cephalopod ink is often through the induction of apoptosis and is often associated with different chemicals in this ink. The compounds associated with the cephalopod ink and their anticancer effects are given below.

i) The tyrosinase extracted from the melanin-free fraction of the cephalopod ink has been reported to be toxic to transformed human cell lines. It is also believed that this apoptotic effect is largely due to the production of dopaquinone, which is known to interact with nucleophiles to produce protein-bound DOPA through a 5-S-cysteinyldopa residue, which, in turn, oxidatively damages cellular molecules.

ii) The peptidoglycans of the squid and cuttlefish ink possess anti-tumor effects by affecting the cell division. The mechanism relating to the effects of these peptidoglycans includes fragmentation of DNA and apoptosis thereby resulting in the inhibition of embryonic development.

iii) The polysaccharide derived by the enzymatic digestion of the peptidoglycans of *Sepiella inermis (= Sepiella maindroni)* ink when treated with chlorosulfonic acid yielded a sulfated SIP, called SIP-SII possessing anti-cancer activity. The mechanisms associated with this activity include a) suppression of the invasion and migration of carcinoma cells through the inhibition of matrix metall opro teinase- 2; b) suppression of melanoma metastasis through the inhibition of tumor adhesion which is mediated by intercellular adhesion molecule 1; and c) inhibition of angiogenesis which is mediated by basic fibroblast growth factor.

iv) The oligopeptide extracted from enzymatically digested Sepia ink sacs possesses anticancer activity. Its mechanism of action in prostate cancer cells is by the induction of apoptosis through the activation of caspase-3 and elevation of the ratio of Bax/Bcl-2.

Anti-inflammatory Activity

The anti-inflammatory activity of the squid ink is due to its inhibition of gastric secretion.

Antioxidant Activity

The melanin and melanin-free fractions of cephalopod ink possess anti-oxidant activity.

Anti-hypertensive Activity

An angiotensin-converting enzyme purified from the squid ink has been reported to cause dilation of blood vessels, thereby resulting in lower blood pressure. The bioactivity may be due to the peptide derivative of ~294 Da present in this ink. This feature represents a potential treatment of hypertension.

Anti-retroviral Activity

The ink of *Loligo duvauceli* and *Sepiella inermis* has been reported to possess anti-retroviral activity.

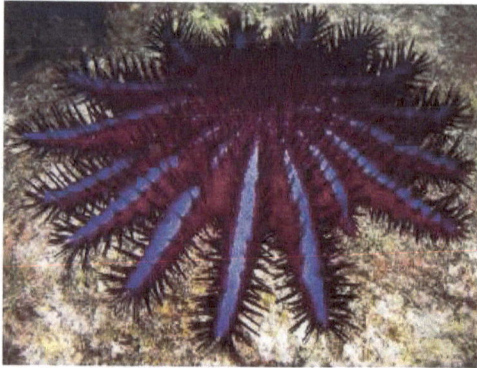

Fig. (57). *Acanthaster planci.*

Anti-ulcerogenic Activity

As the ink from squid and octopus is known to inhibit gastric secretion of rats, this ink has the potential in the development of anti-ulcerogenic drugs. This activity is mainly due to the active fraction of the ink containing an unidentified low molecular weight melanoprotein, which is believed to be responsible for this activity, by enhancing the glycoprotein activity in the gastric mucosa.

Hematopoietic Effects

The cuttlefish ink has been reported to enhance immune responses by affecting hematopoiesis. For example, this ink promotes the proliferation and differentiation of granulocyte-monocyte progenitor cells.

Echinoderms

The phylum Echinodermata has about 7000 species which are exclusively marine without any freshwater or terrestrial members. These echinoderms live on ocean floors in their adult form and they play an important role in the food chain of benthic ecosystems. The echinoderms fall into five clades *viz.* Asteroidea (sea stars, starfish), Ophiuroidea (brittle stars), Echinoidea (sea urchins), Crinoidea (sea lilies, feather stars) and Holothuroidea (sea cucumbers). Echinoderms produce mainly bioactive glycosylated metabolites, dominated by steroidal and sulphated metabolites, saponins and glycolipids. Among the different classes of Echinodermata, Asteroidea, Echinoidea and Holothuroidea have been reported to be therapeutically important. Starfish-derived compounds include mainly asterosaponins and polyhydroxy steroid glycosides with promising anticancer, anti-inflammatory agents, neuritogenic, and antimicrobial properties. Sea urchins are known for their antimicrobial compounds such as peptides including short cationic peptides with positively-charged amino acid residues like strongylocins, centrocin 1 and 2 or their analogues and paracentrin 1. Further, sea urchin pigments, which are found in their test spines, coelomocytes or gonad yield powerful antioxidant compounds. The body wall of sea cucumbers contains mainly polysaccharides and collagen, which are known to display anticancer, anti-hypertensive, anti-angiogenic, anti-inflammatory, anti-diabetic, anti-coagulation, anti-microbial, anti-oxidant, and anti-osteoclastogenic properties. Further, these animals contain saponins, cerebrosides and gangliosides with numerous biological activities. Overall, this phylum exhibits a great variety of bioactive compounds *viz.* cytotoxic or anti-proliferative (38%); anticoagulant (16%); antimicrobial (9%) and antioxidant (7%) [11, 98].

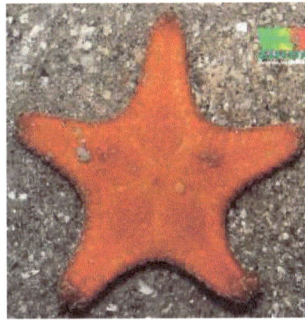

Fig. (58). *Anthenea aspera.*

Biopharmaceutically Important Sea Stars and Starfish (Class: Asteroidea)

Acanthaster planci, Anthenea aspera, Aphelasterias japonica, Archaster typicus, Asterias amurensis, Asterias microdiscus, Patiria pectinifera (= Asterina pectinifera), Asteropsis carinifera), Astropecten polyacanthus, Ceramaster patagonicus, Choriaster granulatus, Craspidaster sp., *Ctenodiscus crispatus, Culcita novaeguineae, Diplasterias brucei, Echinaster luzonicus, Leptasterias* sp., *Lethasterias* sp., *Narcissia canariensis. Patiria pectinifera, Pentaceraster regulus,* and *Solaster* sp. (Figs. **57-76**).

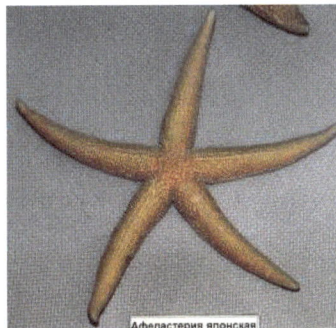

Fig. (59). *Aphelasterias japonica.*

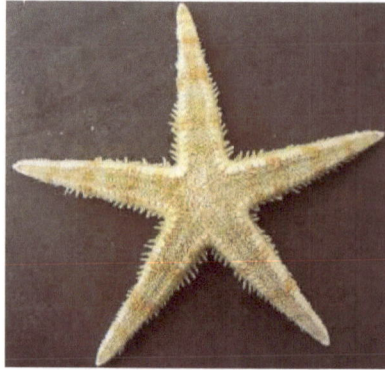

Fig. (60). *Anthenea aspera.*

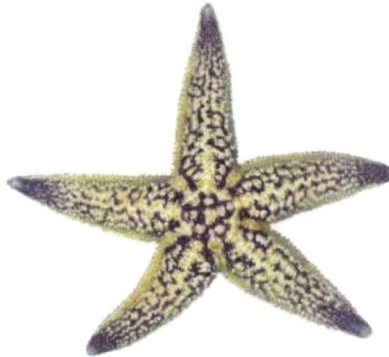

Fig. (61). *Asterias amurensis.*

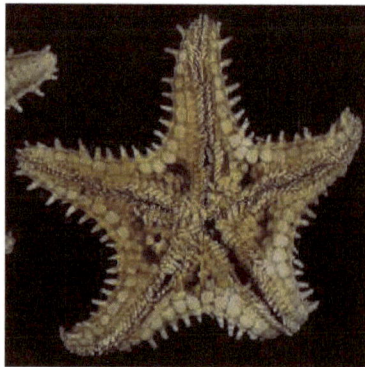

Fig. (62). *Asteropsis carinifera.*

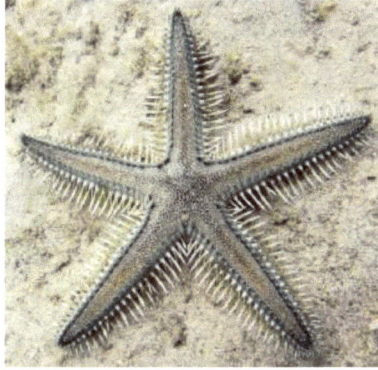

Fig. (63). *Astropecten polyacanthus.*

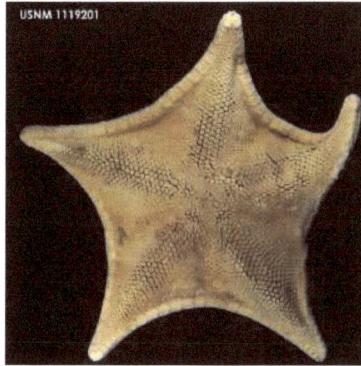

Fig. (64). *Ceramaster patagonicus.*

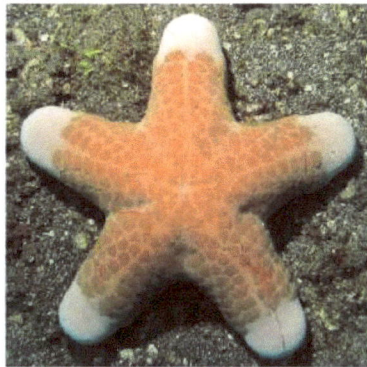

Fig. (65). *Choriaster granulatus.*

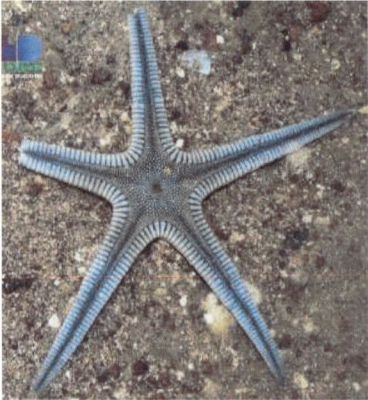

Fig. (66). *Craspidaster* sp.

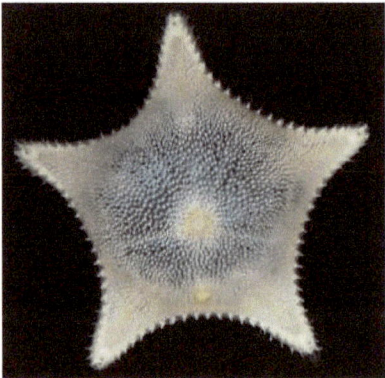

Fig. (67). *Ctenodiscus crispatus*.

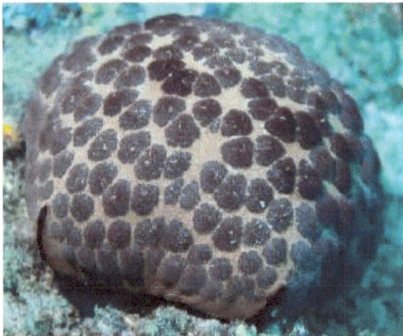

Fig. (68). *Culcita novaeguineae*.

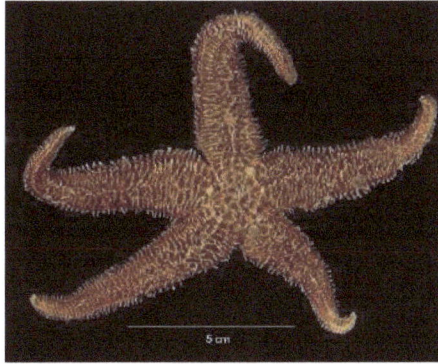

Fig. (69). *Diplasterias brucei.*

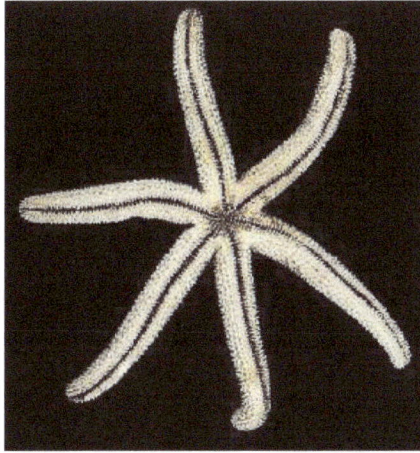

Fig. (70). *Echinaster luzonicus.*

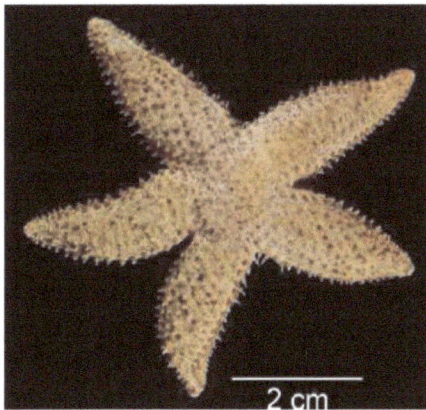

Fig. (71). *Leptasterias* sp.

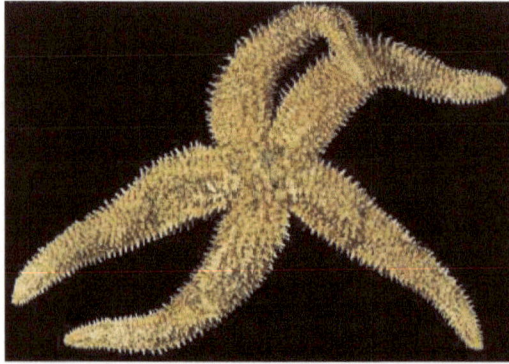

Fig. (72). *Lethasterias* sp.

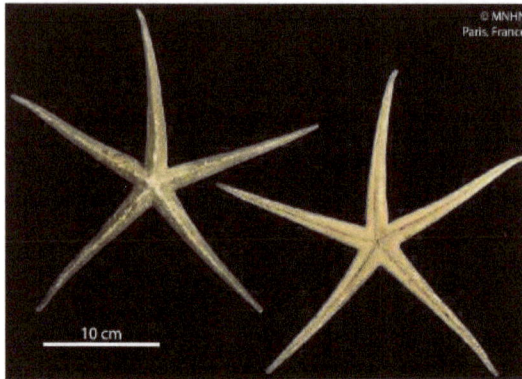

Fig. (73). .*Narcissia canariensis.*

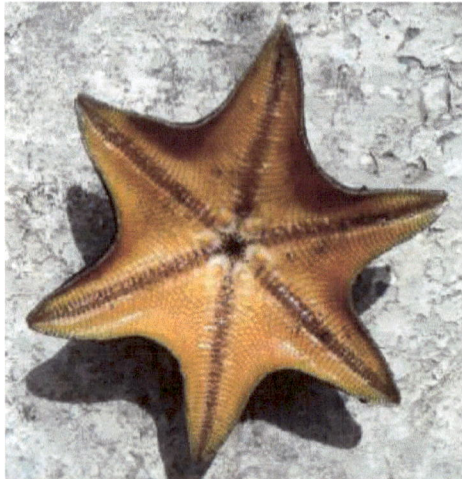

Fig. (74). *Patiria pectinifera.*

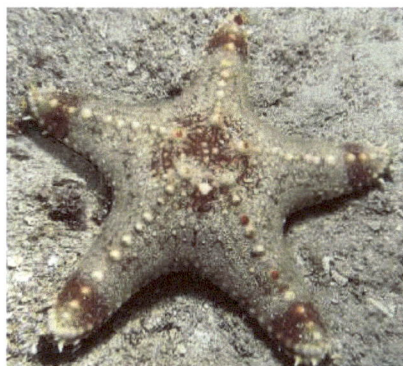

Fig. (75). *Pentaceraster regulus.*

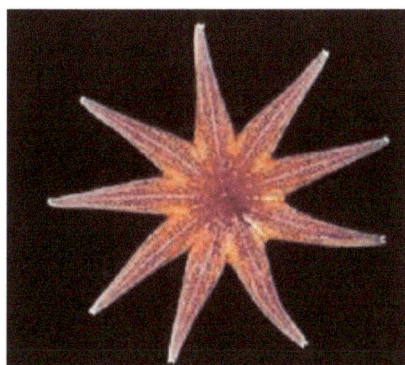

Fig. (76). *Solaster* sp.

Image credit: 57, 60, 64, 66, 68, 69, 71, 72, 76: Wikipedia; 59, 61-63, 65, 70, 74, 75: Wikimedia commons; 67, 73: Wikidata.

The species of starfish have been reported to possess promising anticancer/ cytotoxic and anti-inflammatory compounds as shown in Tables **4** and **5**.

Table 4. Anticancer/cytotoxic compounds of sea stars and starfish [11].

Species	Compound (s)	Chemistry	Mechanism
Acanthaster planci	Acanthaglycoside A,G; maculatoside (or luidiaglycoside B)	Asterosaponins; steroidal glycosides	Inhibition of cell migration and colony formation.
Acanthaster planci	Planciside A-C;	Steroid biglycosides	Cytotoxic; antiproliferative.
Acanthaster planci	Plancitoxin I	Protein	Cytotoxic; antiproliferative.

Species	Compound (s)	Chemistry	Mechanism
Acanthaster planci	Polyhydroxylated steroid	-	Inhibition of cell migration and colony formation.
Anthenea aspera	Anthenoside A1, A2	Polyhydroxysteroidal glycosides	Cytotoxic
Aphelasterias japonica	Aphelasteroside F	Asterosaponin	Cytotoxic
Archaster typicus	Archasteroside A,B; regularoside A	Asterosaponins;	Cytotoxic
Asterias amurensis	Gangliosides LLG-3	Lipids/ Glycolipid	Apoptosis induction ; antiproliferative
Asterias microdiscus	Thornasteroside A ; versicoside A	Asterosaponin; lignin glyocoside	Cytotoxic
Asterina pectinifera	(25S)-5alpha-cholestane-3beta,6alpha,7al-pha,8,15alpha,16beta-hexahydroxyl-26- O-14'Z-eicosenoate	Polyhydroxylated steroid	Cytotoxic
Asterina pectinifera	Asterosaponins P1	Monoglycoside	Cytotoxic
Asterina pectinifera	Asteropsiside A, regularoside A and thornasteroside A	Asterosaponins;	Cytotoxic
Astropecten monacanthus	Astrosterioside D	Asterosaponin	Cytotoxic
Astropecten polyacanthus	(20R,24S)-3β,6α,8,15β,24-pentahydroxy- 5α-cholestane	Polar steroid	Cytotoxic
Astropecten polyacanthus	Polyacanthoside A	Steroid derivative	Cytotoxic
Astropecten polyacanthus	5α-cholest-7-ene-3β,6α-diol (5),3) 5α-cho-lest8(14)-ene-3β,7α-diol (6),4) and 5α-cholest-7,9(11)-diene-3β-ol	Sterols	Apoptosis induction in leukemia related cells
Ceramaster patagonicus	Esters of polyhydroxysteroids	-	Inhibition of colony formation and migration
Choriaster granulatus	Granulatosides D, echinasterosides B and F and laeviuscoloside D	Polyhydroxylated steroids	Cytotoxic
Craspidaster hesperus	Ovaeguinoside A; hesperuside A, B, C	Polyhydroxysteroidal glycosides	Cytotoxic
Ctenodiscus crispatus.	(25S)-5α5α-cholestane-3β3β,5,6β6β,15α15α,16β16β,26-hexaol	Steroid; asterogenin	Cytotoxic

(Table 4) cont.....

Species	Compound (s)	Chemistry	Mechanism
Culcita novaeguineae	Culcinosides A–D, echinasteroside C, linckoside F and linckoside L3	Polyhydroxy steroidal glycosides	Cytotoxic
Culcita novaeguineae	Novaeguinosides I and II	Asterosaponins,	Cytotoxic
Diplasterias brucei	Diplasteriosides A and B	Steroidal glycosides; Asterosaponins,	Cytotoxic
Echinaster luzonicus	Luzonicoside	Polyhydroxylated steroid	Cytotoxic
Lethasterias fusca	Lethasteriosides A	Asterosaponin	Cytotoxic
Leptasterias ochotensis	Leptasteriosides A-F	Asterosaponins	Cytotoxic
Leptasterias ochotensis	Leptaochotensoside A	Sulfated stroid monoglycoside	Inhibition of colony formation
Narcissia canariensis	Peracetylated derivatives	Lipids/Glycolipid	Cytotoxic
Pentaceraster gracilis.	Maculatoside	Steroid glycoside	Cytotoxic
Pentaceraster regulus.	Pentaregulosides A	Asterosaponin	Cytotoxic
Solaster pacificus	Cucumariosides C1, C2, and A10	Triterpene glycosides	Cytotoxic
Solaster pacificus	Pacificusosides C, cucumariosides C1, C2 and A10	Triterpene glycosides	Inhibition of colony formation

Table 5. Anti-inflammatory compounds of starfish [99].

Species	Compound (s)	Chemistry	Mechanism
Acanthaster planci	Plancipyrrosides A and B	Pyrrole oligoglycosides,	Reduction of ROS formation and NO production
Anthenea aspera	Anthenoside O	Polyhydroxysteroidal glycoside	Reduction of ROS formation and NO production
Asterina batheri	Astebatheriosides B-D	Glycosides	Inhibitionnof IL-12 p40 production
Asterias amurensis	Fatty acids	-	Downregulating expression of inflammatory genes
Astropecten monacanthus	Astrosteriosides A and D	Asterosaponins,	Inhibiting secretion of proinflammatory cytokines
Astropecten polyacanthus	Steroids	-	Inhibiting production of IL-12 p40, IL-6 and TNFα

(Table 5) cont.....

Species	Compound (s)	Chemistry	Mechanism
Marthasterias glacialis	cis 11-eicosenoic and cis 11,14 eicosadienoic acids	Fatty acid methyl ester	Downregulating inflammatory gene expression: iNOS, COX-2, IKB-α and CHOP and NF-κB
Pentaceraster regulus	Pentareguloside C, D,E	Asterosaponins,	Reduction of ROS formation and NO production
Protoreaster lincki	Protolinckiosides A-D	Steroidal glycosides	Reduction of ROS formation and NO production
Protoreaster nodosus	Steroid Derivatives	-	Inhibiting secretion of proinflammatory cytokines IL-12 p40, IL-6 and TNFα

Biopharmaceutically Important Brittle Stars (Class: Ophiuroidea)

Astrotoma agassizi, Breviturma dentata, Ophiarachna incrassata, Ophioderma longicauda, Ophiocoma erinaceus, Ophiocoma scolopendrina, Ophiolepis superba, Ophiomastix sp., *Ophiopholis aculeata, Ophioplocus japonicus, Ophiothrix fragilis, Ophiura* sp. (Figs. **77-88**).

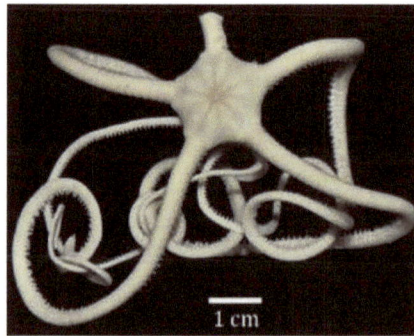

Fig. (77). *Astrotoma agassizi.*

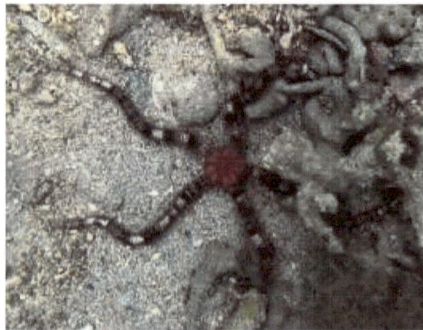

Fig. (78). *Breviturma dentata.*

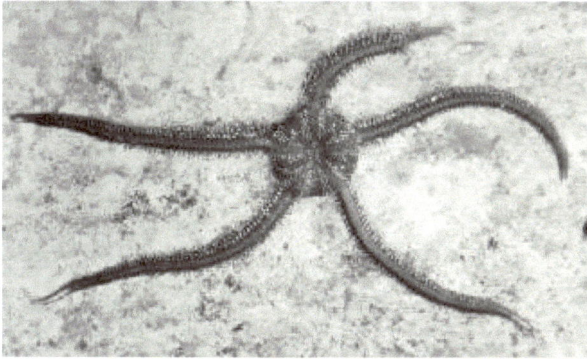

Fig. (79). *Ophiarachna incrassata.*

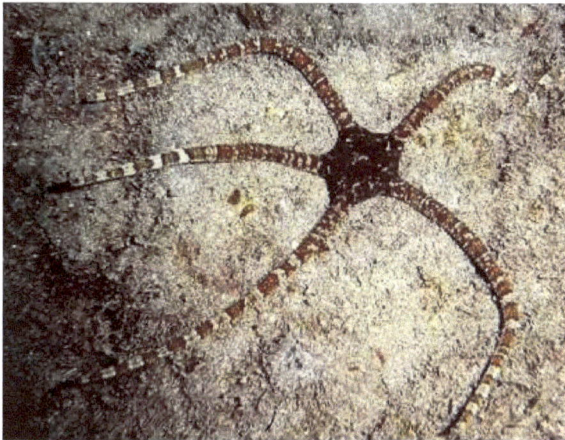

Fig. (80). *Ophioderma longicauda.*

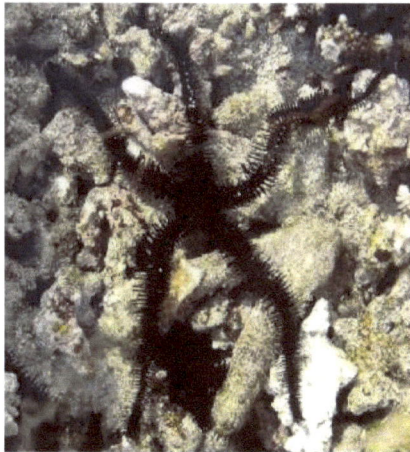

Fig. (81). *Ophiocoma erinaceus.*

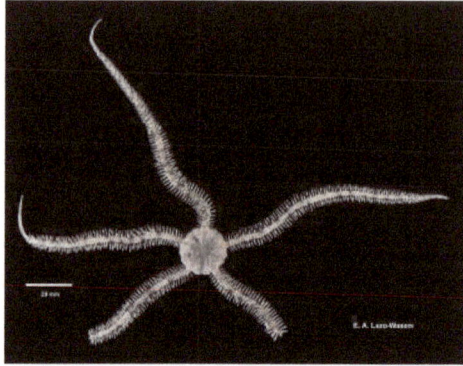

Fig. (82). *Ophiocoma scolopendrina.*

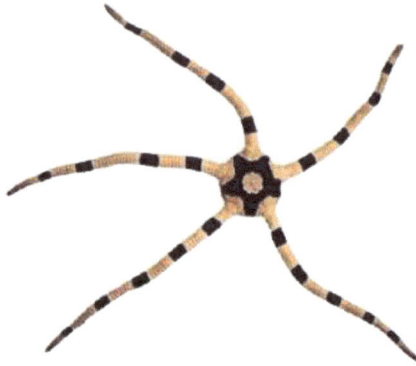

Fig. (83). *Ophiolepis superba.*

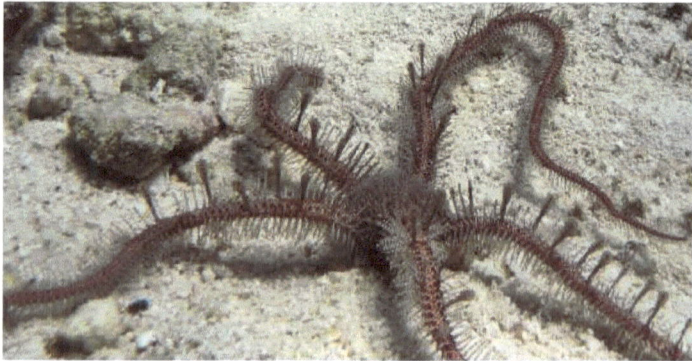

Fig. (84). *Ophiomastix* sp.

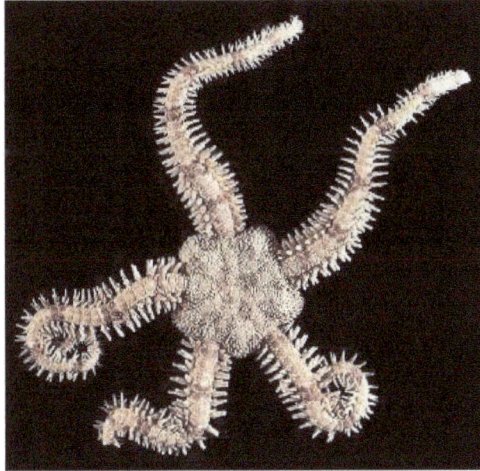

Fig. (85). *Ophiopholis aculeata.*

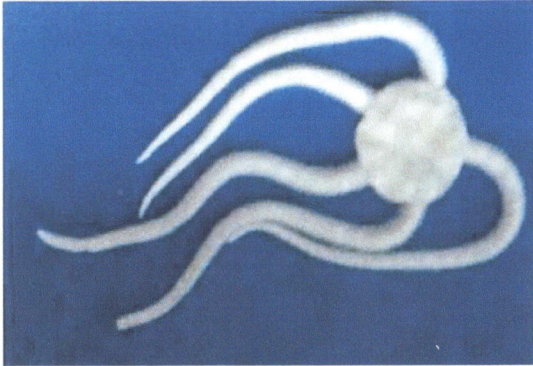

Fig. (86). *Ophioplocus japonicus.*

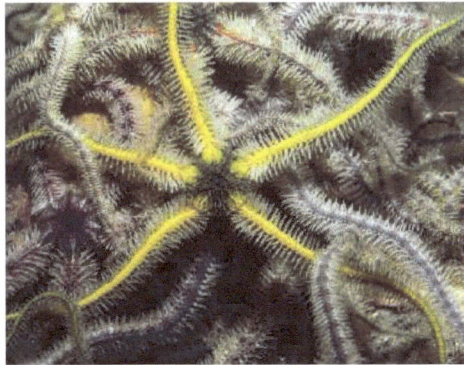

Fig. (87). *Ophiothrix fragilis.*

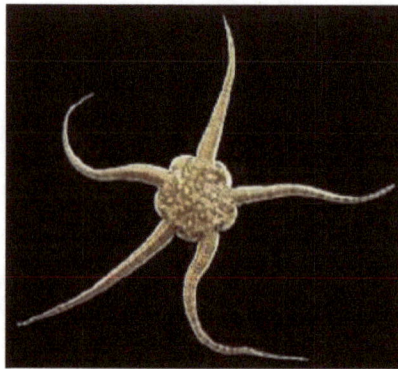

Fig. (88). *Ophiura* sp.

Image credit: 77, 85, 86; Wikidata; 78: Wikispecies; 79, 81, 84, 87, 88: Wikipedia; 80, 82, 83: Wikipedia commons.

The bioactive compounds of several species of brittle stars have shown antiviral, anticancer, antioxidant and hemolytic activities as shown in Table **6**.

Table 6. Biopharmaceutical compounds of brittle stars and their therapeutic values [98].

Species	Compound/extract	Chemistry	Bioactivity
Astrotoma agassizi	Sulphated sterols	-	Against HSV-2,JV-341 and PV-3
Breviturma dentata	Sulphated sterols	-	HIV-1 and HIV-2 inhibition; IC_{50}, >313 and >157 uM
Ophiarachna incrassata	Sulphated sterols	-	HIV-1 and HIV-2 inhibition; IC_{50}, >313 and >157 uM
Ophioderma longicauda	Cholest-5ene-2α,3α,4β,21-tetraol 3,,21-disulphate and cholest-5-ene-2β,3α,21-triol 2,21-disulphate; Sulphated sterols	Sulphated polyhydroxysteroids	Cytotoxic and cytoprotective against HIV-1; HIV-1 and HIV-2 inhibition; IC_{50}, >152-312 to 152-156 uM
Ophiocoma erinaceus	Saponin, Polysaccharide, phenol and flavonoids	-	Saponin-against Hela-S3 (IC_{50}, 23.4 ug/mL); Polysaccharide- against HeLa; Phenol and flavonoids- Antioxidant and Anti-inflammatory
Ophiocoma scolopendrina	Curacin E; ophiodilactone A,B	Hybrid polyketide synthase ; phenylpropanoids	Inhibition of P388
Ophiolepis superba	Sulphated sterols	-	HIV-1 and HIV-2 inhibition; IC_{50}, 157-161uM

(Table 6) cont.....

Species	Compound/extract	Chemistry	Bioactivity
Ophiomastix brocki	Sulphated sterols	-	HIV-1 and HIV-2 inhibition; IC_{50}, >313 and >157uM
Ophiomastix mixta	Butenolide	Lactone	Cytotoxicity against tumor cell lines
Ophiopholis aculeata	Disulphated polyhydroxysteroids	-	Cardiovascular
Ophiopholis mirabilis	Ophiurasaponin		Antioxidant; IC_{50},hydroxyl-radicals,25.5mg/mL
Ophioplocus japonicus	10-acetoxy-18-hydroxy-2,7-dolabelladiene, dihydroxycrenulide, dictyolactone, pachydictyol, dictyol,	Terpenes	Cytotoxicity against human solid tumor cell lines
Ophiosparte gigas	2 Sulphated sterols	-	1: HIV-1 and HIV-2 inhibition; IC_{50}, >161 and >161uM; 2: HIV-1, IC_{50}, <0.02uM
Ophiothrix fragilis	Sulphated sterols	-	HIV-1 and HIV-2 inhibition; IC_{50}, >322 and 161uM
Ophiura leptoctenia	(20R)-cholest-5-ene3a,4b,21-triol 3-sulphate and (20R)-5acholestane-3a,-1-diol dislphate	-	Not known
Ophiura sarsii	Cholest-5-ene-3a,4b,21-triol 3,21-disulphate	Steroidal disulphate	Hemolytic activity

Biopharmaceutically Important Sea Urchins (Class: Echinoidea)

Arbacia lixula, Diadema savignyi, Echinometra lucunter, Echinometra mathaei, Lytechinus variegatus, Mesocentrotus franciscanus. Mesocentrotus nudus, Paracentrotus lividus, Scaphechinus mirabilis, Strongylocentrotus purpuratus, Toxopneustes pileolus, and *Tripneustes gratilla*. (Figs. **89-100**).

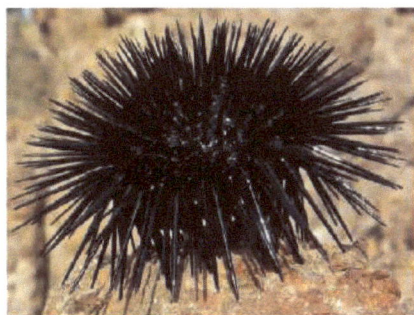

Fig. (89). *Arbacia lixula.*

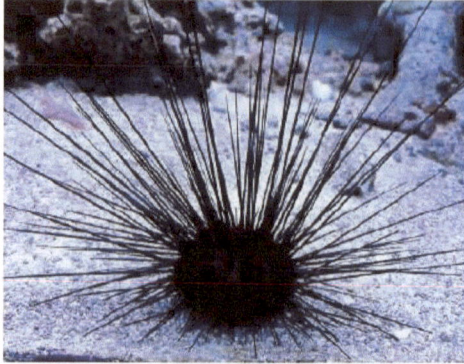

Fig. (90). *Ophiura* sp.

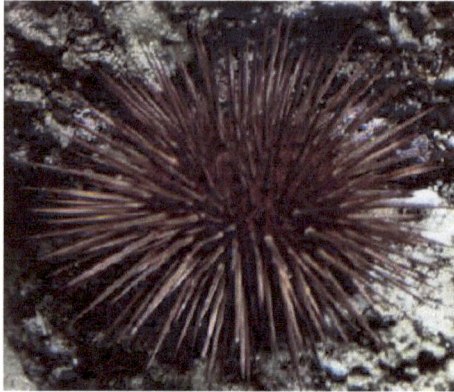

Fig. (91). *Echinometra lucunter.*

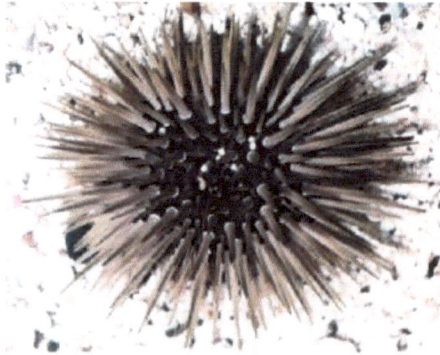

Fig. (92). *Echinometra mathaei.*

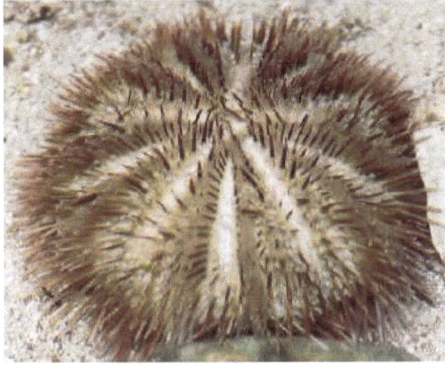

Fig. (93). Lytechinus variegatus.

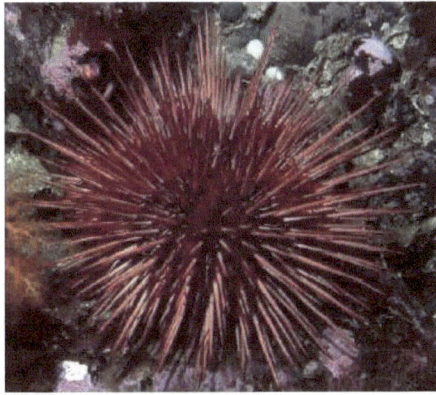

Fig. (94). *Mesocentrotus franciscanus.*

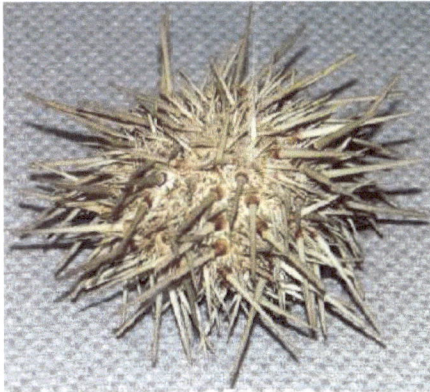

Fig. (95). *Mesocentrotus nudus.*

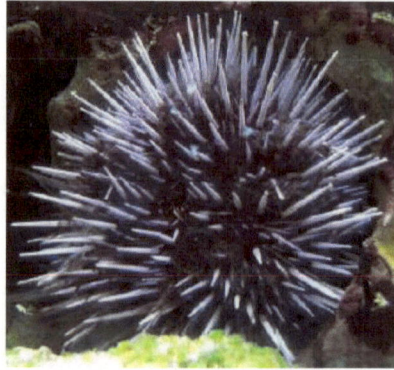

Fig. (96). *Paracentrotus lividus.*

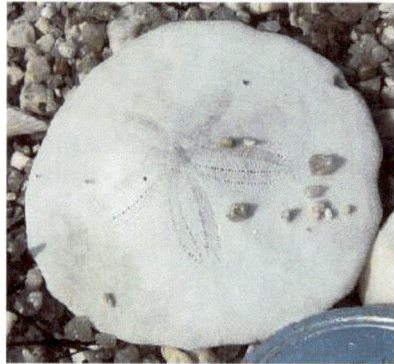

Fig. (97). *Scaphechinus mirabilis.*

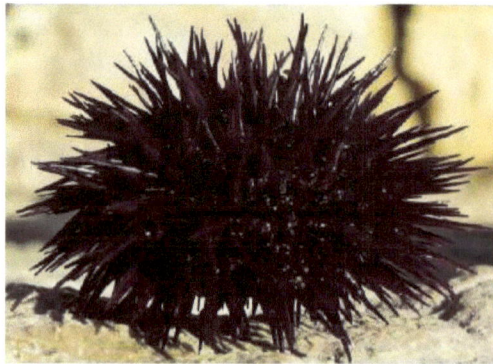

Fig. (98). *Strongylocentrotus purpuratus.*

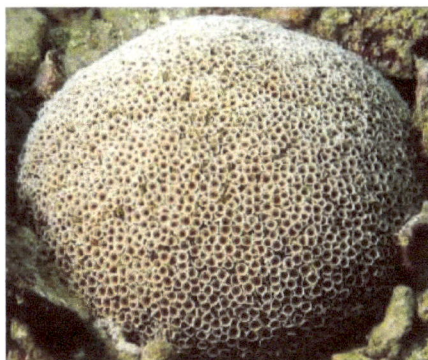

Fig. (99). *Toxopneustes pileolus.*

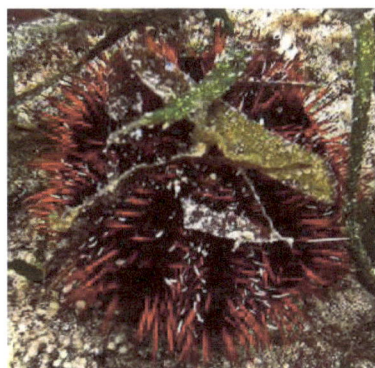

Fig. (100). *Tripneustes gratilla.*

Image credit: 89, 91-94, 96-100: Wikipedia; 90, 95: Wikipedia commons.

The biopharmaceutical compounds of sea urchin species have been reported to possess promising anti-inflammatory compounds. The mode of action of such compounds is shown in Table **7**.

Table 7. Anti-inflammatory compounds of sea urchins [99].

Species	Compound (s)	Chemistry	Mechanism
Anthocidaris crassispina	Gonad polysaccharide	-	Reducing NO production.
Brisaster latifrons	(Z)-4-methylundeca-1,9-diene-6-sulfonic acid	Sulphonic acid derivative	Inhibiting proinflammatory cytokines.

(Table 7) cont.....

Species	Compound (s)	Chemistry	Mechanism
Echinometra mathaei, Diadema savignyi, Tripneustes gratilla and *Toxopneustes pileolus*	Spinochromes and EchA	Pigments, (polyhydroxynaphthoquinones); polyhydroxylated 1,4-naphthoquinone	Reducing TNFα production.
Hemicentrotus pulcherrimus and *Diadema setosum*	Hp-s1 ganglioside	Synthetic analog	Reducing iNOS and COX-2 expression; suppressing cytokine production; and downregulating NF-κB and JNK/p38 MAPK signaling pathway.
Paracentrotus lividus	Sulfated polysaccharide	-	Reducing paw-edema
Paracentrotus lividus	EchA	Pigment (polyhydroxylated 1,4-naphthoquinone)	Stabilizing human RBCs; and suppressing IL-6 and TNFα.
Salmacis bicolor	Salmachroman	Polyketide	Inhibiting COX-2 and 5-LOX.
Salmacis bicolor	Salmacembranes A and B	Polyoxygenated furanocembranoids,	Inhibiting COX-1, COX-2, and 5-LOX
Scaphechinus mirabilis	Spinochromes A and B	Polyhydroxynaphthoquinones	Reducing chronic inflammation.
Scaphechinus mirabilis	EchA	Polyhydroxylated 1,4-naphthoquinone	Attenuating macrophage activation and infiltrating (neutrophils); and inhibiting production of TNFα and IFNγ.
Scaphechinus mirabilis	EchA	Polyhydroxylated 1,4-naphthoquinone	Reducing TNFα, NF-κB antibody positive cells and ROS.

(Table 7) cont.....

Species	Compound (s)	Chemistry	Mechanism
Scaphechinus mirabilis	Histochrome® (1% EchA)	Polyhydroxylated 1,4-naphthoquinone	Reducing MMPs expression and collagen degradation.
Stomopneustes variolaris	Cembrane type of diterpenoid	-	Inhibiting 5-LOX, high COX-1/COX-2 ratio.
Stomopneustes variolaris	Stomopneulactones D	Macrocyclic lactone	Inhibiting COX-2 and 5-LOX; reducing iNOS and intracellular ROS.
Stomopneustes variolaris	Stomopnolides A and B	Macrocyclic pyrone derivatives	Inhibiting 5-LOX
Strongylocentrotus droebachiensis	Fatty acid derivatives	-	Inhibiting COX-1 and COX-2.
Strongylocentrotus droebachiensis	Centrocin 1 (CEN1HC-Br)	Peptide	Reducing expression of inflammatory cytokines *viz.* IL-12p40, IL-6, IL-1β, TNFα
Strongylocentrotus nudus	Spines and shells pigments	-	Reducing NO, IL-6, TNFα, PGE2 and 6-keto-PGF 1α

Other Bioactivities of Sea Urchins

Arbacia lixula

The aqueous ethanol extract of this species has been reported to possess a high concentration of astaxanthin(carotenoid) (27 μg/mg) which displayed marked reducing activity toward radical species with 2,2-diphenyl-1-picrylhydrazyl (DPPH) radical scavenging ability. At concentrations of 0.1, 1, and 10 μg/mL, this extract showed reduction at 7.1.%, 10.3% and 86.4%, respectively [100].

Diadema savignyi

The polyhydroxylated naphthoquinone *viz.* spinochrome of this species displayed cytotoxicity. Further, its extract showed antioxidant activity with DPPH radical scavenging activity which increased significantly in a concentration-dependent manner (12.5–300 µg/ml) [101].

Echinometra mathaei

The Polyhydroxylated naphthoquinone *viz.* spinochrome of this species displayed cytotoxicity. Further, the ethyl acetate extract of this species showed both antidiabetic and antioxidant properties. The shell and Aristotle's lantern extract of this species exhibited the highest α-glucosidase inhibition with IC_{50} values of 3.7 and 4 mg/mL, respectively. Further, its shell extract displayed the highest ABTS (IC_{50}= 183 µg/mL) and DPPH (IC_{50}= 208 µg/mL) radicals scavenging, respectively. Furthermore, its gonad extract showed the highest antioxidant potential by the FRAP method (1140 µg ASA/mg) and NO radical scavenging (70.68%), respectively [102].

Mesocentrotus nudus

The poly Hydroxy Naphtho Quinone (PHNQ) pigments *viz.* spinochromes B and E of this species has been reported to possess a wide range of pharmacological activities including cytotoxic, antioxidant, anti-allergic, antidiabetic and cardioprotective. [103].

Paracentrotus lividus

The carotenoid pigment *viz.* echinenone (β-Caroten-4-one) isolated from the gonad of this species revealed powerful antioxidant activity (Cirino *et al.*, 2017) Further, ovothiols (π-methyl-5-thiohistidines) present in the eggs of this species have been reported to possess powerful ROS scavenging activities [104].

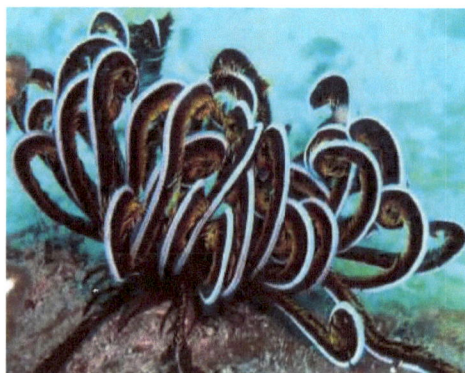

Fig. (101). *Anneissia bennetti.*

Scaphechinus mirabilis

The poly Hydroxy Naphtho Quinone (PHNQ) pigments *viz.* echinochrome A and echinamines A and B (3) of this species has been reported to possess a wide range of pharmacological activities including cytotoxic, antioxidant, anti-allergic, antidiabetic and cardioprotective [103].

Strongylocentrotus franciscanus Lytechinus variegatus, and Echinometra lucunter

The 2-sulfated fucan from *Strongylocentrotus franciscanus*, 4-sulfated fucan from Lytechinus variegatus, and the 2-sulfated galactan from *Echinometra lucunter* have been reported to possess anticoagulant and antithrombotic properties. *Lytechinus variegatus, Strongylocentrotus franciscanus* and *Echinometra lacunter* showed the capacity to inhibit 20%, 25% and 50% of the thrombus weight at the doses of 1.0, 0.5 and 0.25 mg·kg−1, respectively [105].

Strongylocentrotus nudus

A polysaccharide derived from the eggs of this species (SEP) displayed anticancer activity by pancreatic cancer growth by activating NK cells *in vitro/vivovia* TLR4/MAPKs/NF-κB signaling pathway. The values of tumor inhibitory rate were 44.5% and 50.8% at a dose of 40 mg/kg in Bxpc-3 and SW1990 nude mice, respectively. These results suggested that the pancreatic cancer could be effectively inhibited by SEP-enhanced NK cytotoxicity mediated primarily through TLR4/MAPKs/NF-κB signaling pathway. Further, the polysaccharide of this species could represent a potential immunotherapy candidate for the treatment of pancreatic cancer [106].

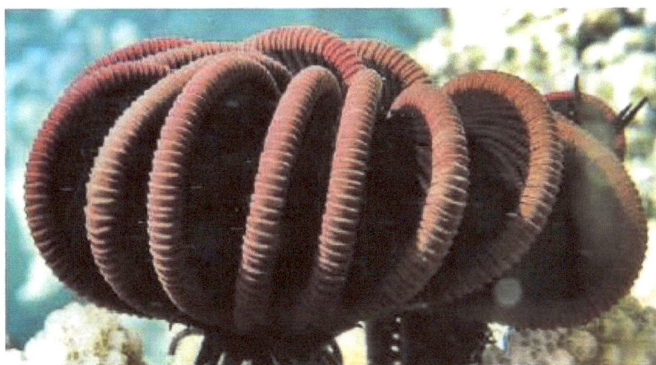

Fig. (102). *Capillaster multiradiatus.*

Strongylocentrotus purpuratus

The rhamnose-binding lectin of this species displayed anticancer activity by apoptosis induction in cancer cells [107].

Toxopneustes pileolus

The polyhydroxylated naphthoquinone *viz.* spinochrome (quinoid pigment) of this species has been reported to display cytotoxicity. Further, this pigment exhibited antimicrobial activities [108].

Tripneustes gratilla

The polyhydroxylated naphthoquinone *viz.* spinochrome present in the nonpolar extracts of gonad and body wall of this species has been reported to possess cytotoxic and antiproliferative effects on most tumor cells. Further, these extracts also showed various antioxidant activities [109].

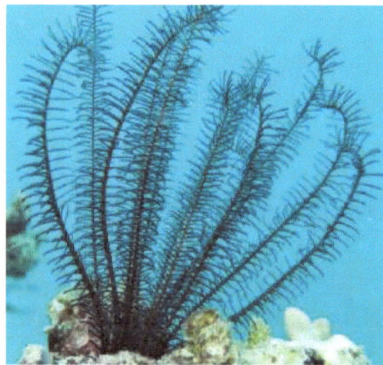

Fig. (103). *Comanthus parvicirrus*.

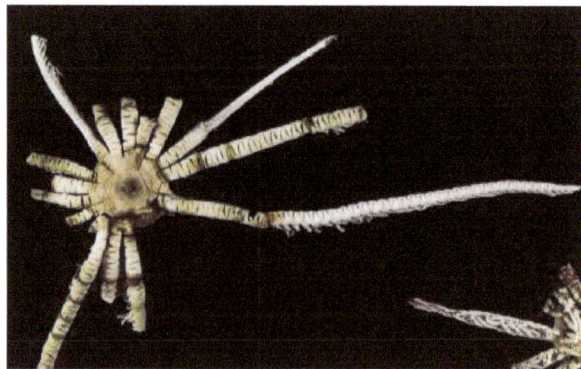

Fig. (104). *Comatula (Validia) rotalari*.

Biopharmaceutically Important Crinoids (Class: Crinoidea)

While the marine invertebrates, such as sponges and cnidarians have been well explored for their bioactive compounds, the echinoderms fairly remain under investigated for their chemistry. Further, among the echinoderms, Crinoids (both stalked sea lilies and unstalked feather stars) have been rarely investigated and only 36 bioactive compounds of 700 species have been chemically investigated to date. Intensive research is therefore needed for the discovery of new chemistry and potential bioactive agents from these echinoderms.

Biopharmaceutically Important Crinoid Species

Anneissia bennetti, Capillaster multiradiatus, Comanthus parvicirrus, Comatula (Validia) rotalaria and *Dichrometra flagellate* (Figs. **101 - 105**).

Image credit: 101, 102: Wikipedia; 103, 105: Wikipedia commons; 104 National. D'Histoire Naturelle (CC).

Biopharmaceutical Compounds of Crinoids and their Therapeutic Activities

Capillaster multiradiatus

The pyrano[2,3-f]chromene, capillasterin A (1) and seven naphthopyrones *viz.* comaparvin (2), TMC-256C1 (3), 6-methoxycomaparvin 5- methyl ether (4), 5,8 - di hydroxy -6- methoxy -2-propyl -4H- naphtho [2, 3-b] pyran-4- one (5), 5, 8- dihydroxy -6,10- dimethoxy -2-propyl -4H-naphtho [2,3-b] pyran-4- one (6), TMC256A1 (7) and 6-methoxycomaparvin (8) have been derived from the EtOH/H2O extract this species. Of these compounds, compounds 2-6 displayed moderate antiviral activity by inhibiting *in vitro* HIV-1 replication in a T cell line with EC50 values ranging from 7.5 to 25.5 μM [110].

Comantheria rotula

This species yielded seven benzo[g]chromen-4-one and benzo[h]chromen-4-one pigments *viz.* 9,9'-oxybis-neocomantherin (1), neocomantherin (2), comantherin (3), 5,8-dihydroxy-6-methoxy-2-propyl-4H-benzo[g]chromen-4-one (4), TMC-256A1 (6), and 8-O-methylneocomantherin (7). Among these compounds, compound 1 exhibited antitumor activity by inhibiting tumor cell growth in the NCI 60-cell line panel with GI50 values ranging from 1.6 to 18.2 μM. On the other hand, compound 6 was found to show tumor cell growth suppression in 5 cell lines with GI50 values ranging from 0.3 to 47 μM. Further, all the above compounds were found to show antioxidant activity by scavenging radicals in a modified DPPH assay [111].

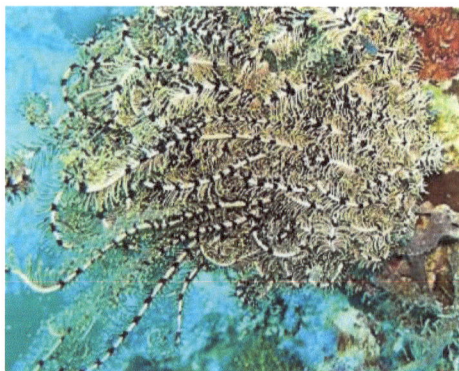

Fig. (105). *Dichrometra flagellata.*

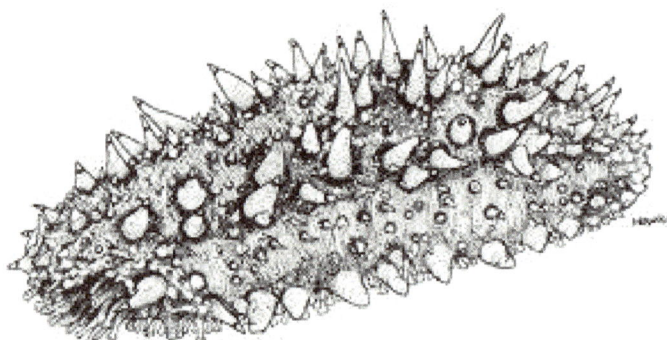

Fig. (106). *Apostichopus japonicus.*

Comanthus parvicirrus

This species yielded naphthopyrones *viz.* 8-hydroxy-5,6,9,10-tetrametho-y-2-methyl-4H-benzo[h]chromen-4-one (1). Xomaparvin (2) and 6-methoxycomaparvin-5-methyl ether (3). Among these compounds, compound 3 displayed potent anti-inflammatory activity in lipopolysaccharide (LPS)-induced RAW264.7 mouse macrophages by reducing the expression of the inducible nitric oxide synthase (iNOS) proteins [112].

Comanthus sp.

Anthraquinone derivatives *viz.* 1' -de oxyrho doptilo metrin and (S)-(-)-rhodop tilometrin derived from this species showed cytotoxic effects toward two tumor cell lines, C6 glioma and Hct116 colon carcinoma. Among these compounds, the first one showed an IC_{50} value of 13.1 µM in Hct116 cells [113].

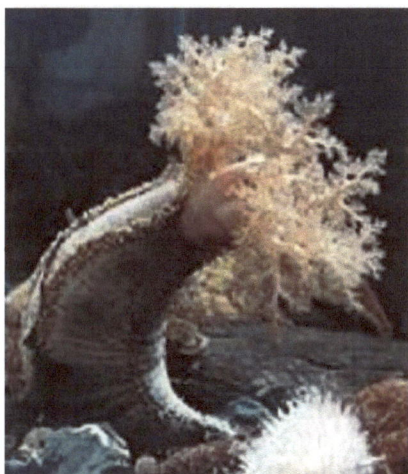

Fig. (107). *Cucumaria* sp.

Comatula rotalaria

Conjugated anthraquinones, comatulins A–E; and a naphthopyrone derivative, 6-methoxycomaparvin 5,8-dimethyl ether have been obtained from this species. Among them, 6- methoxycomaparvin 5,8-dimethyl ether showed antiparasitic activity against the exsheathed third-stage larvae of Haemonchus contortus, a highly pathogenic parasite nematode with an IC_{50} value of 30 µM [114].

Dichrometra flagellata

The sulphated compound, 5,10-dihydroxy-6–methoxy-8- sulphate-2-propyl-4H-naphtho[2,3-b]pyran-4-one has been isolated from this species and its bioactivity is yet to be known [114].

Biopharmaceutically Important Sea Cucumbers (Class: Holothuroidea)

Apostichopus japonicus, Cucumaria spp., Holothuria (Metriatyla) albiventer (= Holothuria albiventer), Holothuria (Halodeima) edulis (= Holothuria edulis), Holothuria (Microthele) fuscopunctata (= Holothuria fuscopunctata), Holothuria (Halodeima) grisea (= Holothuria grisea), Holothuria (Halodeima) mexicana (= Holothuria mexicana), Holothuria (Microthele) nobilis (= Holothuria nobilis), Holothuria (Roweothuria) poli (= Holothuria poli), Holothuria (Metriatyla) scabra (= Holothuria scabra), Isostichopus badionotus, Stichopus horrens (= Stichopus variegatus) and Thelenota ananas (Figs. **106-118**).

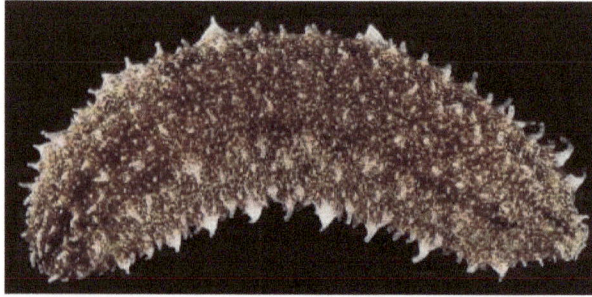

Fig. (108). *Holothuria (Metriatyla) albiventer.*

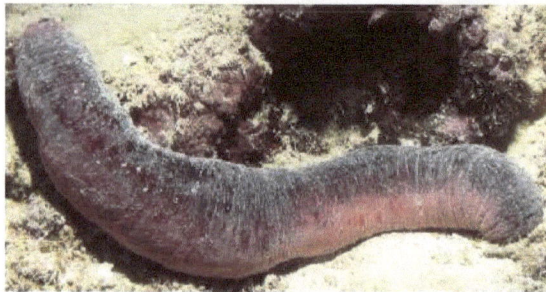

Fig. (109). *Holothuria (Halodeima) edulis.*

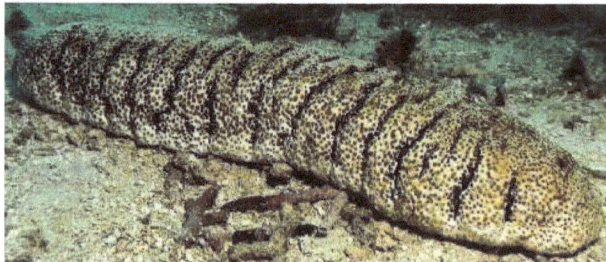

Fig. (110). *Holothuria (Microthele) fuscopunctata.*

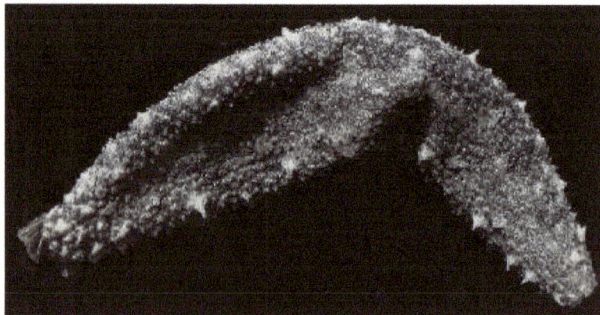

Fig. (111). *Holothuria (Halodeima) grisea.*

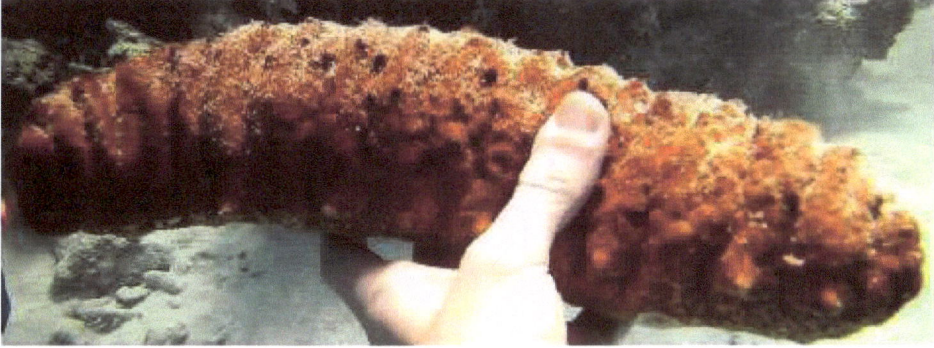

Fig. (112). *Holothuria (Halodeima) mexicana.*

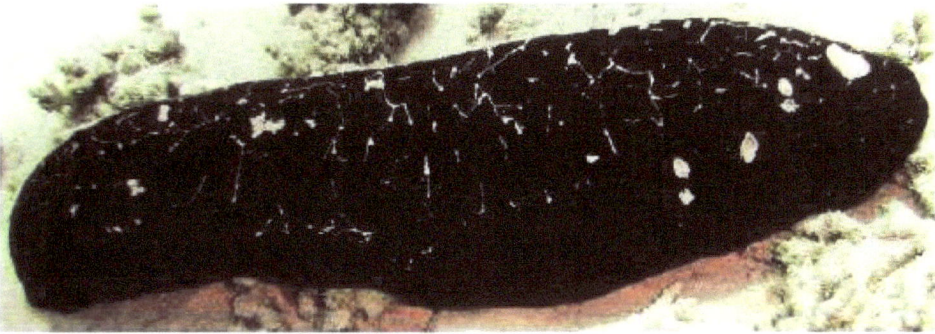

Fig. (113). *Holothuria (Microthele) nobilis.*

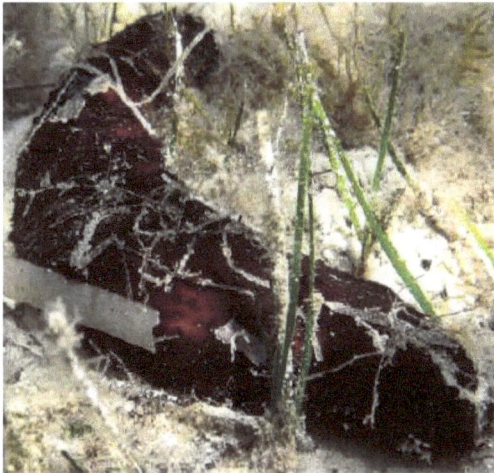

Fig. (114). *Holothuria (Roweothuria) poli.*

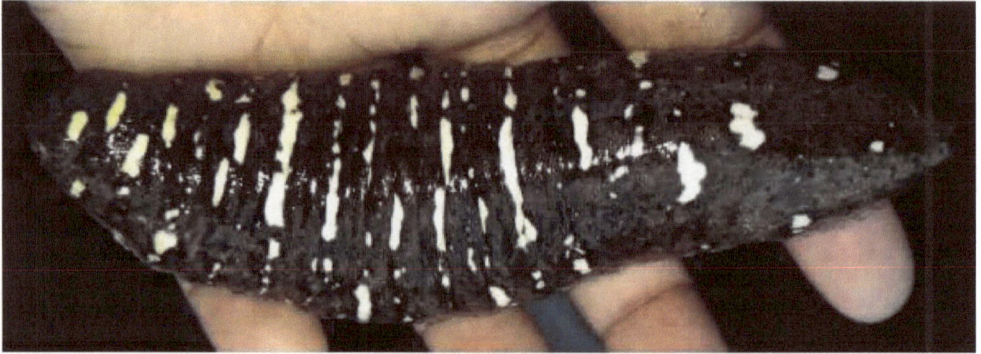

Fig. (115). *Holothuria (Metriatyla) scabra.*

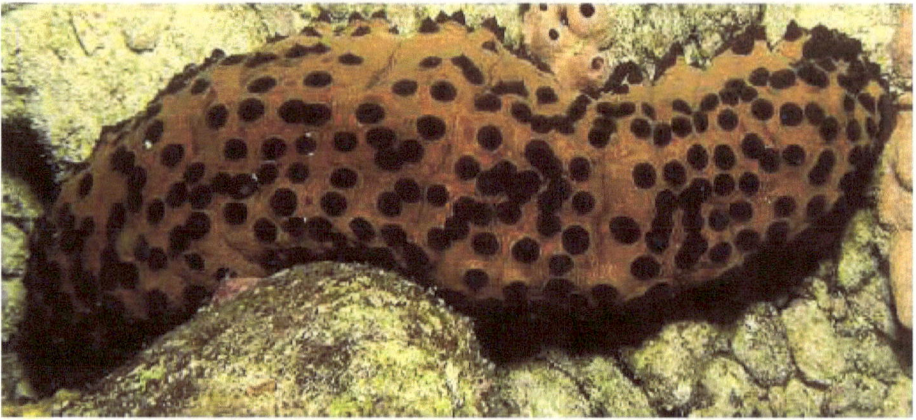

Fig. (116). *Isostichopus badionotus.*

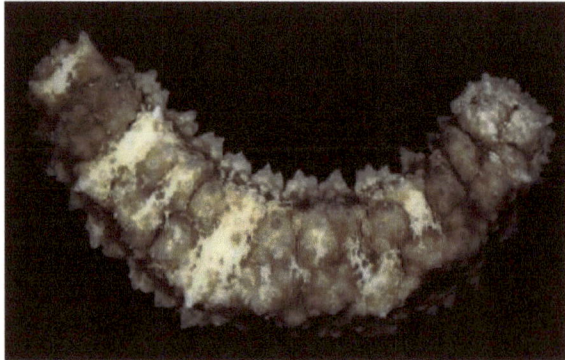

Fig. (117). *Stichopus horrens.*

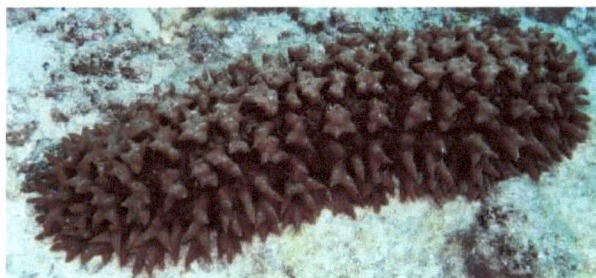

Fig. (118). *Thelenota ananas.*

Image credit: 106, FAO (CC); 107-110, 112-118: Wikipedia; 111: Wikidata.

Several species of sea cucumbers have been reported to possess potential anticancer and anti-inflammatory compounds as shown in Tables **8** and **9**.

Table 8. Anticancer compounds of sea cucumbers.

Species	Compound(s)	Chemistry	Activity	Refs.
Acaudina molpadioides	Cerebrosides	Glycosphingolipids	Antitumor	[115]
Apostichopus japonicus	Intestinal peptides	----	Antitumor/Apoptosis	[115]
Apostichopus japonicus	(5Z)-dec-5-en-1-yl sulfate, (3 E)-dec-3 en-1-yl sulfate, 2,6-dimethylheptyl sulphate, octyl sulfate and decyl sulfate	Alkenes	Cytotoxicity	[11]
Apostichopus japonicus	Holotoxin A1	Triterpene glycoside	Blood leukocyte increase; Anti-carcinogenic	[115]
Colochirus quadrangularis	Coloquadranoside A	Sulphated saponin	Antitumor	[115]
Cucumaria frondosa	Frondoside A	Saponin	Cytotoxicity	[11]
Cucumaria japonica	Cucumarioside A2-2	Saponin	Cytostatic	[11]
Cucumaria japonica	Cumaside	Saponin	Cytotoxicity	[11]
Holothuria fuscopunctata	Fucosylated glycosaminoglycan	Oligosaccharide	Antimetastatic	[11]
Holothuria lessoni	Lessoniosides A-K	Acetylated saponins	Antitumor	[98]
Holothuria moebii	Holothurin A, Moebioside A, Holothurin B, 24-dehydroechinoside B	Sulphated saponins	Antitumor	[115]

(Table 8) cont.....

Species	Compound(s)	Chemistry	Activity	Refs.
Holothuria moebii	Sulphated and non-sulphated saponins	-	Cytotoxicity	[11]
Holothuria poli	Bivittoside	Glycoside	Cytotoxicity	[111]
Pearsonothuria graeffei	Echinoside A	Saponin	Antitumor.	[11]
Stichopus horrens	Stichorrenosides A-D,E	Saponins	Cytotoxicity	[11]
Stichopus japonicus	Acid mucopolysaccharide	-	Anti-metastasis and immunomodulatory	[115]
Stichopus japonicus	Sulphated fucans	Polysaccharides	Cytotoxicity	[11]
Stichopus variegatus	Fucosylated chondroitin sulphates (FCS)	Polysaccharides	Antitumor	[11]
Thelenota anax	Stichoposide C	Triterpene glycoside	Antitumor	[115]

Table 9. Anti-inflammatory compounds of sea cucumbers [99].

Species	Compound(s)	Chemistry	Mechanism
Apostichopus japonicus and *Stichopus chloronotus*	Fucosylated chondroitin sulphate (FCS)	Polysaccharide	Reducing neutrophil migration and paw edema.
Apostichopus japonicus and *Acaudina leucoprocta*	GPSGRP, GPAGPR, PQGETGA, GFDGPEGPR	Peptides	Downregulating proinflammatory cytokines and upregulating anti-inflammatory cytokines, and inhibiting TLR4/MyD88/NF-κB signaling pathway.
Apostichopus japonicus	GL, APA	Peptide	Suppressing leukocyte migration and ACE enzyme inhibition.
Apostichopus japonicus	Hydrolysate	-	Blocking NF-kB activation by suppressing proinflammatory cytokines
Apostichopus japonicus	Fatty acids	-	Reducing eosinophil infiltration and goblet cell hyperplasia,; and attenuating IL-4, IL-5, IL-13, IL-17 and increasing anti-inflammatory cytokines TGFβ and IL-10.
Cucumaria frondosa	Eicosapentaenoic acids	Omega-3 fatty acids	Reducing serum TNFα, IL-6 and MCP-1; attenuaing macrophage infiltration and attenuating phosphorylation of NF-κB in Raw264.7 macrophages.
Cucumaria frondosa	Frondanol	Omega-3 fatty acid	Reducing inflammation in colon in mice; reducing proinflammatory cytokine and mRNA level; and reducing proinflammatory LTB4 levels.

(Table 9) cont.....

Species	Compound(s)	Chemistry	Mechanism
Cucumaria frondosa,	Sphingolipids	Lipids	Reducing serum proinflammatory cytokines IL-1β, IL-6 and TNFα; and increasing anti-inflammatory IL-10.
Cucumaria frondosa	Frondanol A5	Omega-3 fatty acid	Reducing inflammatory cytokines and suppressing mRNA expression of inflammatory markers.
Holothuria albiventer and *Cucumaria frondosa*	Sulfated fucan /FCS	Polysaccharide	Suppressing production of proinflammatory cytokines *viz.* TNFα and IL-6.
Holothuria forskali and *Parastichopus tremulus*	Hydrolysate	----	Reducing VCAM-1, ICAM-1 and IL-6 expression in endothelial cells; and inhibiting ACE-1.
Holothuria thomasi	Triterpenoid Glycoside	----	Reducing serum IL-6, TNFα levels.
Isostichopus badionotus	FCS	Polysaccharide	Suppressing TPA-mediated up-regulation of TNFα, IL-6, NF-κB, iNOS, IL-10, IL-11, COX-2 and STAT3 genes.
Isostichopus badionotus	Fucoidan	Sulphated polysaccharide	Regulating serum inflammatory cytokines (TNFα, CRP, MIP-1, IL-1β, IL-6, and IL-10)
Pearsonothuria graeffei	Triterpenoid glycoside liposomes	-	Reducing TNFα, IL-1β, and IL-6.
Stichopus japonicus	Peptides	-	Suppressing NO production and mRNA expression of inflammatory mediators (iNOS, TNFα, IL-1β and IL-6).
Stichopus japonicus	Collagen	Protein	Suppressing mRNA expression of inflammatory cytokines in synoviocytes.
Stichopus japonicus	Yolk protein	-	Preventing tissue damage, promotes IL-4 and IL-10.

OTHER PROMISING COMPOUNDS OF SEA CUCUMBERS AND THEIR THERAPEUTIC USES

Antihyperglycemic Effects

The fucoidan and FCS derived from the species of sea cucumber, such as *Acaudina molpadioides, Cucumaria frondosa, Isostichopus badionotus* and *Pearsonothuria graeffei* have been reported to possess antihyperglycemic properties [115].

For Treating Insulin Resistance

Fucoidan is derived from *Isostichopus badionotus*; FCS from *Acaudina molpadioides*; fucoidan, EPA-enriched phospholipids and sterol sulphate from *Cucumaria frondosa*; glycosaminoglycan from *Apostichopus japonicus*; and the saponins, holothurin A and echinoside A derived from *Pearsonothuria graeffei* have been reported to treat insulin resistance by inhibiting gluconeogenesis, the promotion of glycogen synthesis [115].

Antidiabetic Activity

Cucumaria frondosa

The oral gavage of the extract of this species into a high-fat-diet (HFD) and streptozotocin (STZ) induced T2DM rat model for 8 weeks led to the amelioration of hyperglycemia, restoration of hypertriglyceridemia and hypercholesterolemia, and reduction in inflammatory status and oxidative stress thereby protecting against liver injury. Further, the intragastrical administration of EPA-enriched phosphatidylcholine derived from this species induced hyperglycemic rat model. Furthermore, the intragastrical administration (at 10mg/kg/day) of glycosphingolipids of this species has been reported to act against type 2 diabetic nephropathy.

Holothuria leucospilota

The polysaccharide of this species has been reported to improve glucose intolerance and regulate blood lipid and hormone levels.

Thelenota ananas and Cucumaria frondosa

The oral gavage of a fucoidan-dominated polysaccharide fraction of *Thelenota ananas* and a FCS dominated polysaccharide fraction of *Cucumaria frondosa* into a HFD and streptozotocin (STZ) induced T2DM rat model for 8 weeks has been reported to ameliorate hyperglycemia, restore hypertriglyceridemia and hypercholesterolemia, decrease inflammatory status and oxidative stress, and protect against liver injury.

Anticoagulant Activity

The polysaccharide compound, fucosylated chondroitin sulphate (FCS) of several species of sea cucumbers such as *Apostichopus japonicus, Cucumaria frondosa, Holothuria mexicana, Holothuria edulis, Holothuria albiventer, Holothuria nobilis, Holothuria fuscopunctata, Holothuria scabra, Holothuria coluber, Isostichopus badionotus, Ludwigothurea grisea, Stichopus japonicus, Stichopus horrens,* and *Thelenota ananas* has been reported to possess anticoagulant activity [11].

Antihyperlipidemic (Dyslipidemic) Activity

Acaudina molpadioides and Isostichopus badionotus

At a dose of 80mg/kg/day, the FCS derived from Acaudina molpadioides displayed anti-obesity activity by reducing body weight gain and adipose weights. Further, the fucoidan of *Acaudina molpadioide* and *Isostichopus badionotus* when administered at 80mg/kg/day exhibited considerable reduction in the subcutaneous, perirenal and epididymal fat content.

Apostichopus japonicus and Holothuria leucospilota

The polysaccharides from these species when orally administrated to an HFD induced rat for 28 days, caused significant reduction in the serum total cholesterol (TC), triglyceride (TG) and low-density lipoprotein (LDL-C).

Cucumaria frondosa

The saponins of this species have been reported to effectively suppress the adipose accumulation and reduce serum and hepatic lipids. Further, its EPA-enriched phospholipids suppressed lipid accumulation and lipid droplets (LDs) in liver and white adipose tissue.

Apostichopus japonicus and Holothuria leucospilota

The polysaccharides of these species when orally administrated to an HFD induced rat for 28 days significantly reduced the serum total cholesterol (TC), triglyceride (TG) and low-density lipoprotein (LDL-C). Further, the saponin-enriched extracts of *Holothuria leucospilota* significantly decreased the fat deposition and triglyceride levels.

Isostichopus badionotus and Pearsonothuria graeffei

When the FCS of *Isostichopus badionotus* was fed at 40mg/kg/day; and fucoidan from *Pearsonothuria graeffei* at 80mg/kg/day for 6 weeks, it was found to inhibit the serum total cholesterol by 25.9% in an HFD-fed mouse model. Further, when the FCS from *Isostichopus badionotus* was fed at the doses of 20mg and 40mg/kg/day for 6 weeks, both doses were found to significantly reduce weight gain.

Pearsonothuria graeffei

The fucoidan from this species gavaged for 6 weeks could dose-dependently reduce the body weight gain, liver, and fat tissue weight. Further, the dietary saponins from this species at 0.03% and 0.1% dose-dependently displayed a weight-loss effect. Furthermore, the saponin liposomes of this species displayed better effects on anti-obesity and anti-hyperlipidemia activities.

Wound and Bone Healing

Stichopus herrmanni

The gamat oil derived from this species has been used as positive control for wound healing products. For bone healing, a mixture of hydroxyapatite obtained from gypsum powder and collagen from this species served as a bone graft substitute.

Stichopus japonicus

At 30 mg/kg, 100mg/kg, and 300mg/kg, when the peptides of this species were fed to mouse for 14 weeks, this administration was found to protect mice from OVX-induced bone loss by increasing bone mineral density, thereby preventing the bone loss Immunological Disorders [115].

Acaudina leucoprocta

The water soluble sulphated fucan derived from this species was reported to have a significant effect on enhancing the immune response.

Apostichopus japonicus

The FCS of this species have been reported to be the stimulators of hematopoiesis. Further, the polysaccharide, glycosaminoglycan of this species showed immunomodulatory activities in cyclophosphamide-induced immunosuppressed mice.

Colochirus quadrangularis

The saponin, coloquadranoside A of this species displayed effective immunomodulation activity.

Holothuria poli and Holothuria tubulosa

The FCSs of these species have shown immune-enhancing capability.

Neurological Diseases

Acaudina molpadioides

Its glycolipid, cerebroside has been reported show bioactivity against Alzheimer's disease.

Cucumaria frondosa

The glycoside, frondoside A derived from this species has been used to treat transgenic *Caenorhabditis elegans* model of Alzheimer's disease. Further, the ethanolamine plasmalogens enriched with EPA (extracted from this species) has been reported to ameliorate memory, learning and cognitive functionalities.

Holothuria fuscopunctata

The derivatives of fucosylated glycosaminoglycan (FG) of this species *viz.* depolymerized FG (dHG) and octasaccharide have been reported to dose-dependently inhibit deep venous thrombosis at concentrations of 4.0-9.0mg/kg and 3.3-7.5mg/kg, respectively.

Thelenota ananas and Holothuria fuscopunctata

The fucosylated glycosaminoglycan of these species have caused significant cardiovascular and respiratory dysfunction.

Thelenota ananas

A depolymerized fragment of native FCS derived from this species exhibited better inhibition of venous thrombus formation.

Pearsonothuria graeffei

A highly purified FCS derived from this species has been reported to selectively inhibit intrinsic factor Xase complex and displayed remarkable antithrombotic activity.

Holothuria poli

At a concentration of 8 mg/kg, the fucoidan of this species was found to reduce platelet aggregation caused by cyclophosphamide.

Ageing and Memory Impairments

Apostichopus japonicus

The protein hydrolysates derived from this species showed anti-ageing properties through antioxidant bioactivity.

Cucumaria frondosa

The EPA-enriched phospholipids derived from this species displayed neuroprotective antioxidant activity in the senescence-accelerated prone mouse model.

Holothuria leucospilota

The saponin-rich extract of this species significantly decreased the accumulation of lipofuscin, which is an ageing-biomarker.

Stichopus japonicus

The protein hydrolysate of this species has been reported to significantly enhance the serum testosterone level in the male rat and this species is considered to be very useful as an andropause-relief agent.

CONCLUSION

Among the marine invertebrates, the marine crustaceans, molluscs and echinoderms constitute the major fisheries resources with significant biodiversity. But pharmaceutically, these groups are not adequately explored except the sea cucumbers of the phylum Echinodermata. Keeping this in view, intensive research is needed to explore the bioactive potential of inadequately explored groups such as marine shrimp, marine crabs, bivalve and cephalopod molluscs, and all the classes of the phylum Echinodermata except the class Holothuroidea.

Promising Pharmaceutical Compounds of Marine Tunicates: Their Chemistry and Therapeutic Applications

Abstract: This chapter deals with the pharmaceutically important species of the subphylum Tunicata of the phylum Chordata; their secondary metabolites and their bioactivities.

Keywords: Tunicates, Ascidians, Urochordates, Secondary metabolites, Bioactivities.

INTRODUCTION

Tunicates (Phylum: Chordata; Subphylum: Tunicata or Urochordates) are marine invertebrate chordates and are considered as the sister group of vertebrates. Their common name is due to the tunic, the external layer of the body. The test or tunic is secreted by the epidermis and is composed of collagen and tunicin (a form of cellulose) fibres. These tunicates include benthic and sessile species of the clade Ascidiacea (ascidians) and pelagic species of the clades Thaliacea and Larvacea or Appendicularia. There are about 3000 species of tunicates living in the seas and oceans of the world and about 2300 of them are represented by ascidians which is the largest and the most studied tunicate group. Among these tunicates, the ascidians possess a great variety of bioactive compounds with cytotoxic, antimitotic, antiviral, and antimicrobial activities and are of great interest to the biomedical field [116]. The most represented chemical class among the bioactive compounds isolated from the tunicates is alkaloids, (50%) followed by polyketides (37%) and peptides (13%). The compounds related to the cytotoxicity against human cancer cell lines and anti-proliferative activity account for 58% of the total number of bioactive compounds isolated from the ascidians and three of these compounds have entered clinical trials [111].

Santhanam Ramesh, Ramasamy Santhanam & Veintramuthu Sankar

Biopharmaceutically Important Ascidians

Aplidium sp., *Ciona savignyi, Cystodytes* sp., *Diazona.*sp., *Didemnum* sp., *Eudistoma* sp., *Herdmania* sp., *Lissoclinum.* sp., *Phallusia nigra, Styela plicata,* and *Synoicum adareanum* (Figs. **1 - 11**).

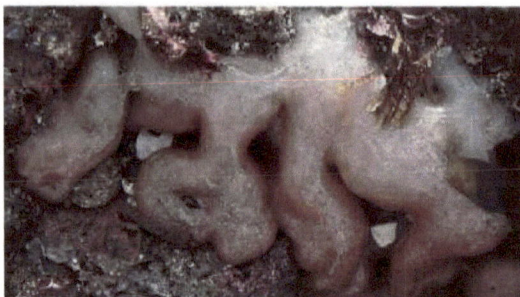

Fig. (1). *Aplidium* sp.

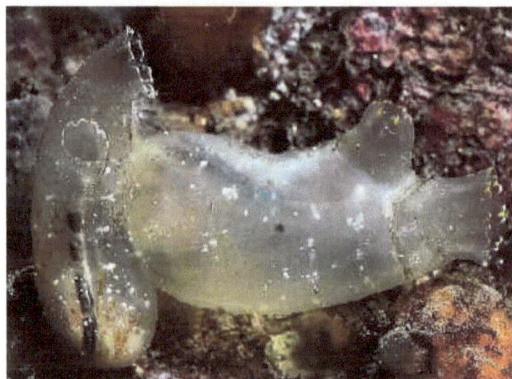

Fig. (2). *Ciona savignyi.*

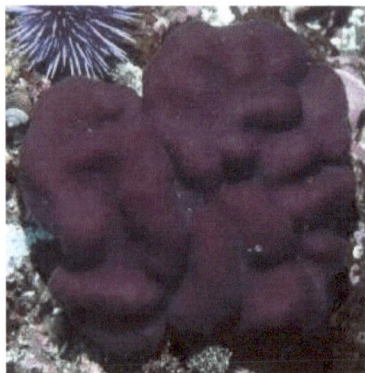

Fig. (3). *Cystodytes* sp.

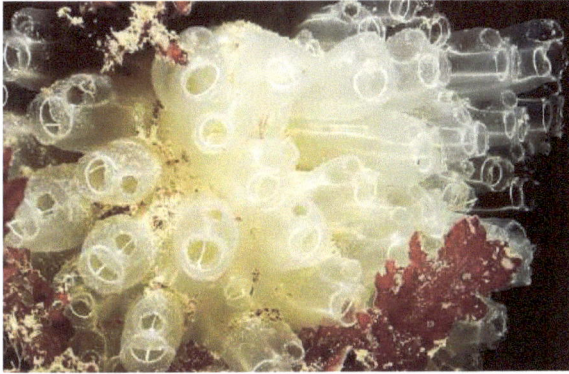

Fig. (4). *Diazona* sp.

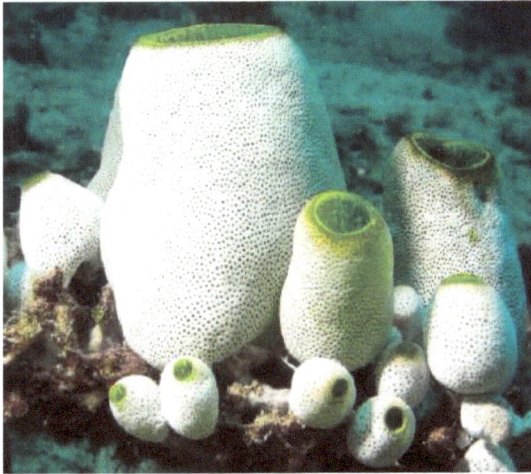

Fig. (5). *Didemnum* sp.

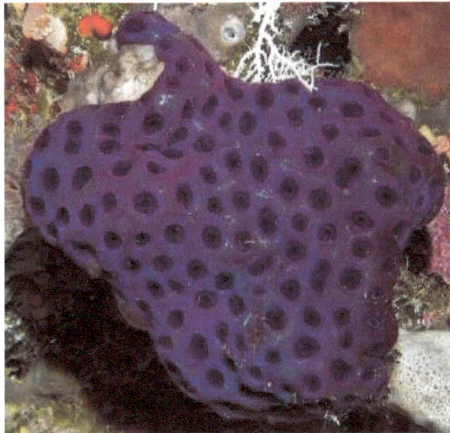

Fig. (6). *Eudistoma* sp.

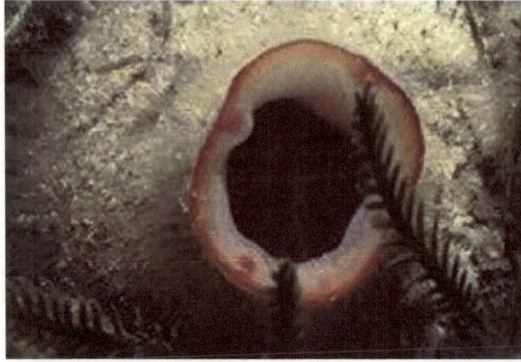

Fig. (7). *Herdmania* sp.

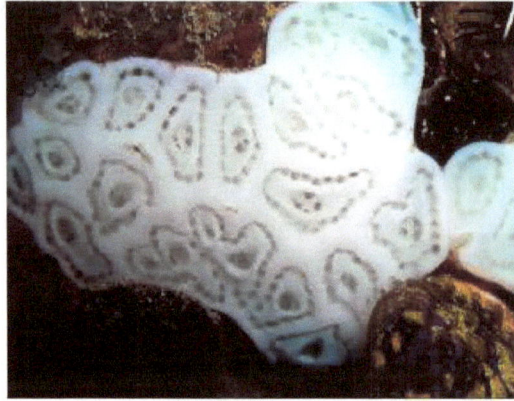

Fig. (8). *Lissoclinum* sp.

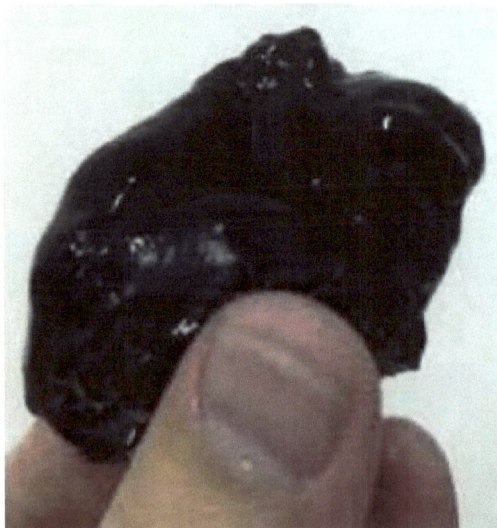

Fig. (9). *Phallusia nigra.*

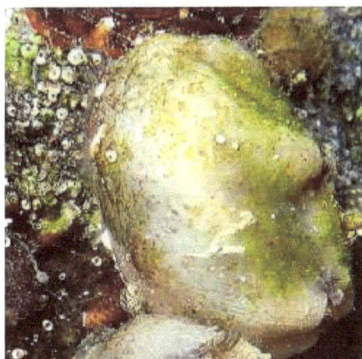

Fig. (10). *Styela plicata.*

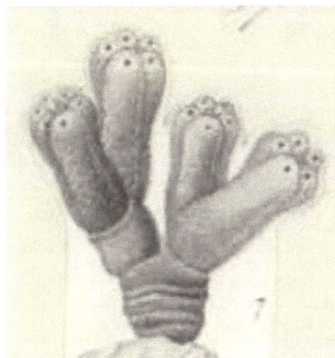

Fig. (11). *Synoicum adareanum.*

Image credit: *Aplidium* sp., *Cystodytes* sp., *Didemnum* sp., *Phallusia nigra* and *Synoicum adareanum:* Wikipedia; *Ciona savignyi:* Wikipedia commons; *Styela plicata*: Wikidata.

The biopharmaceutical compounds of several species of tunicates have been reported to possess potential therapeutic activities such as anticancer, antiviral, anti-inflammatory and antiparasitic and such species are shown in Tables **1** and **2**.

Table 1. Tunicates with anticancer activity.

Species	Compound (s)	Chemistry	Mechanism	Refs.
Aplidium albicans	Aplidin = Dehydrodidemnin B) (plitidepsin)	Depsipeptide	Against Multiple myeloma cell lines, MDA-MB-231 breast cancer cells, A-498 and ACHN cell lines with IC_{50} 1 to 15 nmol/L; against Ehrlich carcinoma cells with 70–90% inhibition.	[117]

(Table 1) cont.....

Species	Compound (s)	Chemistry	Mechanism	Refs.
Aplidium falklandicum and *Aplidium meridianum*	Meridianins	Alkaloids	Anti-proliferative;Apoptosis inducer	[11]
Aplidium glabrum	3-Demethylubiquinone Q2 ; glabruquinone	Quinones	Anticancer, cytotoxic	[117]
Aplidium haouarianum	Haouamine A	Alkaloid	Cytotoxic	[117]
Aplidium meridianum	Meridianins	Alkaloids	Anticancer	[117]
Aplidium sp.	Rossinone, Epoxy- rossinone	Quinones	Cytotoxic	[117]
Ciona savignyi	CS5931	Peptide	Cytotoxic	[117]
Ciona savignyi	Chondromodulin-1	Proteins- glycoprotein	Anti-proliferative	[11]
Clavelina lepadiformis	Lepadins and villatamines	Alkaloids	Anticancer	[117]
Clavelina picta	Clavepictine A,B	Alkaloids	Cytotoxicity; against Murine leukemia and human solid tumor cell lines with IC_{50} 12 μg/mL.	[117]
Cynthia savignyi	Cynthichlorine	Alkaloid	Cytotoxic	[117]
Cystodytes dellechiajei	Cystodytins A-I ; Ascididemin	Alkaloids	Antitumor, cytotoxic	[117]
Diazona formosa	Tanjungide A,B	Alkaloids	Cytotoxic	[11]
Didemnum granulatum	Granulatimide, Isogranulatimide	Alkaloids	Cytotoxicity against MCF-7 mp53 cells; Inhibition of kinases Chk1 and Cdk1.	[50]
Didemnum molle	Mollamide B	Cyclic hexapeptide	Anticancer	[117]
Didemnum psammatodes	Methyl myristate, methyl palmitate, and methyl stearate; and mixture of glyceryl ethers {1,2-propanediol, 3-(heptadecyloxy), batyl alcohol, and 1,2- propanediol, 3-(methyloctadecyl)oxy	Methyl esters	Antiproliferative	[50]
Didemnum psammatodes	Fatty acids	---	Cytotoxicity against leukemia cell lines HL-60, Molt-4, CEM, and K562; and induction of programmed cell death on HL-60 cell line.	[50]
Didemnum proliferum	Shishijimicins	Enediyne antibiotics	Antitumor	[117]
Didemnum ternerratum	Lamellarin sulphates	Sulphated members	Against HCT-116 human colon tumor cells; IC_{50} 9.7 μM.	[117]
Diplosoma virens	Virenamides A–C	Tripeptides	Cytotoxic	[117]
Didemnum sp.-	Tamandarin A, B	Depsipeptides	Inhibition of colony formation of BX-PC3, DU145, and UMSCC10b cells lines.	[118]
Didemnum sp.	3-bromofascaplysin	Alkaloid	Cytotoxic	[11]
Diplosoma sp.	Diplamine	Catecholamine	Cytoytoxic; Leukemia L1210 cells ;IC_{50} 2 × 10−2 μg/mL	[117]
Didemnidae	Siladenoserinol A,B	Bactericidal Gram-positive antibiotics	Antitumor	[117]

(Table 1) cont.....

Species	Compound (s)	Chemistry	Mechanism	Refs.
Ecteinascidia turbinata	Ecteinascidin 743 (Trabectedin)	*Tetrahydroisoquinoline alkaloid*	Against Leukemia L1210 cells; IC_{50} 0.5 µg/mL	[117]
Eudistoma gilboverde	Methyleudistomins	Beta-carboline alkaloids	Antitumor	[117]
Eudistoma glaucus	Lamellarin sulphates	Alkaloids	Cytotoxic	[11]
Eudistoma olivaceum	Eudistomins H	Harmala alkaloid	Against HeLa cell lines ;IC_{50} 0.49 µg/mL	[117]
Eudistoma vannamei	2-hydroxy-7-oxostaurosporine and 3-hydroxy-7-oxostaurosporine	Staurosporine derivatives	Cytotoxicity against HL-60, Molt-4, Jurkat, K562, HCT-8, MDA MB-435, and SF-295 cell lines; IC_{50} 10–58 nM.	[50]
Eudistoma vannamei with *Aspergillus* sp. EV-10	Penicillic acid	Mycotoxin	Cytotoxicity against HCT-8 and MDA-MB-435 cell lines.	[50]
Eudistoma vannamei with *Micromonospora* sp. BRA-006	Antracyclinones (4,6,11-trihydroxy-9-propyltetracene-5,12- dione and 10β-carbomethoxy7,8,9,10-tetrahydro-4,6,7α,9α,11-pentahydroxy-9-propyltetracene5,12-dione)	Antibiotics	Cytotoxicity against HCT-8 cell line.	[50]
Eudistoma vannamei with *Streptomyces* sp. BRA-010	Dithiolpyrrolone	Organic compound	Cytotoxicity against HCT 116, OVCAR-8, NCI-H358, PC-3M, HL-60, and SF-295.	[50]
Eudistoma viride	Eudistomins H	Harmala alkaloid	Anticancer	[117]
Eusynstyela tincta	Kuanoniamine A	Alkaloid	Antitumor	[117]
Halocynthia roretzi.	Halocyamine A,B	Alkaloids	Against Rat neuronal cells, mouse neuroblastoma N-18 cells, and human Hep-G2 cells-	[117]
Lissoclinum badium	Lissoclibadins	Polysulfur aromatic alkaloids	Anticancer	[117]
Lissoclinum fragile	Eudistomin U, Isoeudistomin U	Alkaloids	Cytotoxic	[119]
Lissoclinum patella	Patellazole B,C	Macrolides	Cytotoxic	[117]
Lissoclinum sp.	Mandelalide	Polyketides	Cytotoxic	[11]
Phallusia nigra	Dermatan sulphate	Glycosaminoglycan	Inhibition of LS180 cells ; Heparan sulfate-Polysaccharide- inhibition of LS180 cells.	[50]
Polycarpa clavata	Polycarpine dihydrochloride	Hydrochloride salt	Cytotoxic- against HCT-116 human colon tumor cells ;ED50 1.9 µg/mL.	[117]
Polysyncraton lithostrotum	Namenamicin	Enediyne antibiotic	Cytotoxic, and antitumor against P388 leukemia cells, 3Y1, and HeLa IC_{50} 3.5 nM; IC_{50} 3.3–13 pM.	[117]
Polysyncraton sp.	Mycalamide A	Polyketide	Cytotoxic against cancer cells	[11]
Polyandrocarpa sp.	Polyandrocarpidines	N-alkyl-γ-alkylidene-γ-lactams (Alkaloids)	Cytotoxic	[117]

(Table 1) cont.....

Species	Compound (s)	Chemistry	Mechanism	Refs.
Pycnoclavella kottae	Kottamide D	Alaklaoid	Cytotoxic	[117]
Sidnyum turbinatum	Alkyl sulphates	----	Antiproliferative	[117]
Stolonica sp.	Stolonic acid A,B	Cyclic peroxides	Antiproliferative	[117]
Styela plicata	Dermatan sulphate	Glycosaminoglycan	Inhibition of LS180 cells	[50]
Synoicum adareanum	Palmerolide A	Polyketide	Cytotoxic	[11]
Synoicum adareanum	Hyousterones, Abeohyousterone	Ecdysteroids,	Cytotoxic, Anticancer	[117]
Synoicum sp.	Meridianins	Alkaloids	Anti-proliferative; Apoptosis inducer	[11]
Synoicum sp.	Rossinone, Epoxy- rossinone	Quinones	Cytotoxic	[11]
Trididemnum solidum	Didemnins A-C	Cyclic depsipeptide	Cytotoxic against Leukaemia P388 cells IC_{50} 1.5–25 µg/mL	[117]

Table 2. Tunicates possessing antiviral, anti-inflammatory and antiparasitic activities.

Species	Compound (s)	Chemistry	Activity	Refs.
Didemnum guttatum	Cyclodidemniserinol trisulphate	Sulphated serinolipid	Anti-retroviral	**[117]**
Didemnum molle	Divamide A	Lanthipeptide	Anti-HIV drug	[117]
Eudistoma olivaceum	Eudistomins A, D; G,-J; M,-Q	Alkaloids	Antiviral	[117]
Eudistoma olivaceum	Eudistomins C, E, K, and L	Alkaloids	Antiviral	[117]
Polycarpa clavata	Polycarpaurine A,C	Alkaloids	Antiviral	[117]
Trididemnum solidum	Didemnin A-C	Alkaloids	Antiviral	[117]
Eudistoma olivaceum	Eudistomin A, C,D,E; G-Q	Alkaloids	Antiviral	[117]
Herdmania momus	Herdmanines A-D	Alkaloids	Anti-inflammatory	[11]
Pycnoclavella kottae	Kottamide D	Alkaloid	Anti-inflammatory	[117]
Clavelina lepadiformis	Lepadins, villatamines	Alkaloids	Antiparasitic	[117]
Didemnum sp.	Lepadin D-F	Alkaloids	Antiplasmodial, antitrypanosoma	[117]
Pseudodistoma opacum	Opacaline B,C	Alkaloids	Antimalarial	[11]

CONCLUSION

Tunicates have been serving as an important marine drug reservoir to treat a variety of diseases, including cancer. However, these resources from the from the deep-sea remain largely untapped for drug discovery. Therefore, exploration and exploitation of tunicate resources from such regions would certainly open new insights into drug discovery. Further, intensive research is also needed on the chemical ecology of these organisms as such studies would help in the bioprospecting of marine drugs from this unique group of marine organisms.

CHAPTER 10

Promising Pharmaceutical Compounds of Marine Fishes: Their Chemistry and Therapeutic Applications

Abstract: This chapter deals with the bioactive potential of the different groups of marine fishes *viz.* cartilaginous, bony, and jawless fish species.

Keywords: Cartilaginous fish, Bony fish, Jawless fish, Eicosapentaenoic acid, Docosahexaenoic acid.

INTRODUCTION

According to available reports, the total number of fish species ranges is about 35000 and about 28,600 fish species have been found to be valid. Of these total fishes, 95% are bony fishes (mostly teleosts), about 50 species are agnathas (jawless fishes) and about 800 species are cartilaginous fishes. Further, 58% of fish species are marine; 41% are freshwater fish; and the remaining 1.0% are diadromous (travel between salt water and fresh water as part of their life cycle). Fish are nutritionally, medically and economically important owing to their rich protein and beneficial liver oils known as omega-3 fatty acids. The most vital omega-3 fatty acids present in fish oil are Eicosapentaenoic acid (EPA) and Docosahexaenoic acid (DHA) which are seen in adequate quantities in fishes like mackerel, salmon, tuna, sturgeon, bluefish, mullet, sardines, anchovy, menhaden trout, and herring. All these fish are known to be rich in Omega-3 fatty acid and every 85 g of fish provide 1 gram of omega-3 fatty acids. Ullah and Ahmad [120] reported on the medicinal importance of fish as food and fish oil as detailed below.

i) Fish oil is used for a wide range of diseased conditions including ailments associated with the heart and blood system for which it truly lowers high triglyceride level.

Santhanam Ramesh, Ramasamy Santhanam & Veintramuthu Sankar

ii) Fish is also considered "brain food" because they can treat Alzheimer's disease, psychosis, attention deficit-hyperactivity disorder (ADHD), and other cognitive problems.

iii) Fish oil may also be used for dry eyes glaucoma; and age-related macular degeneration (AMD).

iv) Women may use fish oil to prevent menstrual pain (dysmenorrheal), and breast pain. Fish oil is also beneficial for complications associated with pregnancy such as early delivery, miscarriage, and high blood pressure late in pregnancy.

v) Fish oil is used for diabetes, asthma, kidney disease, movement disorders, disorders, obesity, dyslexia, developmental coordination, certain diseases associated with pain and swelling including psoriasis, and avert weight loss caused by the use of some cancer drugs.

vi) It is also used for rheumatoid arthritis, weak bones (osteoporosis), stroke, and Raynaud's syndrome (Raynaud's (ray-NOSE) disease causes some areas of the body such as fingers and toes to feel numb and cold in response to cold temperatures or stress).

vii) Fish oil is used for complications arising due to surgery itself or some drugs *i.e.* after heart transplant surgery to preclude high blood pressure and kidney damage. It is also used to reduce the chances for the body to reject the new heart. Sometimes fish oil is used following coronary artery bypass surgery.

viii) Fish oil is known to assist hardening of the arteries (atherosclerosis), bipolar disorders, psychosis and kidney problems.

ix) Fish oil is believed to be handy for endometrial (uterus) cancer and weight loss. It reduces the risk of blood vessel re-blockage after heart bypass surgery or "balloon" catheterization (balloon angioplasty) and Age-related eye disease (age-related macular degeneration, abbreviated as AMD).

x) Fish oil has been reported to be efficient for recurrent miscarriage in pregnant women with high blood pressure, anti-phospholipid syndrome, and kidney problems after heart transplant. It also puts off damage to kidneys and high blood pressure caused by cyclosporine drugs.

xi) Fish oil is useful for movement disorders in children, known as dyspraxia. It is often used for preventing blockage of grafts used in kidney dialysis, developmental coordination disorder and psoriasis.

xii) It is extensively used to lower high cholesterol levels, coronary artery bypass surgery, asthma and cancer-related weight loss.

Pharmaceutically Important Bony Fishes

The therapeutically important marine teleost fish possessing promising bioactive compounds are: Bony fishes (Class: Osteichthyes): *Anguilla japonica, Cynoglossu semilaevis, Epinephelus coioides, Hippoglossus hippoglossus, Lagocephalus slatus, Lateolabrax japonicus, Limanda aspera, Miichthys miiuy, Pagru major, Pardachirus marmoratus, Pleuronectes latessa, Pseudopleuronectes ameri, Sarda orientalis, Seriola lalandi,* and *Tachysurus fulvidraco* (Figs. **1-14**).

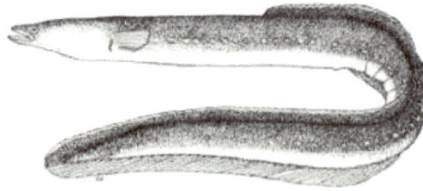

Fig. (1). *Anguilla japonica.*

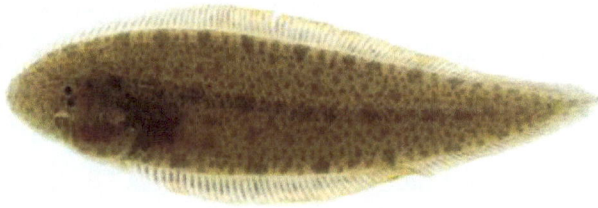

Fig. (2). *Cynoglossus* sp.

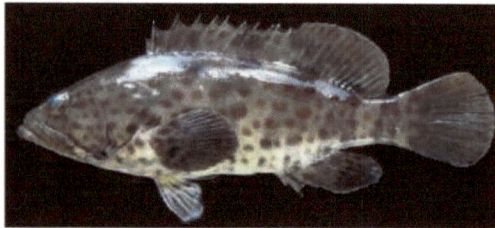

Fig. (3). *Epinephelus coioides.*

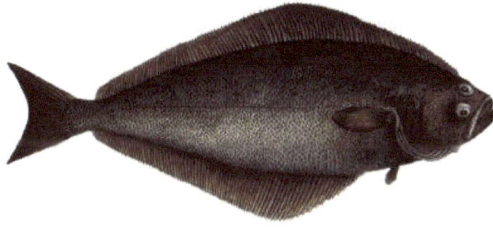

Fig. (4). *Hippoglossus hippoglossus.*

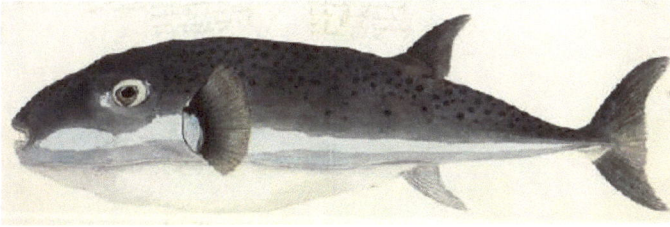

Fig. (5). *Lagocephalus sceleratus.*

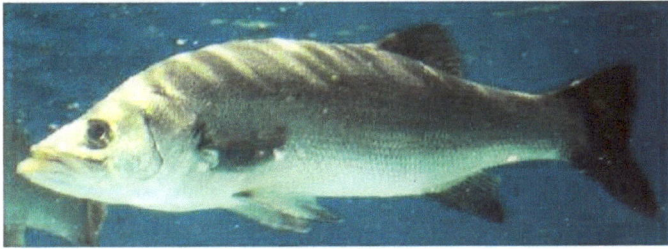

Fig. (6). *Lateolabrax japonicus.*

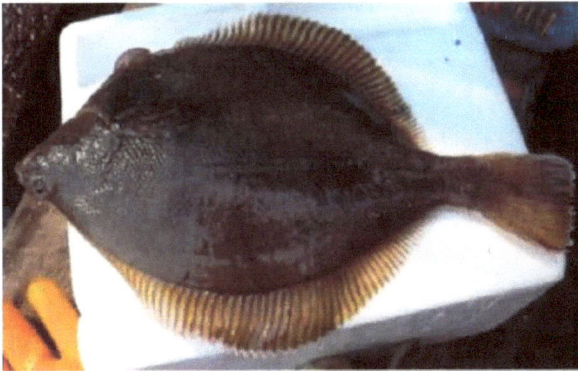

Fig. (7). *Limanda aspera.*

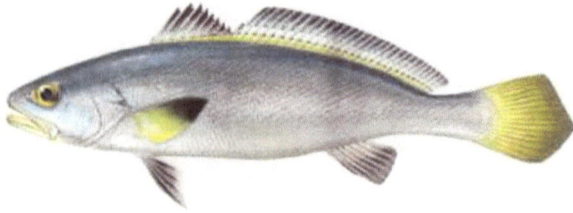

Fig. (8). *Miichthys miiuy.*

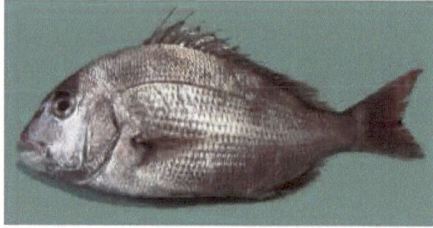

Fig. (9). *Pagrus major.*

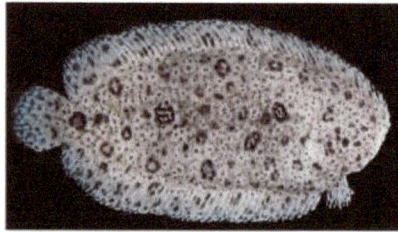

Fig. (10). *Pardachirus marmoratus.*

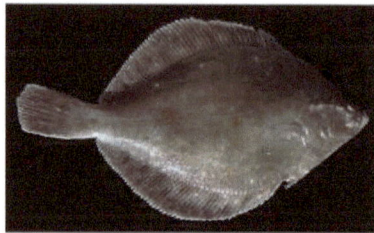

Fig. (11). *Pleuronectes platessa.*

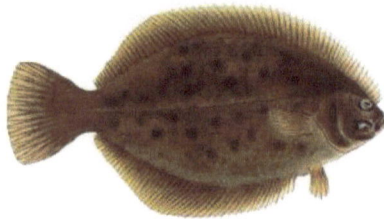

Fig. (12). *Pseudopleuronectes americanus.*

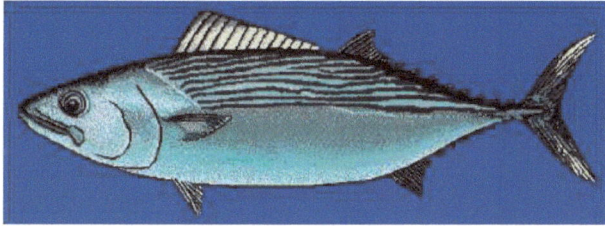

Fig. (13). *Sarda orientalis.*

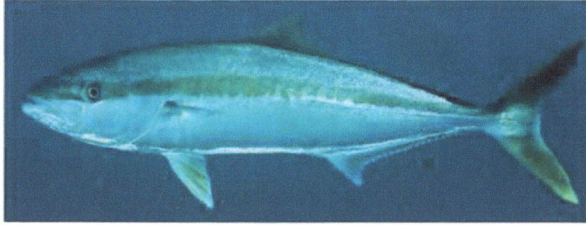

Fig. (14). *Seriola lalandi.*

Image credit; *Anguilla japonica,* FAO (CC); *Cynoglossus semilaevis,* Wikipedia; *Epinephelus coioides,* Wikipedia; *Hippoglossus hippoglossus,* Wikipedia; *Lagocephalus sceleratus,* Wikipedia commons; *Lateolabrax japonicus* – Fishes of Australia. (CC) *Limanda aspera* - Wikipedia commons; *Miichthys miiuy* – EOL (Applied for permission); *Pagrus major,* Wikipedia; *Pardachirus marmoratus-* India Biodiversity Portal (applied for permission) *Pleuronectes platessa,* Wikipedia; *Pseudopleuronectes americanus,* Wikipedia; *Sarda orientalis,* Wikipedia; *Seriola lalandi.* - Fishes of Australia (CC).

BIOPHARMACEUTICALS FROM MARINE FISHES

Bony Fishes (Class: Osteichthyes)

Anguilla japonica

The peptide of this species *viz.* cathelicidin 1 displayed antimicrobial activity. Further, the promising compounds present in the diethyl extracts of its skin and flesh exhibited DPPH radical scavenging activity with 89.2 and 61.5%, respectively [121].

Cynoglossu semilaevis

The peptide NKLP27 isolated form this species showed both antiviral and antibacterial activity [121].

Epinephelus coioides

A truncated peptide of this species viz.epinecidin-1 (Epi-1) showed several bioactivities [121] as listed below.

Anticancer Activity

At a concentration of 2.5ug/mL, the Epi-1 displayed anticancer activity against U937 cell line by suppressing the proliferation of cells through apoptosis. Further, this compound has been reported to inhibit about 90% of the growth of A549, HeLa and HT1080 cell lines.

Antiviral Activity

At a high concentration of 125ug/mL, its Epi-1 exhibited antiviral activity against foot-mouth disease virus. In-vitro studies have shown that Epi-1 acted against Japanese encephalitis virus with 40% and 50% at concentrations of 0.5 ug/mL and 1.0ug/mL, respectively.

Antibacterial Activity

Its Epi-1 displayed significant antibacterial activity against Gram negative bacteria such as *Morganella morganii, Escherichia coli, Vibrio alginolyticus, Vibrio parahaemolyticus, Pasturella mutocida, Aeromonas hdrophial, Aeromonas sobrio* and *Flavobacterium meningosepticum* with an MBC of less than 2 ug/mL; and weak activity against Gram- negative *Pseudomonas fluorescens* and *Vibrio vulnificus* with MBC values of 4.2ug/mL and 67.0ug/mL, respectively.

Antifungal Activity

Epi-1 displayed antifungal activity against *Candida albicans, Microsporosis canis, Trichophytonsis mentagrophytes* and *Cylindrocarpon* sp. with MIC values of 25.0,16.8, 33.5 and 33.5 ug/mL, respectively.

Immunomodulatory Effects

In experimental zebra fishes, its Epi-1 showed immunomodulatory effects by gamma-modulating the expression of immune-responsive genes like IL-10, IL-1, and TNF. Further, the Epi-1 has been reported to inhibit the production of some cytokines which slow down the immune system.

Wound Healing Property

Epi-1 has been reported to heal methicillin-resistant *Staphylococcus aureus* (MRSA) – associated heat burn injuries. This compound has also been reported to repair neurological injury by inducing the production of glial fibrillary acidic protein.

Hippoglossus hippoglossus

The peptide hipposin derived from the skin mucus of this species displayed activity against both Gram-negative and Gram-positive bacteria at concentrations less than 0.3um [121].

Lagocephalus scleratus

The crude tetrodotoxin (TTX) derived from the skin of this pufferfish displayed antimicrobial activity against pathogenic bacteria such as *Escherichia coli, Salmonella typhi, Staphylococcus aureus, Bbacillus subtilis, Streptococcus agalactiae, Vibrio cholerae* and *Aeromonas veronii* with the inhibition zone diameter (IZD) values ranging from 8.5 to 20.2 mm; and against pathogenic fungi such as *Aspergillus fumigatus, Trichophyton rubrum* and *Candida albicans* with IZD values 17.1,5.3 amnd 13.2 mm, respectively [121].

Lateolabrax japonicus

The hepcidin-like peptide derived from the extract of this species displayed antimicrobial activity [121].

Limanda aspera

A peptide (with the amino-acid sequence Met-Ile- Phe,-Pro-Gly-Ala-Gl- -Gly-Pro-Glu-Leu) isolated from the protein hydrolysate of this species showed ACE-inhibitory activity with an IC_{50} value of 28.7ug/mL. Further, at a concentration of 1.0uM, an unidentified protein of this species displayed anticoagulant activity by inhibiting the activated coagulation factor XII [120]. One unidentified peptide derived from the hydrolysis of frame protein of this species showed antioxidant activity [122].

Miichthys miiuy

The pepsin-soluble collagen (PSC) derived from the extract of this species displayed significant DPPH, ABTS, hydroxyl radical and superoxide anion radical scavenging activities. Further, its collagen which has shown anti-aging property by safeguarding human skin from UV damage may be of great use in the manufacture of cosmeceuticals. Furthermore, the synthetic form of its peptide, hepcidin isoform -1 has shown antibacterial activity against the Gram- positive *Staphylococcus aureus* and Gram – negative *Escherichia coli* and *Aeromonas hydrophila* [121].

Pagrus major

Its cationic peptide *viz.* chrysophsin-1 showed weak cytotoxic activity against human gingival fibroblasts (HGFs) which are believed to respond with inflammatory protein. Further, this compound showed broad-spectrum bactericidal activity against both Gram-negative and Gram-positive bacteria. It also showed potential lethal effect against *Streptococcus mutans* biofilms which are the causative factors for dental caries and pulpal diseases. Furthermore all its chrysophsin-1,2 and 3 have been reported to display antibacterial activity against Gram-negative and Gram-positive bacteria [121]

Pardachirus marmoratus

A 33-amino-acid pore-forming polypeptide toxin *viz.* pardaxin derived from this species showed activity against pathogenic bacteria such as *Escherichia coli, Pseudomonas aeruginosa* and *Bacillus subtilis* with MIC values of 13,25 and 5 uM, respectively [121].

Pleuronectes platessa

The protein hydrolysate of this species displayed antiproliferative activity by inducing growth inhibition on two human breast cancer cell lines *viz.* MDA-M--231 and MCF-7/6. Further, its protein which is designated as KilC (bacterial killing metalloprotease C) isolated from this species displayed significant antibacterial activity (74%) against *Staphylococcus aureus, Escherichia coli, Bacillus subtilis* and *Pseudomonas aeruginosa* [121].

Pseudopleuronectes americanus

Its purified peptide *viz.* pleurocidin derived from the skin mucus secretion of this species showed antibacterial activity against *Staphylococcus aureus, Escherichia coli,* and *Bacillus subtilis* with MIC values of 17.7, 2.2 and 1.1 ug/mL, respectively [121].

Sarda orientalis

The promising peptides of this species have shown ACE-inhibitory activity. Clinical observations suggest that these peptides incorporated as nutritional supplements may help improve borderline blood pressure and mild hypertensive patients. Further, two peptides *viz.* LKPNM and LKP derived from the thermolysin digest of the dried bonito displayed significant anti-hypertensive (66% and 91% respectively) and weak ACE-inhibitory (0.92% and 7.73% respectively) activities [121].

Seriola lalandi

Two peptides *viz.* piscidin and hepcidin derived from the protein hydrolysate of this species displayed antibacterial activity against several pathogenic bacteria [121].

Tachysurus fulvidraco

A peptide named pelteobagrin isolated from this species displayed antimicrobial activity against *Escherichia coli, Bacillus subtilis, Staphylococcus aureus* and *Candida albicans* with MIC values of 16,2,4 and 64 uM, respectively [121].

Pharmaceutically Important Cartilaginous Fish (Class: Chondrichthyes)

Squalus acanthias

The steroid, squalamine derived from the shark, *Squalus acanthias* (Fig. **15**) has shown several bioactivities as detailed below.

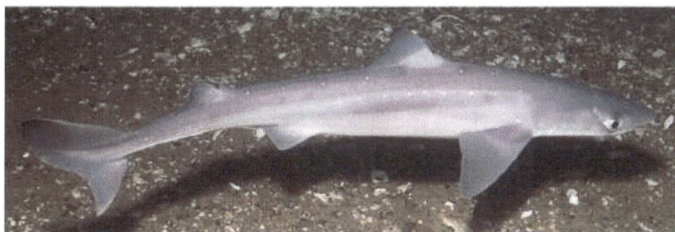

Fig. (15). *Squalus acanthias.* Image credit: Wikipedia

Anticancer Activity

The squalamine of this species displayed significant anticancer activity.

Continuous squalamine treatment at 192 mg/m^2/day for 120 h developed hepatotoxicity in patients with advanced lung and ovarian cancers. Further, this compound has been reported to stop the function of Mitogen-activated protein (MAP) kinase and associated cell proliferation in vascular endothelial cells. It is also suggested that this compound may be of great use in chemotherapy [121].

Antiviral Activity

The squalamine of this species showed both dengue virus Den V2 and human hepatitis B virus inhibitory activities. At a concentration of 100g/mL, this compound showed 100% DenV2 inhibition. On the other hand, at concentrations of 2,6 and 20 ug/mL, squalamine inhibited hepatitis B virus with 14,54 and 84%, respectively [121].

Pharmaceutically Important Jawless Fish (Class: Agnatha)

Myxine glutinosa

An antimicrobial peptide, myxinidin derived from the epidermal mucus extract of the jawless fish species, *Myxine glutinosa* (Fig. **16**) exhibited activity against pathogenic bacteria *viz. Escherichia coli D31, Salmonella enterica serovar typhimurium* C610, *Aeromonas salmonicida* A449 and *Listonella anguillarum* 02-11 with MBC values ranging from 1.0 to 2.5 ug/mL; and against *Staphylococcus epidermis* C621 and *Candida albicans* with an MBC value of 10.0ug/m [121].

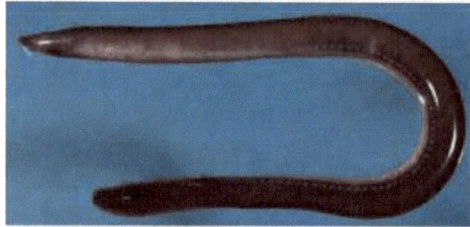

Fig. (16). *Myxine glutinosa.* Image credit: Wikipedia

CONCLUSION

It is understood from the published reports that among the different constituents of marine life, only marine sponges and marine cnidarians have yielded more than 60% of the promising bioactive compounds and there is a big gap on the collection and identification of the therapeutically important species of several marine invertebrate phyla in general and fishes among the phylum Chordata in particular. This calls for intensive and coordinated investigation on the left-out pharmaceutical marine fishes with advanced deep-sea collection methods.

CHAPTER 11

Marine Biopharmaceutical Compounds against SARS-CoV-2

Abstract: This chapter deals with the marine biopharmaceutical compounds acting against SARS-CoV-2. The promising compounds derived for anti-coronal activity were from marine plants such as cyanobacteria (blue-green algae), green algae, brown algae, and red algae. Among marine invertebrates, only sponges and soft corals contributed with their active bioactive compounds. The chemistry and mechanism of action of the different bioactive compounds have also been dealt with.

Keywords: SARS-CoV-2, Cyanobacteria, Seaweeds, Marine sponges, Marine soft corals, Bioactive compounds against SARS-CoV-2, Mechanism of action of anti-coronal compounds.

INTRODUCTION

Nowadays, among the several infections which threat people, viruses pose a very serious danger, with devastating global pandemics. The huge population growth, urbanization and local environments have been reported to be largely responsible for the emergence and spread of these viral diseases especially in many developing countries. The ongoing outbreak of pneumonia which was first identified in Wuhan, China at the end of 2019 was found to be caused by a novel virus known as 2019-novel coronavirus (2019-nCoV). As the International Committee on Taxonomy of Viruses related this virus with acute respiratory syndrome coronavirus 2, it was designated as SARS-CoV-2. Subsequently, on 11 February 2020, the WHO officially named it Coronavirus Disease 2019 (COVID 19) as it was caused by 2019-nCoV, and on 11 March 2020, this viral disease was announced as a pandemic [122]. Among all the SARS-CoV-2 variants, Omicron is the most recent one and it has been reported to harbor several mutations which yield the viral particles an improved ability to infect and transmit between hosts. Further, such viral particles may avoid immune protection even after vaccination. Newly developed therapeutics from different sources have started entering the market and many such therapeutics are still in preclinical phases only. Though considerable progress has been made in immunization and drug development, prophylactic vaccines and effective antiviral therapies for these coronavirus

Santhanam Ramesh, Ramasamy Santhanam & Veintramuthu Sankar

infections are still wanting and therefore, the search for new antiviral substances is the need of the hour. The world experience of marine pharmacy has already testified the marine biota as sources of potential bioactive compounds for developing new and novel pharmaceutical substances and drugs for treating several diseases including cancer. In this connection, the bioactive compounds derived from marine invertebrates could be of great value with their ability to halt or treat corona viral infection. Metabolites derived from the marine biota capable of inhibiting coronaviruses include polysaccharides, terpenoids, steroids, alkaloids, peptides, *etc*. These compounds are not only environmentally friendly, metabolically compatible, and possess little (or no) toxins but are also able to prevent viral entry, viral replication, and protein synthesis, thus completely halting the viral life cycle [123, 124].

POTENTIAL MARINE BIOTA FOR THE PREVENTION/TREATMENT OF SARS-COV-2 VARIANTS

Seaweeds

Dictyosphaeria versluyii

The decalactone dictyospheric acid A, a compound of coumarin class derived from this green alga inhibits TMPRSS2, the priming agent of SARS-CoV-2 [124].

Dictyota pfaffii

New diterpenes dolabelladienols A–C derived from this Brazilian brown alga serve as promising protease inhibitors of SARS-Cov-2 Mpro [124].

Ecklonia cava

A total of 8 phlorotannins derived from this edible brown alga possess SARS-CoV3CLpro inhibitory properties in a dose-dependent and competitive manner. Of these phlorotannins, Dieckol and 6,6'-bieckol exhibited the most potent SARS-CoV3CLpro trans/cis-cleavage and Mpro inhibitory effects [124].

Saccharina japonica

The sulphated polysaccharide RPI-27 derived from this brown alga has been reported to strongly bind to the S-protein SARS-CoV-2 *in vitro*. This polysaccharide may be used *via* a nasal spray, metered dose inhaler, or oral delivery [124].

Sargassum spinuligerum

The phlorotannins and flavonoids, apigenin-7-O-neohesperidoside, and luteolin-7-rutinoside derived from this brown alga have been reported to be the most promising inhibitors of SARS-CoV-2Mpro [124].

Sargassum wightii

Two organic compounds *viz.* caffeic acid hexoside and phloretin isolated from this brown algal species have been reported to serve as inhibitors of the omicron variant. These compounds inhibited important residues necessary for ACE-2 interaction (ASN417, SER496, TYR501, and HIS505) [123].

Sargassum sp.

The drug-like compound, NPC163169 extracted from this brown alga inhibits the transmembrane protease serine 2 (TMPRSS2), the priming agent of SARS-CoV-2 [124].

Corallina officinalis

The cholesterol derivative cholestan-3-ol and 2-methylene derived from the red alga *Corallina officinalis* was found to serve as the inhibitor of the omicron variant. This compound inhibited the novel mutated residues, LEU452 and ALA484 on the RBD of the spike protein [123].

Chondrus crispus and Euchema cottonii

The polysaccharide, lambda-carrageenan derived from these red algae has been reported to possess inhibitory activity against influenza virus and SARS-CoV-2 viral replication dose-dependently [123].

Marine Sponges

The inorganic polyphosphate which is abundantly present in marine sponges has been reported to bind RBD of SARS-CoV-2 and prevent ACE-2 binding. Further, the alkaloids bromotyrosines derived from certain species of marine sponges have been reported to be promising compounds to investigate for SARS-CoV-2 infection blockade [123].

Agelas oroides

The alkaloid compound, (11R)-11-epi-Fistularin-3 isolated from the sponge *Agelas oroides* is a promising inhibitor of COVID-19 [124].

Axinella cf. corrugata

Two coumarin derivatives *viz.* esculetin-4-carboxylic acid methyl ester and esculetin-4-carboxylic acid ethyl ester, derived from this sponge species inhibited SARS-CoV3CLpro *in vitro* and SARS-CoV replication in Vero cells [124].

Axinellae polypoides

The bacterium *Streptomyces axinellae* associated with this sponge produced tetronic acid-based antibiotic teromycins which showed inhibitory activity against cathepsin L [124].

Petrosia strongylophora

The terpene puupehedione derived from this sponge species displayed a good interaction with viral Mpro [124].

Plakortis halichondroides

The compound, placortide E derived from this species showed inhibitory activity against cathepsin-like cysteine proteases [124].

Theonella spp.

A tetrapeptide molecule with the alpha-carboxylic aziridine acid moiety *viz.* miraziridine A isolated from the species of *Theonella aff. mirabilis* and *Theonella swinhoei* demonstrated inhibitory activities against trypsin-like serine proteases, pepsin-like aspartyl proteases and papain-like cysteine proteases. Further, the peptides Pseudoteonamide D and pseudotheonamide C derived from *Theonella swinhoei* displayed activity against SARS-CoV-2Mpro. Furthermore, the aldehyde, tokaramide A of *Theonella* aff. *mirabilis* acted as the lysosomal protease cathepsin B inhibitor [124]. Cathepsin B is primarily involved in the degradation of lysosomal proteins and it plays key roles in the lifecycle of several viruses.

Sea sponges of the family Aplysinidae: The alkaloid, fistularin-3/11-epifistular-n-3 isolated from these unidentified species of marine sponges has shown the maximum ability to bind to SARS-COV-2Mpro [124].

Soft Corals

Briareum sp.

The diterpene excavatolide M, derived from this soft coral has been reported to inhibit TMPRSS2, which is believed to be responsible for proteolytic priming of the SARS-CoV-2 spike protein. This bioactive compound therefore represents a potential tool for the prevention and treatment of COVID-19 [124].

Pterogorgia citrina

The marine lipids of this species affect the major protease of SARS-CoV-2 [124].

The anti-CoV effects of marine biopharmaceutical compounds and their sources and modes of action are shown in Table **1**.

Table 1. Anti-CoV effects of Marine Biopharmaceutical compounds [124].

Source species	Taxonomic Group	Compound	Chemical Class	Mechanism of Action
Schizothrix sp. [125]	Cyanobacteria	Gallinamide A (Fig. **1**)	Peptide	A potent inhibitor of cathepsin L with an IC_{50} value of 17.6 pM.
Lyngbya confervoides	Cyanobacteria (Blue-green alga)	Grassistatin A (Fig. **2**)	Peptide	Inhibits cathepsins D and E; IC_{50} = 26.5 nM; 886 pM
Lyngbya confervoides	Cyanobacteria (Blue-green alga)	Grassistatin B (Fig. **3**)	-	Inhibits cathepsins D and E; IC_{50} = 7.3 nM; 354 pM
Lyngbya confervoides	Cyanobacteria (Blue-green alga)	Grassistatin C (Fig. **4**)	-	Inhibits cathepsins D and E; IC_{50} = 71.6nM; 42.9 pM
Dictyosphaeria versluyii	Green alga	Dictyosphaeric acid A (Fig. **5**)	Coumarin	Binds with TMPRSS2 (2), $\Delta GB = -14.02$
Ecklonia cava	Brown alga	Dioxinodehydroeckol (Fig. **6**)	Phlorotanni	Inhibits SARS-COV-2 3CLpro, IC_{50} = 146.5 µM
Ecklonia cava	Brown alga	Dieckol (Fig. **7**)	Phlorotannin	Inhibits SARS-COV-2 3CLpro, IC_{50} = 68.1 µM
Ecklonia cava	Brown alga	2-phloroeckol (Fig. **8**)	Phlorotannin	Inhibits SARS-COV-2 3CLpro, IC_{50} = 112.2 µM

Source species	Taxonomic Group	Compound	Chemical Class	Mechanism of Action
Ecklonia cava	Brown alga	7-phloroeckol (Fig. **9**)	Phlorotannin	Inhibits SARS-COV-2 3CLpro, $IC_{50} = 112.0\ \mu M$
Ecklonia cava	Brown alga	Fucodiphloroethol G (Fig. **10**)	Phlorotannin	Inhibits SARS-COV-2 3CLpro, $IC_{50} = 177.1\ \mu M$
Saccharina japonica	Brown alga	Sulphated polysaccharide RPI27	Polysaccharide	Binds to the S-protein SARS-CoV-2, EC50 = 8.3μg/mL
Saccharina japonica	Brown alga	Sulphated polysaccharide RPI28	Polysaccharide	Binds to the S-protein SARS-CoV-2, EC50 = 1.2 μM
Sargassum spinuligerum	Brown alga	Apigenin-7-Oneohesperidoside (Fig. **11**)	Flavonoid	Binds with SARS-COV-2 Mpro, ΔGB = −12,4 kcal/mol
Sargassum spinuligerum	Brown alga	Luteolin-7-rutinoside (Fig. **12**)	Flavonoid	Binds with SARS-COV-2 Mpro, ΔGB = −12,1 kcal/mol
Sargassum spinuligerum	Brown alga	Resinoside (Fig. **13**)	Flavonoid	Binds with SARS-COV-2 Mpro, ΔGB = −12,2 kcal/mol
Griffithsia sp.	Red alga	Griffithsin	Lectin	Inhibits viral replication and the cytopathicity induced by SARS, EC50 = 0,28 μM
Griffithsia sp.	Red alga	Griffithsin	Lectin	Binds with SARS-CoV (Urbani strain), EC50 = 0.61 μg/mL
Red algae (Unidentified)	-	Iota-carrageenan (Fig. **14**)	Polysaccharide	Inhibits SARS-CoV-2 replication, $IC_{50} = 2.58\ \mu g/mL$; Inhibis HCoV OC43 (2) replication, IC5 = 0.33 μg/mL

(Table 1) cont.....

Source species	Taxonomic Group	Compound	Chemical Class	Mechanism of Action
Red algae (Unidentified)	-	Kappa-carrageenan (Fig. 15)	Polysaccharide	Inhibis SARS-CoV-2 replication, $IC_{50} > 10$ µg/mL ; Inhibis hCoV OC43 replication, $IC_{50} > 100$ µg/mL
Axinella corrugata	Marine sponge	Esculetin-4-carboxylic acid ethyl ester (Fig. 16)	Coumarin	Inhibits SARS-COV-2 3CLpro, ID50 = 46 mmol/L
Petrosia strongylophora.	Marine sponge	15-α-methoxypuupehenol	Phenol	Binds with SARS-COV-2 Mpro, E score = −7,26
Petrosia strongylophora.	Marine sponge	Puupehedione	Terpene	Binds with SARS-COV-2 Mpro, E score = −7,26
Plakortis halichondroides	Marine sponge	Plakortide E (Fig. 17)	Dioxolan	At 100 µg/mL inhibits SARS PLpro, 68%; cathepsin B, 90%; cathepsins L,85%; SARSMpro, 30%
Theonella mirabilis	Marine sponge	Tokaramide A (Fig. 18)	Peptide	Inhibits cathepsin B, IC_{50}= 29.0 ng/mL
Theonella swinhoei	Marine sponge	Miraziridine A (Fig. 19)	Peptide	Inhibits cathepsin L, 60% inhibition at 100 µg/m L
Agelas oroides	Marine sponge	Fistularin-3/11-epi-fistularin-3	Alkaloid	Binds with SARS-COV-2 Mpro, E_score2 = −7,8
Aplysinidae (Unidentified)	Marine sponge	15-methyl-9(Z)-hexadecenoic acid (Fig. 20)	Lipid	Binds with SARS-COV-2 Mpro, E_score2 = −7,5
Axinella polypoides with *Streptomyces axinellae*	Marine sponge	Tetromycin B (Fig. 21)	Tetronic acid-based Antibiotic	Inhibits cathepsin L, IC_{50} = 32.50 µM
Briareum sp.	Soft coral	Excavatolide (Fig. 22)	Terpene	Binds with TMPRSS2, ΔGB = −14.38
Pterogorgia citrina	Soft coral	(Hexadecyloxy) propane,1,2-diol (Fig. 23)	Lipid	Binds with SARS-COV-2 Mpro, E_score2 = −7,54

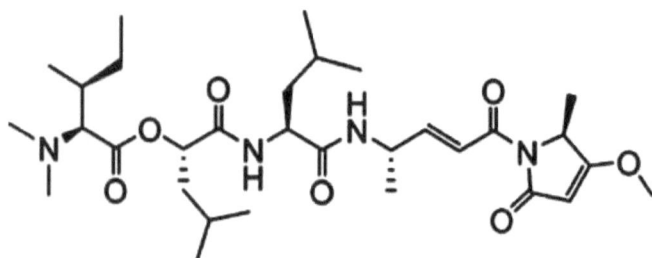

Fig. (1). Gallinamide A.

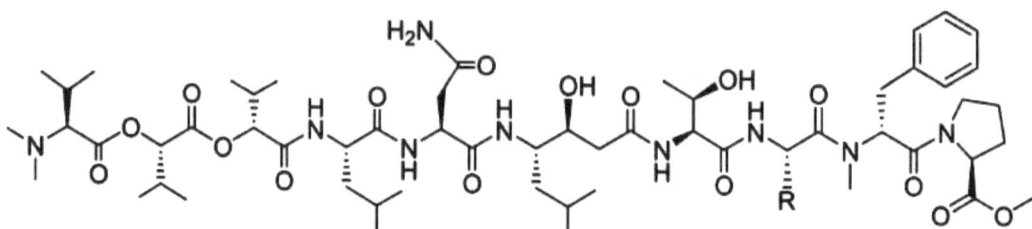

Fig. (2). Grassistatin A (R=Me).

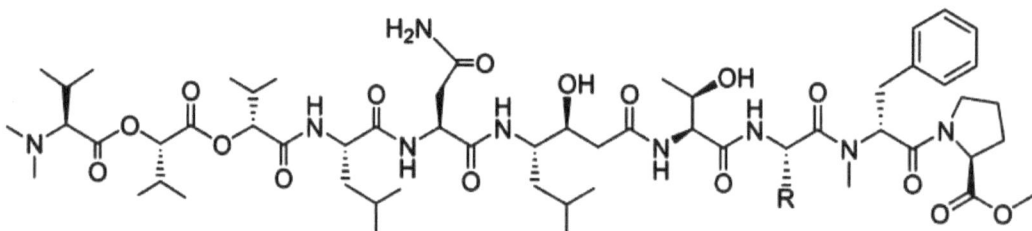

Fig. (3). Grassistatin B (R=Et).

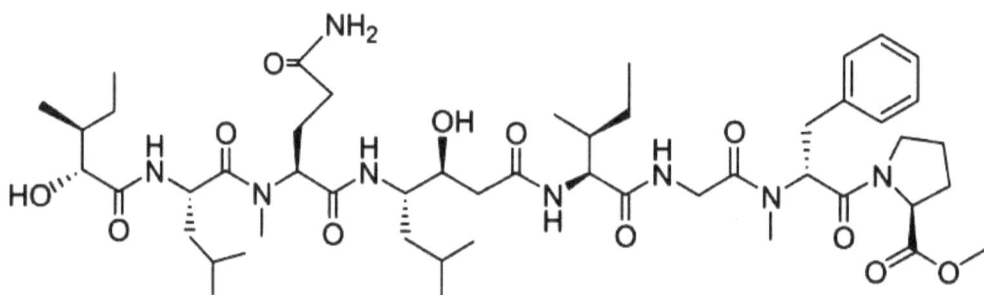

Fig. (4). Grassistatin C.

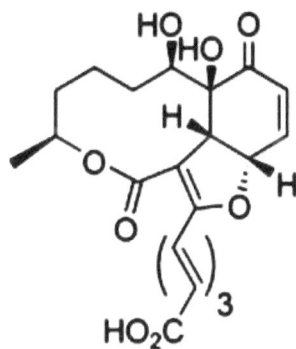

Fig. (5). Dictyosphaeric acid A.

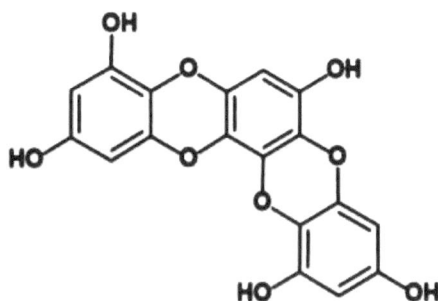

Fig. (6). Dioxinodehydroeckol.

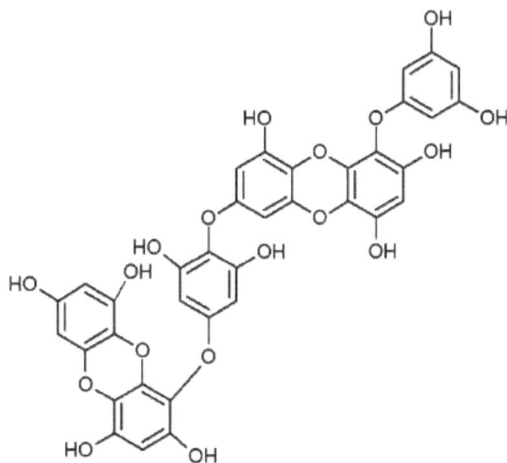

Fig. (7). Dieckol.

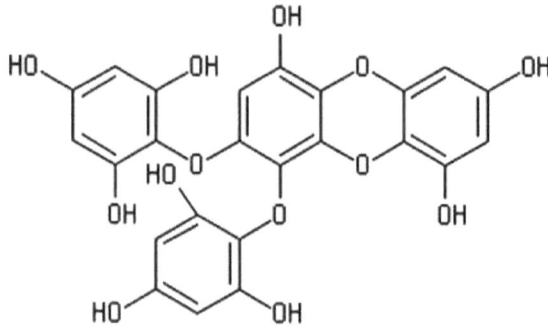

Fig. (8). 2-phloroeckol.

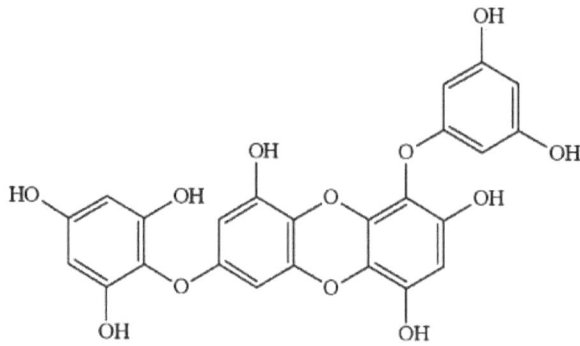

Fig. (9). 7-phloroeckol.

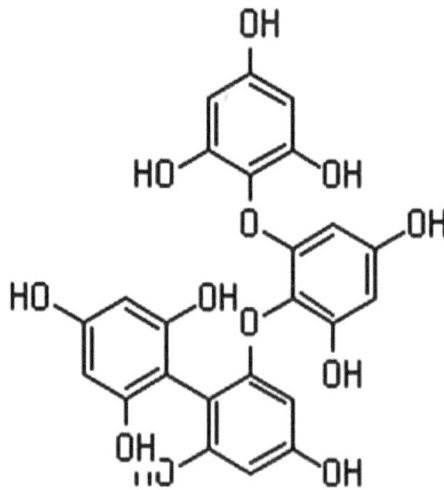

Fig. (10). Fucodiphloroethol.

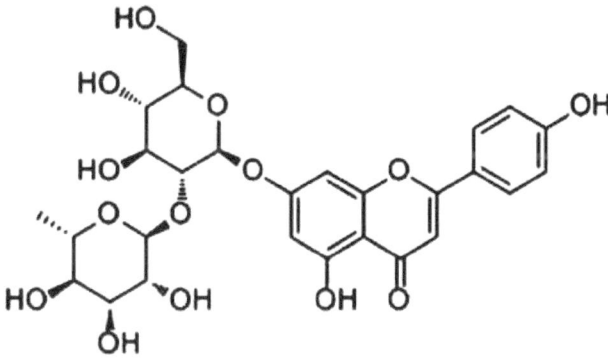

Fig. (11). Apigenin-7-Oneohesperidoside.

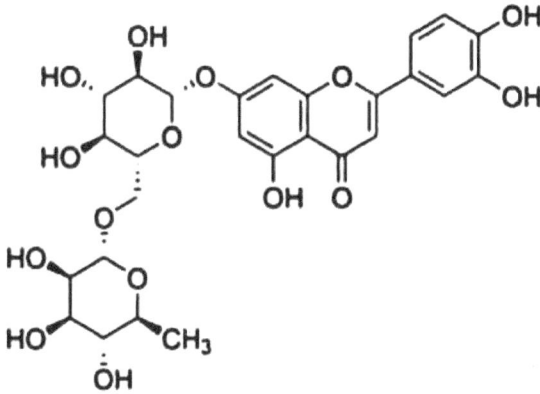

Fig. (12). Luteolin-7-rutinoside.

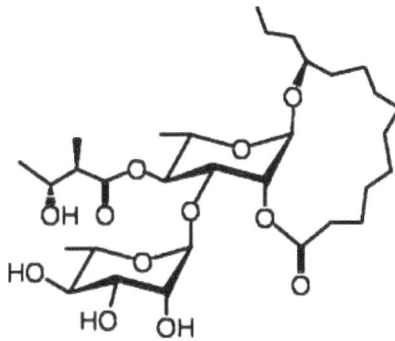

Fig. (13). Resinoside.

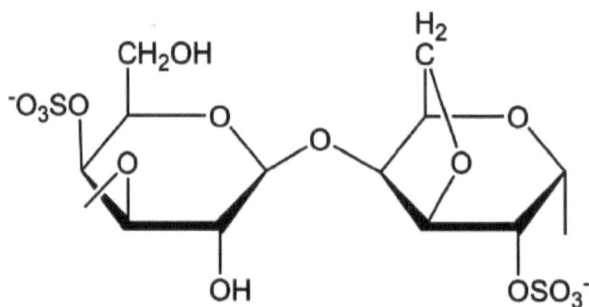

Fig. (14). Iota-carrageenan.

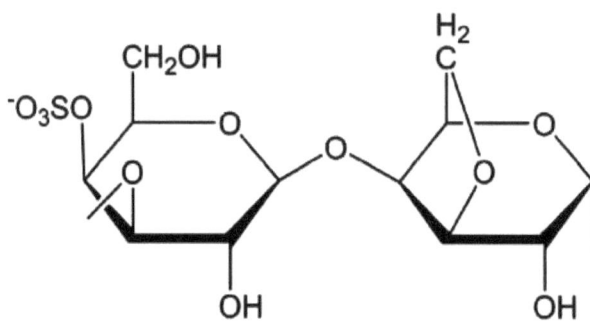

Fig. (15). Kappa-carrageenan.

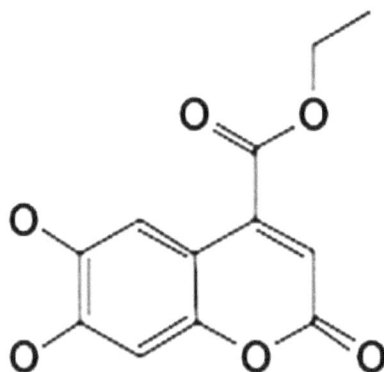

Fig. (16). Esculetin-4-carboxylic acid ethyl ester.

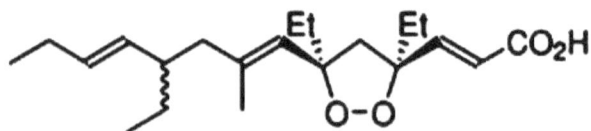

Fig. (17). Plakortide E.

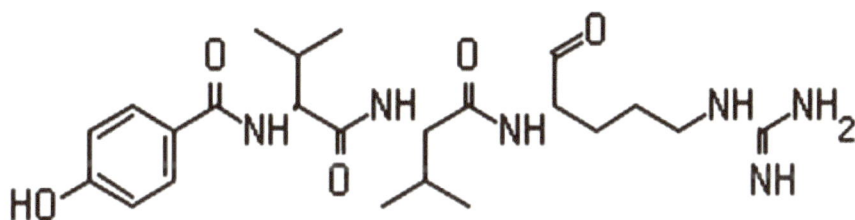

Fig. (18). Tokaramide A.

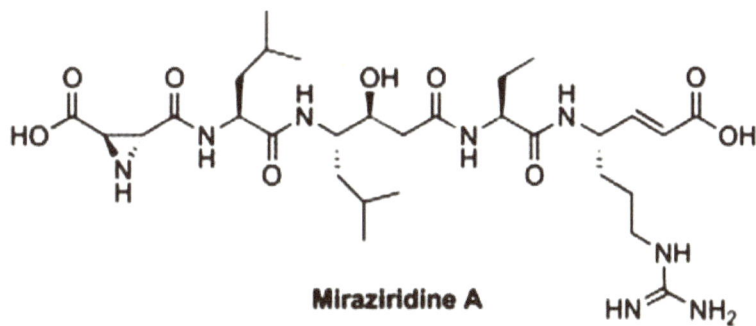

Miraziridine A

Fig. (19). Mirqziridine A.

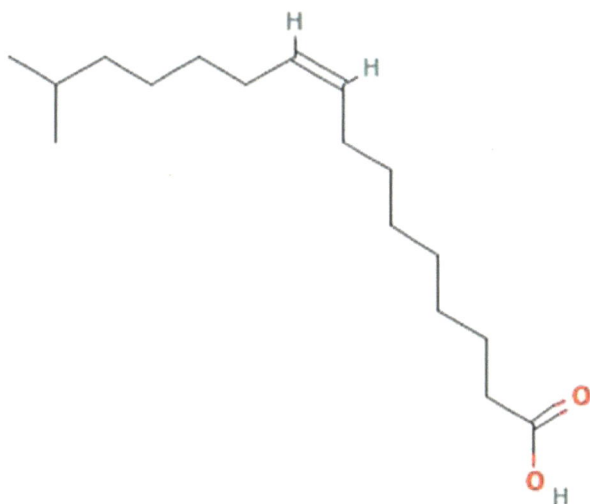

Fig. (20). 15-methyl-9(Z)-hexadecenoic acid.

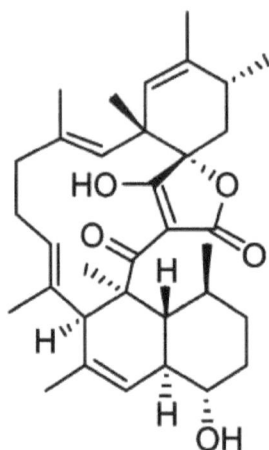

Fig. (21). Tetromycin B.

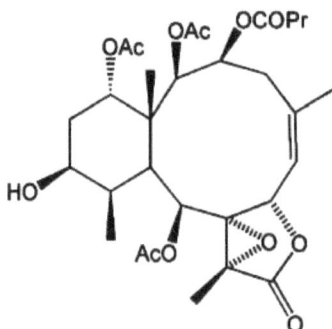

Fig. (22). Excavatolide.

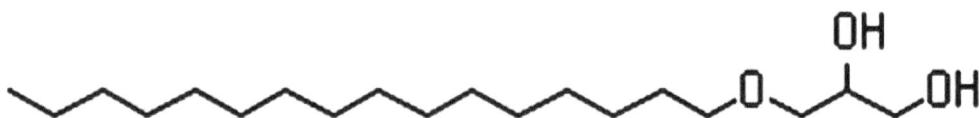

Fig. (23). Hexadecyloxy) propane,1,2- diol.

CONCLUSION

Most of the presently available antiviral drugs have been designed to block the function of critical viral proteins, which is, however, believed to be a unique particular virus or family of viruses. Furthermore, the absence of broad-spectrum antiviral drugs for blocking the targets of host cells and inhibiting the replication of many viruses makes a large gap in the preparedness for emergency situations relating to viral infectious diseases. Screening of the naturally derived bioactive compounds in clinical studies is an important frontline of controlling the coronaviruses pandemic. It is also to be remembered that the high structural similarity between the different viruses *viz.* SARS-CoV-2 and SARS-CoV or MERS-CoV make these viruses respond in a more or less similar way to all the available therapeutic drugs. The diversity of bioactive compounds isolated from the marine biota could be of great value to meet the impending problems. These compounds are only known to inhibit both RNA and DNA viruses but are also able to block the penetration of coronavirus into the cell and disrupt the replication of the viral genome. Several marine biota- derived compounds belonging to flavonoids, alkaloids, lectins, terpenes, polysaccharides, GAGs and peptides, have been successfully tested against COVID-19 and many of them were found to inhibit coronaviruses. These research results give immense hope that biologically active substances of marine origin could form the basis for new anti-coronavirus strategies. It is also hoped that such clinically proven compounds could be important complementary drugs to fight against corona viruses due to their safety and low cost compared to the presently available synthetic drugs. By organizing networked scientific research involving pharmacologists, marine biologists, organic chemists and other related scientists, the problems could be solved greatly.

CHAPTER 12

Marine Biopharmaceuticals in Pipeline

Abstract: This chapter deals with the marine biopharmaceuticals in the pipeline *i.e.* year-wise number of approved marine drugs during the period 1969-2021 and their clinical uses; approved and marketed drugs up to 2021; marine biota-derived drug candidates under the different phases of clinical trials up to 2021; and marine biotaderived clinical level compounds against SARS-CoV-2.

Keywords: Marine biopharmaceuticals in the pipeline, Year-wise approved marine drugs, Clinical uses of approved marine drugs, Marketed marine drugs up to 2021, and clinically tested marine compounds against SARS-CoV-2.

INTRODUCTION

In the urgent need for new pharmaceuticals, the marine biota-based drug discovery has progressed significantly over the past several decades and we now largely benefit from a series of approved marine drugs (= biopharmaceuticals) to treat cancer and pain while a number of promising drug candidates are in clinical trials. However, the discovery of marine biota-based pharmaceuticals has always been challenging and this is due to several constraints including supply problems in pharmaceutically important biota; and lack of advanced technologies, collaboration between academics and pharmaceutical industries and adequate fund support. The development of new and improved organic synthesis methods made possible the synthesis of promising active compounds in the amounts required for further preclinical and clinical studies. Further, tremendous progress in the clinical development of marine-derived drugs has been achieved over the past 20 years. It is interesting to note that in the terrestrial environment, the plant kingdom is the main source of bioactive compounds. On the other hand, in the marine environment, the animals are the primary source of marketed drugs. Further, most of these animals, are heterotrophic, benthic invertebrates with little or no movement and living in symbiosis with microorganisms, which are believed to be the real producers of drug candidates with more relevance in drug discovery.

Santhanam Ramesh, Ramasamy Santhanam & Veintramuthu Sankar

APPROVED AND MARKETED MARINE BIOTA - DERIVED DRUGS

Between 1969 and 2021, 19 marine-derived drugs have been approved. Among these compounds, 13 (68%) belong to cancer; 3 for hyperglyceridemia; 1 for virus; and 1 for chronic pain. The details relating to the year-wise approved marine drugs are given in Table **1**.

Table 1. Year-wise Number of Approved Marine Biota- derived Drugs and their Clinical Uses [126, 127].

Year of Approval	Approved	Clinical Use
1969	1	Leukemia
1976	1	Virus
1992, 1994	1	Leukemia
2004, 2005	1	Chronic Pain
2004, 2005	1	Hypertriglyceridemia
2005,2007	1	Leukemia
2007, 2015	1	Ovarian Cancer
2010, 2011	1	Breast Cancer
2011, 2012	1	Lymphoma
2012	1	Hypertriglyceridemia
2014	1	Hypertriglyceridemia
2015	1	Cancer
2018	1	Cancer
2019, 2020	1	Breast Cancer
2020	1	Ovarian Cancer
2019, 2021	1	Urothelial Cancer
2020	1	Multiple Myeloma
2021	2	Cancer

ADC: Antibody Drug Conjugate; FDA: Food and Drug Administration; EMA: European Medicines Agency.

Approved Drugs

The approved and marketed marine drugs up to 2021 and their brand names, approved agencies, source species, chemical classes, and clinical uses are given in Table **2**.

Table 2. Approved and Marketed Marine Biota-derived Drugs up to 2021 [126, 127].

Generic Name	Brand Name (s)	Approved Yr/Agency	Source/Group	Chemical Class	Clinical Use
Cytarabine (Fig. 1)	Cytosar-U Aracytin, C-Hospira	1969 (FDA)	*Tectitethya cripta* (Sponge)	Nucleoside	Leukemia
Vidarabine (Fig. 2)	Vira-A	1976 (FDA)	*Tethya crypta.* (Sponge)	Nucleoside	Virus
Fludarabine (Fig. 3)	Fludara	1992 (FDA); 1994 (EMA)	Sponge	Nucleoside	Leukemia
Ziconotide (Fig. 4)	Prialt	2004 (FDA); 2005 (EMA)	*Conus magus* (Mollusk)	Peptide	Chronic pain
Omega-3 acid ethyl esters (Fig. 5)	Lovaza (US) Eskim (EU) and others	2004 (FDA) ; 2005 (EMA)	Tuna, Salmon, Herring, Sardines, Mackeral (Fish)	PUFA	Hypertriglyceridemia
Omega-3 acid ethyl esters	Vascepa	2012 (FDA)	Tuna, Salmon, Herring, Sardines, Mackeral (Fish)	PUFA	Hypertriglyceridemia
Omega-3 acid ethyl esters	Epanova	2014 (FDA)	Tuna, Salmon, Herring, Sardines, Mackeral (Fish)	PUFA	Hypertriglyceridemia
Nelarabine (Fig. 6)	Arranon (US) Atriance (EU)	2005 (FDA) ; 2007 (EMA)	Sponge	Nucleoside	Leukemia
Eribulin (Fig. 7)	Halaven	2010 (FDA); 2011 (EMA)	*Lissodendoryx* sp. (Sponge)	Macrolide	Breast cancer
Trabectedin (Fig. 8)	Yondelis	2007 (EMA) ; 2015 (FDA)	*Ecteinascidia turbinata* (Tunicate)	Alkaloid	Ovarian cancer, soft tissue sarcoma
Brentuximab vedotin)	Adcetris	2011 (FDA) 2012 (EMA)	*Dolabella auricularia* (Mollusk)/ *Lyngbya majuscuae, Symploca* spp. (Cyanobacteria)	ADC	Lymphomas
Panobinostat (Fig. 9)	Farydak	2015 (FDA)	-	cinnamic hydroxamic acid analogue	Cancer (antineoplastic activity.)
Plitidepsin (Fig. 10)	Aplidine	2018(Auistralia)	*Aplidium albicans* (Tunicate)	Depsipeptide	Cancer

(Table 2) cont.....

Generic Name	Brand Name (s)	Approved Yr/Agency	Source/Group	Chemical Class	Clinical Use
Polatuzumab vedotin (Fig. 11)	Polivy	2019 (FDA) ; 2020 (EMA)	*Dolabella auricularia* (Mollusk)/ *Symploca* sp. (Cyanobacterium)	ADC	Breast cancer
Lurbinectedin (Fig. 12)	Zepzelca	2020 (FDA)	*Ecteinascidia turbinata* (Tunicate)	Alkaloid	Ovarian cancer
Enfortumab vedotin	Padcev	2019 (FDA) ;2021 (EMA)	*Dolabella auricularia,* (Mollusk)/ *Symploca* sp. (Cyanobacterium)	ADC	Urothelial cancer
Belantamab mafodotin (Fig. 13)	Blenrep	2020 (FDA) ;2020 (EMA)	*Lyngbya* sp. (Cyanobacterium)	ADC	Multiple myeloma
Disitamab vedotin (Fig. 14)	Aidixi	2021 (China)	Fungi	ADC	Cancer
Tisotumab vidotin	Tivdak	2021 (FDA)	Mollusk/Cyanobacterium	ADC	Cancer

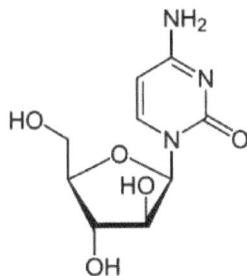

Fig. (1). Cytarabine.

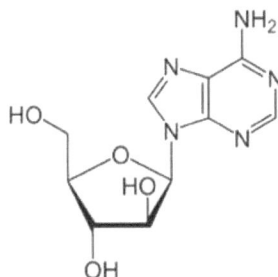

Fig. (2). Vidarabine.

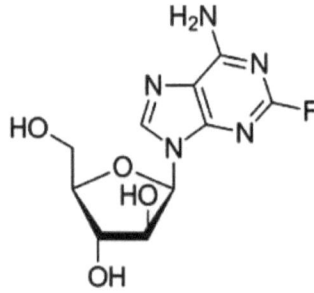

Fig. (3). Fludarabine.

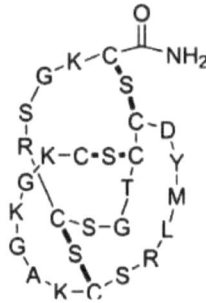

Fig.(4). Ziconotide.

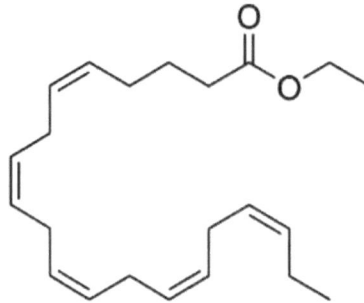

Fig. (5). Omega-3 acid ethyl ester.

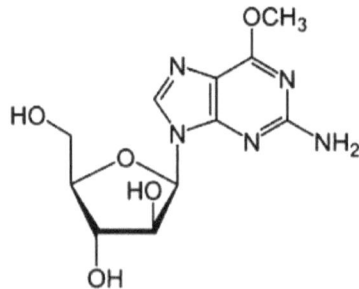

Fig. (6). Nelarabine.

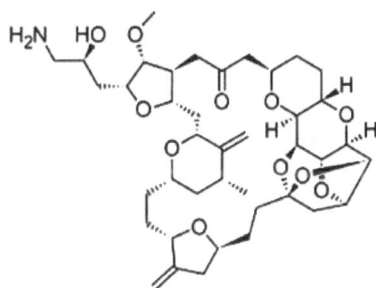

Fig. (7). Eribulin.

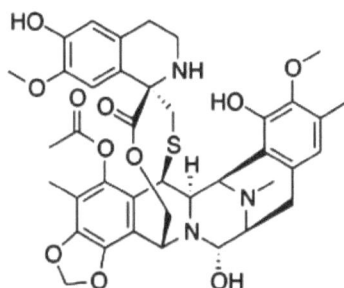

Fig. (8). Trabectedin.

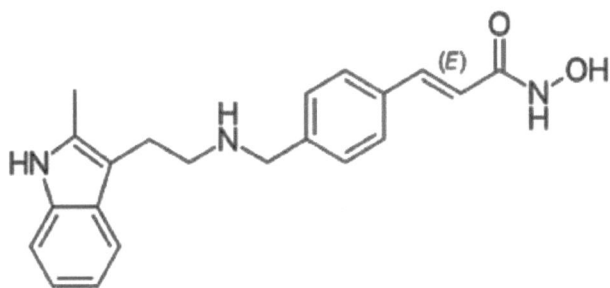

Fig. (9). Panobinostat.

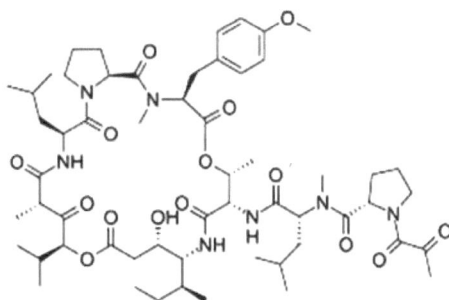

Fig. (10). Plitidepsin.

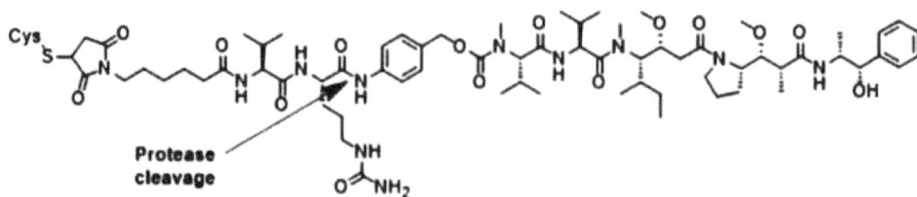

Fig. (11). Polatuzumab vedotin.

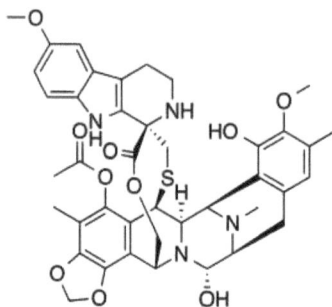

Fig. (12). Lurbinectedin.

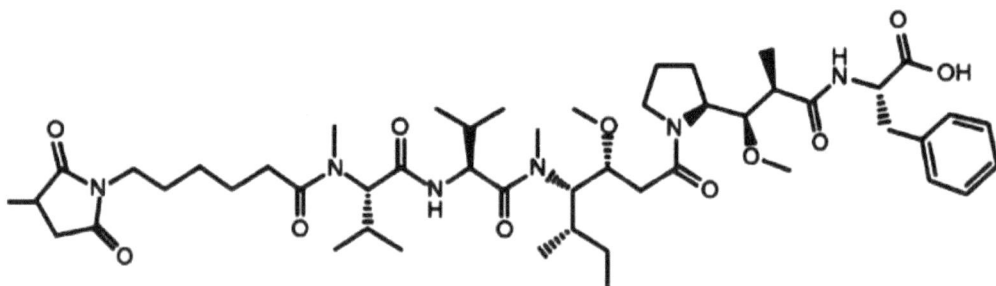

Fig. (13). Belantamab mafodotin.

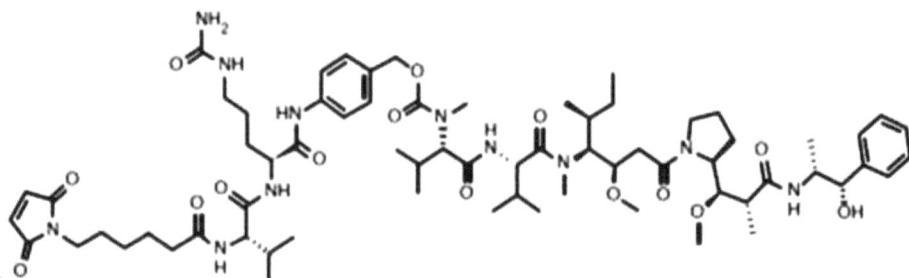

Fig. (14). Disitamab vedotin.

MARINE BIOTA -DERIVED DRUG CANDIDATES UNDER CLINICAL TRIALS

Marine Biota -derived Drug Candidates Under Clinical Trials up to 2021

In regard to marine-derived drug candidates under clinical trials, a total of 65 compounds are under trials up to 2021 (9 in phase III, 20 in phase II and 36 in Phase I) [126, 127]. The number of marine-derived drug candidates under the different phases of clinical trials and their clinical uses are given in Table **3**.

Table 3. Marine Drug Candidates under Clinical Trials up to 2021 [126, 127].

Year	Phase III	Phase II	Phase I	Clinical Use
Up to 2020	2	7	18	Cancer
Up to 2020	1	-	-	COVID-19
Up to 2020	1	-	-	Chronic Pain
Up to 2020	-	-	1	Obesity
Up to 2020	-	1	-	Alzheimer
Up to 2020	-	-	1	Amyloidosis*
2021	5	12	16	-

* Abnormal protein called amyloid builds up in human tissues and organs.

The drug candidates (selected up to 2020) undergoing clinical trials of III, II and I phases and their source species, chemical classes, and clinical uses are shown below (Tables **4-6**).

Table 4. Marine Biota-derived Drug Candidates under III Phase Clinical Trials up to 2020 [126, 127].

Generic Name	Source sp./Group	Chemical Class	Clinical Use
Tetrodotoxin (Fig. **15**)	*Lagocephalus lunaris.* (Pufferfish)	Alkaloid	Chronic pain
Plinabulin (Fig. **16**)	*Aspergillus* sp. (Fungus)	Diketopiperazine	Cancer
Marizomib (Fig. **17**) (salinosporamide A)	*Salinospora* sp. *(*Actinomycete*)*	γ-lactam-β-lactone	Cancer
Aplidin (Plitidepsin)	*Aplidium albicans* ()Tunicate	Depsipeptide	COVID-19

Table 5. Marine Biota- derived Drug Candidates under II Phase Clinical Trials up to 2020 [126, 127].

Generic Name	Source sp./Group	Chemical Class	Clinical Use
Bryostatin (Fig. **18**)	*Bugula neritina* (Bryozoan)	Macrolide lactone	Alzheimer
Plocabulin (PM060184) (Fig. **19**)	*Lithoplocamia lithiostoides.*(Sponge)	Polyketide	Cancer

(Table 5) cont.....

Generic Name	Source sp./Group	Chemical Class	Clinical Use
Ladiratuzumab vedotin (SGN-LIV1A)	Mollusk/Cyanobacterium	ADC	Cancer
Telisotuzumab vedotin	Mollusk/Cyanobacterium	ADC	Cancer
CAB-ROR2 (BA-3021)	Mollusk/Cyanobacterium	ADC	Cancer
CX-2029	Mollusk/Cyanobacterium	PDC	Cancer
W0101	Mollusk/Cyanobacterium	ADC	Cancer

Table 6. Marine Biota- derived Drug Candidates under I Phase Clinical Trials up to 2020 [126, 127].

Generic Name	Source sp./Group	Chemical class	Clinical use
GTS-21 (DMXBA) (Fig. **20**)	*Amphiporus lactifloreus* (Ribbon Worm)	Alkaloid	Obesity
Samrotamab vedotin	Mollusk/cyanobacterium	ADC	Cancer
Sirtratumab vedotin (ASG-15ME)	Mollusk/cyanobacterium	ADC	Cancer
SGN-CD48A	Mollusk/cyanobacterium	ADC	Cancer
ALT-P7	Mollusk/cyanobacterium	ADC	Cancer
ARX788	Mollusk/cyanobacterium	ADC	Cancer
Upifitamab rilsodotin (XMT-1536)	Mollusk/cyanobacterium	ADC	Cancer
AGS62P1	Mollusk/cyanobacterium	ADC	Cancer
PF-06804103	Mollusk/cyanobacterium	ADC	Cancer
Cofetuzumab pelidotin (ABBV-647) (Fig. **21**)	Mollusk/cyanobacterium	ADC	Cancer
ZW-49	Mollusk/cyanobacterium	ADC	Cancer
MRG003	Mollusk/cyanobacterium	ADC	Cancer
STRO-002	Mollusk/cyanobacterium	ADC	Cancer
MORAb-202	Mollusk/cyanobacterium	ADC	Cancer
RC-88	Mollusk/cyanobacterium	ADC	Cancer
SGN-B6A	Mollusk/cyanobacterium	ADC	Cancer
SGN-CD228A	Mollusk/cyanobacterium	ADC	Cancer
FOR-46	Mollusk/cyanobacterium	ADC	Cancer
A-166	Mollusk/cyanobacterium	ADC	Cancer
STI-6129	Mollusk/cyanobacterium	ADC	Amyloidosis

ADC: Antibody Drug Conjugate; PDC: Probody Drug Conjugate.

Marine Drug Candidates Under III Phase Clinical Trials

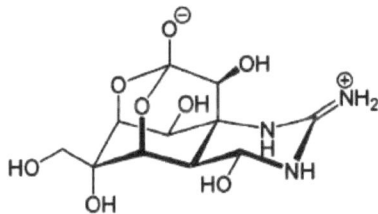

Fig. (15). Tetrodotoxin.

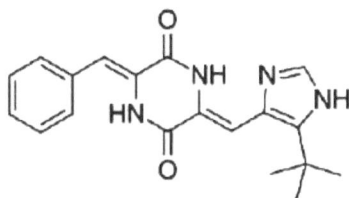

Fig. (16). Plinabulin.

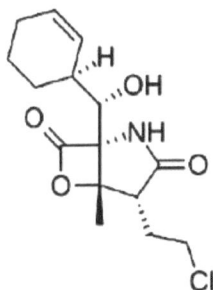

Fig. (17). Salinosporamide A.

Marine Drug Candidates Under II Phase Clinical Trials

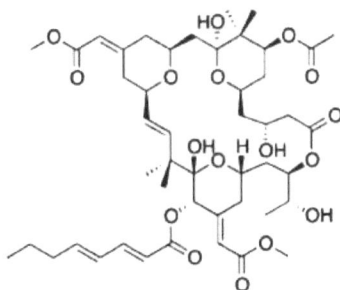

Fig. (18). Bryostatin.

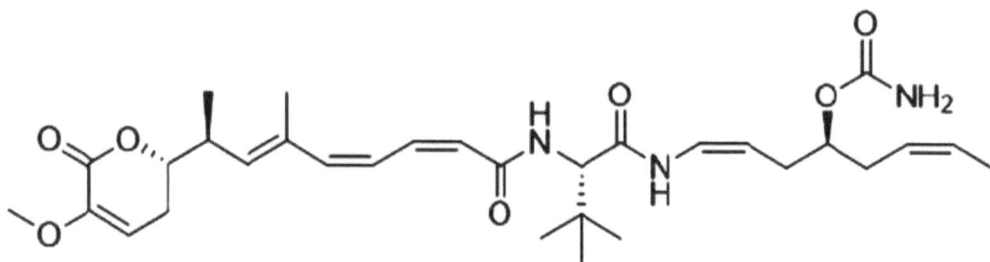

Fig. (19). Plocabulin.

Marine Drug Candidates Under I Phase Clinical Trials

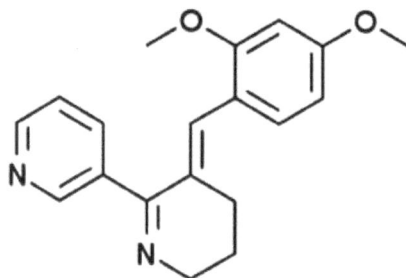

Fig. (20). GTS-21.

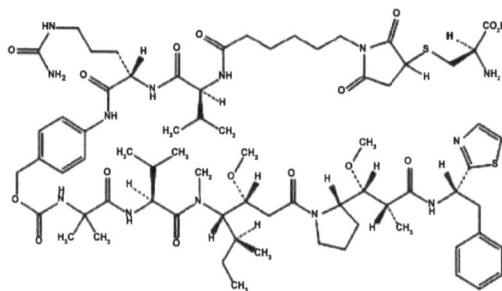

Fig. (21). Cofetuzumab pelidotin.

Marine Biota -derived Clinical Level Compounds against SARS-CoV-2

About 20 clinical level compounds have been identified for clinical trials to serve against SARS-CoV-2 [126, 128]. Such compounds are listed in Table **7**.

Table 7. Marine Biota -derived Clinical Level Compounds against SARS-CoV-2 [126, 128].

Compound Name	Chemical Class
Aplidin (Plitidepsin)	Depsipeptide
Bromophycolide (Fig. **22**)	Terpene
Capnellene (Fig. **23**)	Terpene

(Table 7) cont.....

Compound Name	Chemical Class
Chrysophaentin A (Fig. **24**)	Shikimate
Cytarabine, ara-C	Nucleoside
DMXBA (GTS-21)	Alkaloid
Dysidine (Fig. **25**)	Terpene
Geodisterol sulphate (Fig. **26**)	Steroid
HCQ (Fig. **27**)	Standard drug
Homogentisic acid (Fig. **28**)	Phenolics
Hymenidin (Fig. **29**)	Alkaloid
Paracetamol (Fig. **30**)	Standard drug
Phenethylamine (Fig. **31**)	Alkaloid
Plakortin (Fig. **32**)	Polyketide
Plinabulin	Alkaloid
Pseudopterosin A (Fig. **33**)	Glycoside
Pulicatin A (Fig. **34**)	Alkaloid
Tetrodotoxin	Alkaloid
Vidarabine, ara-A	Nucleoside

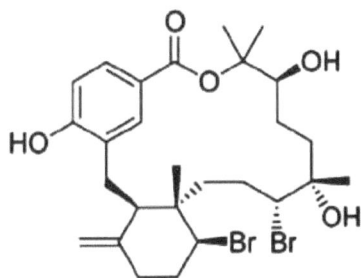

Fig. (22). Bromophycolide.

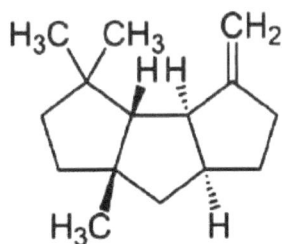

Fig. (23). Capnellene.

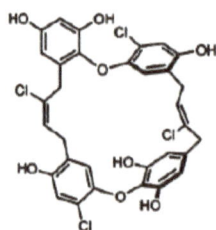

Fig. (24). Chrysophaentin A.

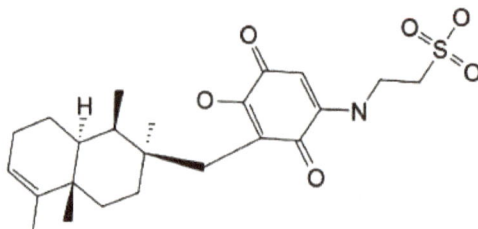

Fig. (25). Dysidine.

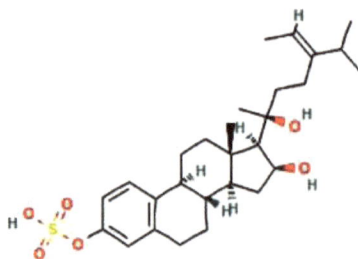

Fig. (26). Geodisterol sulphate.

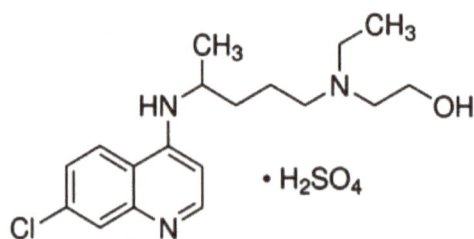

Fig. (27). Hydroxychloroquine sulphate.

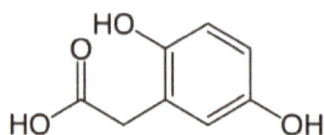

Fig. (28). Homogentisic acid.

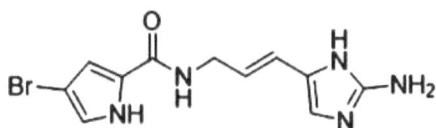

Fig. (29). Hymenidin.

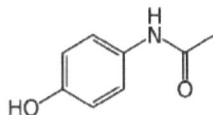

Fig. (30). Paracetamol.

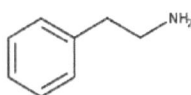

Fig. (31). Phenethylamine.

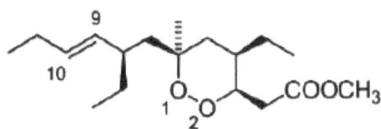

Fig. (32). Plakortin.

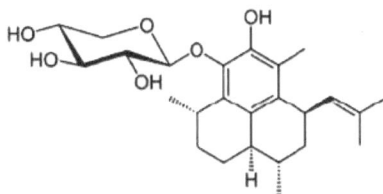

Fig. (33). Pseudopterosin A.

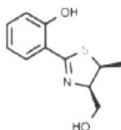

Fig. (34). Pulicatin A.

During the last decade, the number of marine drugs on the USA and/or EU drug market has almost duplicated. Further, a significant increase of clinical trials has been registered, especially in the first two phases. Furthermore, most of the marine drug candidates both in clinical use and under trial are for the anticancer treatment (Fig. **35A** and **B**) and most of them are antibody drug conjugates (ADCs) (Fig. **35**) [126].

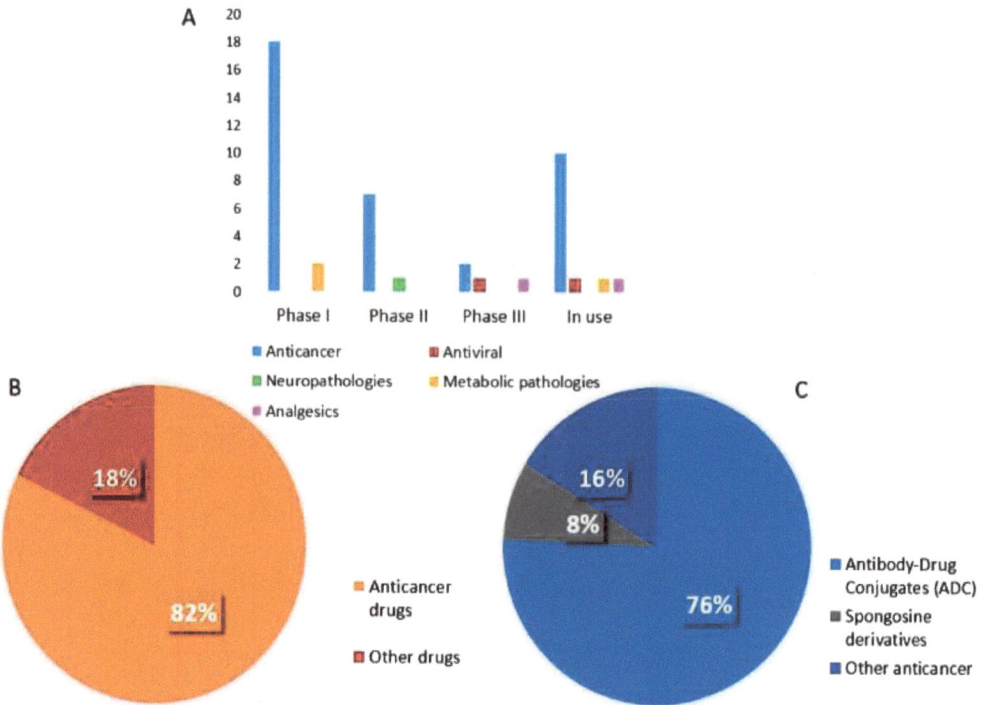

Fig. (35). Anticancer marine drug candidates and antibody drug conjugates for clinical use and under trial. A. A number of marine-derived drugs marketed and under clinical trials as per activity; B. Percentage distribution of cancer and non-cancer marine drugs (marketed and under clinical trials); C. Percentage distribution of anticancer agents (marketed and under clinical trials) in different typology. Image credit: Cappello and Nieri (CC).

CONCLUSION

Most of the presently available and marketable drugs developed from natural sources including marine life are used for only cancer treatment and this is largely due to importance and fund support available to offer to this ailment. Though the seas and oceans possess unique bioactive compounds for treating various diseases like diabetes, and cardiovascular and neurodegenerative diseases, intensive research on this aspect is lacking. A coordinated approach between different target groups is therefore required to discover more number of marine biota-derived drug candidates for clinical trials and resulting marketable, cost-effective drugs.

CHAPTER 13

New PG Degree Course, Marine Bio-Pharmacy: Scope and Career Prospects

Abstract: This chapter deals with the importance and recent status of marine biopharmaceuticals and the need for popularizing this aspect; the introduction and scope of Marine Bio-Pharmacy as an interdisciplinary PG course; suggested syllabus for taught program and practicals in the event of its introduction; and career opportunities for the Marine Bio-Pharmacy graduates.

Keywords: Recent status of marine biopharmaceuticals, Marine bio-Pharmacy, Marine biopharmaceutical sciences, Suggested PG syllabus, Career opportunities for the marine bio-pharmacy graduates.

INTRODUCTION

The industry sector involved in land-based biopharmaceutical development, manufacture and marketing is about 25 years old (or several hundred years old, depending on the type of definition followed) with more than 350 marketed products (or thousands, depending on the definition followed). However, these biopharmaceuticals still remain a small and distinct subset (generally ~15%) of the pharmaceutical industry in terms of products, R&D, companies, revenue or other parameters. For example, the worldwide annual biotechnology-based biopharmaceutical revenues are now only about $100 billion, compared with $650+ billion for all pharmaceuticals [129].

Marine Biopharmaceuticals

Although marine biopharmaceuticals are very recent in their derivation, they have been reported to be very promising for disease control and prevention due to their characteristics and multiple advantages over chemical-based synthetic drugs. Apart from the approved marine biopharmaceuticals (so-called marine drugs), many novel marine biopharmaceuticals are under clinical trials and they may be applied for clinical application in the near future, though some scientific and regulatory issues are yet to be solved. More intensive research works including the discovery, production, applications, prospects, and challenges of marine

Santhanam Ramesh, Ramasamy Santhanam & Veintramuthu Sankar

biopharmaceuticals are expected in the future to gain a fruitful outcome and have a great impact on humans. As land-based biopharmaceuticals, the marine biopharmaceutical industry which is an important part of the marine biological resources development has also not attained significant progress and this is largely due to the incomplete Industry-University-Research cooperation. It is worth mentioning here that the course Bachelor of Marine Pharmaceutical Science is presently offered only at the College of Food and Pharmaceutical Sciences at Ningbo University (Zhejiang, China) [130]. Considering the vast scope and career prospects of such academic programs there is an urgent need for starting PG degree programs in all universities worldwide. In this regard, a postgraduate degree program in Marine Bio-Pharmacy (= Marine Biopharmaceutical Sciences) would take care of this long felt need. Through innovative coursework and independent research opportunities, this interdisciplinary program may instill younger generations with skills in pharmaceutical sciences, medical product development business, marketing, *etc.*

Marine Bio-Pharmacy (=Marine Biopharmaceutical Sciences or Pharmaceutical Marine Biology, an Interdisciplinary PG Course)

The concept of Marine Bio-Pharmacy, Marine Pharmacology, or Marine Pharmacognosy is either new to the world or in an infant stage. Although the pharmaceutically important marine species diversity is enormous, no intensive research has been carried out on this aspect due to the absence of an inter-disciplinary approach. Although research papers on marine natural products and their bioactivities appear every now and then, there is no coordinated approach between Marine Biologists and Scientists of Pharmaceutical Sciences. As a result, the number of new marine bioactive compounds and drugs developed is almost nil in developing countries. This calls for an integrated approach among the concerned stakeholders so that the information and skills can be applied to novel and complex issues or challenges associated with the development of new marine drugs.

This applied course may involve disciplines such as, Marine Pharmacy, Marine Pharmaceutical Chemistry, Marine Pharmaceutical Biology, Marine Pharmaceutical Microbiology and Marine Pharmaceutical Biotechnology which are required to design and develop medicines from marine organisms. Courses focus on sub-disciplines of pharmaceutical sciences—including the study of the chemical and physical properties of drugs and their biological effects—and link these systems to the discovery, development and commercialization of pharmaceuticals for the advancement of human health. Courses also explore the business and marketing aspects of the pharmaceutical industry. In paramedical colleges, the master's degree program in Marine Bio-Pharmacy may be offered as a full-fledged course similar to the ongoing M.Pharm. course. As the newly designed course is of an interdisciplinary nature, it is advisable to include staff with other specializations like Marine Biology, Marine Biochemistry, Marine Microbiology and Marine Biotechnology apart from the regular Pharmacy Faculty.

Suggested Syllabus for the Master's Degree Program in "Marine Bio-Pharmacy (Marine Biopharmaceutical Sciences)"

Taught Program

i) Pharmaceutical Marine Life of World Seas and Oceans: Pharmaceutical Marine Biodiversity and its Ecology and Biology

ii) Pharmaceutical-yielding Marine Plant and Animal Sources: Collection, Taxonomy, and Storage

iii) Development of Chemical Processes/Technologies (Extraction, Isolation, Purification and Quantification for Pharmaceutical Compounds from Marine Organisms.

iv) Chemistry of Marine Pharmaceutical Compounds from Marine Life (Alkaloids, Peptides, Nucleosides, Prostaglandins, *etc.*): Chemistry, Medicinal Chemistry, Bioorganic Chemistry, Chemical Biology, Chemical Ecology and Synthesis.

v) Marine Microbial Pharmacognosy- Bacteria, Fungi, and Symbiotic Microbes; Pharmaceutical Compounds; and their Anticancer, Antimicrobial and Photoprotective Activities

vi) Pharmaceutical Compounds from the Different Groups of Marine Plants and Animals; and their Bioactivities such as Antimicrobial, Antiviral, Anti-tumor, Antioxidant, Antiprotozoal, Antihelmintic, Antidiabetic, Anti-inflammatory, Wound-healing, Lipid-lowering, Cytotoxic, Analgesic, Anticoagulant, Hypolipidemic, Antidiarrheal, Hepatoprotective, Neuroprotective, *etc.*

vii) Marine Biotoxins and their Therapeutic Activities

viii) Marine Drugs: Present status (Approved and under Clinical trials)

ix) Supply Problems in Marine Biopharmaceutical Compounds and Remedial Measures: Chemical Synthesis; Semisynthesis; Biotechnological Techniques; and Cultivation (Aquaculture) of need-based Marine Plants and Animals of Pharmaceutical Value.

Practicals

i) Collection of pharmaceutically important Marine Species from the nearby Sea.

ii) Identification of collected Marine Organisms.

iii) Preparation of collected materials for extraction.

iv) Preparation of extracts by green processing methods.

v) Isolation of bioactive compounds and identification of their chemical class.

vi) Determination bioactivity of compounds isolated from different constituents of marine life.

Pharmaceutical Marine Biology, an Interdisciplinary Course

As marine biopharmaceuticals possess immense employment potential both in the research sector and pharmaceutical industries, a course titled " Pharmaceutical Marine Biology" may be started in Conventional colleges and Professional colleges like Fisheries Colleges.

As this newly designed course is also of interdisciplinary nature, it is advisable to include staff with other specializations like Marine Biology, Marine Biochemistry, and Pharmaceutical Sciences apart from the regular Marine Biology/ Fisheries Science Faculty.

Syllabus for the Taught Program

i) Pharmaceutical Marine Life of World Seas and Oceans: Pharmaceutical Marine Biodiversity and its Ecology and Biology.

ii) Collection of Pharmaceutical-yielding Species of Marine Microbiota *viz.* Bacteria, Fungi, and Microalgae, such as Diatoms, Dinoflagellates, and Cyanobacteria (Blue-green Algae) in different Marine Ecosystems; and Taxonomic Identification.

iii) Collection of Pharmaceutical-yielding Species of Marine Plants such as Macroalgae (Sea Weeds), Seagrass, and Mangroves in different Marine Ecosystems; and Taxonomic Identification.

iv) Collection of Pharmaceutical-yielding Species of Marine Invertebrates in different Marine Ecosystems; and Taxonomic Identification.

v) Collection of Pharmaceutical - yielding Species of Marine Fishes in different Marine Ecosystems; and Taxonomic Identification.

vi) Purification and Drying of collected Specimens for further Analysis.

vii) Development of Chemical Processes/Technologies (Extraction, Isolation, Purification and Quantification for Pharmaceutical Compounds from Marine Organisms.

viii) Chemical Classes of Marine Pharmaceutical Compounds derived from the different Groups of Marine Life.

Suggested Practicals

i) Collection of pharmaceutically important Marine Species from different Marine Ecosystems.

ii) Identification of collected Marine Organisms from different Marine Ecosystems.

iii) Assessment of Pharmaceutical Biodiversity of different Marine Ecosystems.

iv) Preparation of Extracts by using Green Processing Methods.

v) Isolation of Bioactive Compounds and Identification of their Chemical Class.

vi) Determination of Bioactivity of Compounds isolated from different Constituents of Marine Life.

Career Opportunities for the Marine Bio-Pharmacy Graduates

Graduates qualified with Marine Bio-Pharmacy can be engaged in scientific research departments, universities, pharmaceutical companies, hospitals, and government departments for scientific research, teaching, drug production, management technology, drug testing, drug marketing, quality control, drug management, *etc*.

CONCLUSION

It is known from the research reports that only about 0.5% of the total marine biopharmaceutical compounds isolated during the last five decades have seen the market. This is largely due to the lack of awareness about drug candidate-yielding marine life among the target groups *viz*. researchers, drug companies and governmental agencies. Further, at present, there are no universities offering PG courses on Marine Bio-Pharmacy or Marine Biopharmaceutical Sciences. Keeping these in view, there is an urgent need to initiate this venture as an interdisciplinary program.

REFERENCES

[1]   Available From: https://www.fauna-flora.org/environments/marine/

[2]   Lomartire S, Gonçalves AMM. An overview of potential seaweed-derived bioactive compounds for pharmaceutical applications. Mar Drugs 2022; 20(2): 141.
[http://dx.doi.org/10.3390/md20020141] [PMID: 35200670]

[3]   Catanesi M, Caioni G, Castelli V, Benedetti E, d'Angelo M, Cimini A. Benefits under the Sea: The role of marine compounds in neurodegenerative disorders. Mar Drugs 2021; 19(1): 24.
[http://dx.doi.org/10.3390/md19010024] [PMID: 33430021]

[4]   Available From: https://oceanexplorer.noaa.gov/facts/medicinesfromsea.html

[5]   Sankar V, Ramesh S, Santhanam R. Marine bio-pharmacy: Scope and career prospects. Pharm Times 2022; 54: 14-6.

[6]   Albini A. From sea bed to bedside: Tapping the cancer pharmacy beneath the waves. 2021. Available From: https://cancerworld. net/from -sea-bed-to-bedside-tapping-the-cancer- pharmacy-beneath- the-waves/

[7]   Korsmo KA. Isolation and characterization of bioactive compounds from the marine hydrozoans *Halecium muricatum* and *Halecium beanie*. Master of Pharmacy Thesis 2012.

[8]   Available From: https://www.earthreminder.com/marine-ecosystem-characteristics-types/

[9]   Stonik VA. Marine natural products: A way to new drugs. Acta Nat 2009; 1(2): 15-25.
[http://dx.doi.org/10.32607/20758251-2009-1-2-15-25] [PMID: 22649599]

[10]   Aguiar ACC, Parisi JR, Granito RN, de Sousa LRF, Renno ACM, Gazarini ML. Metabolites from marine sponges and their potential to treat malarial protozoan parasites infection: A systematic review. Mar Drugs 2021; 19(3): 134.
[http://dx.doi.org/10.3390/md19030134] [PMID: 33670878]

[11]   Romano G, Almeida M, Varela Coelho A, *et al.* Biomaterials and bioactive natural products from marine invertebrates: from basic research to innovative applications. Mar Drugs 2022; 20(4): 219.
[http://dx.doi.org/10.3390/md20040219] [PMID: 35447892]

[12]   Ghosh S, Sarkar T, Pati S, Kari ZA, Edinur HA, Chakraborty R. Novel bioactive compounds from marine sources as a tool for functional food development. Front Mar Sci 2022; 9: 832957.
[http://dx.doi.org/10.3389/fmars.2022.832957]

[13]   Kesik-Brodacka M. Progress in biopharmaceutical development. Biotechnol Appl Biochem 2018; 65(3): 306-322 .
[http://dx.doi.org/10.1002/bab.1617] [PMID: 28972297]

[14]   Santhanam R, Ramesh S, Suleria HAR. Biology and Ecology of Pharmaceutical Marine Plants CRC Press 2018; 504.
[http://dx.doi.org/10.1201/9781351187114]

[15]   Cotas J, Pacheco D, Gonçalves AMM, Silva P, Carvalho LG, Pereira L. Seaweeds' nutraceutical and biomedical potential in cancer therapy: A concise review. J Cancer Metastasis Treat 2021; 2021: 13.
[http://dx.doi.org/10.20517/2394-4722.2020.134]

[16]   Nho JA, Shin YS, Jeong H, *et al.* Neuroprotective effects of phlorotannin-rich extract from brown seaweed *ecklonia cava* on neuronal pc-12 and sh-sy5y cells with oxidative stress. J microbiol biotechnol 2020; 30(3): 359-67.
[PMID: 9728360]

[17]   Jha R, Zi-rong X. Biomedical compounds from marine organisms. Mar Drugs 2004; 2(3): 123-46.
[http://dx.doi.org/10.3390/md203123]

[18] Vajiravelu S, Subbiah M, Sundaresan B, Natarajan TS. *In vitro* cytotoxic studies of red algae *Portieria hornemannii* and *Spyridia fusiformis* against Dalton's lymphoma ascite and Ehrlich ascite carcinoma cell lines. J Coastal Life Med 2016; 4: 949-52.
[http://dx.doi.org/10.12980/jclm.4.2016J6-208]

[19] Kang C, Jin YB, Lee H, *et al.* Brown alga *Ecklonia cava* attenuates type 1 diabetes by activating AMPK and Akt signaling pathways. Food Chem Toxicol 2010; 48(2): 509-16.
[http://dx.doi.org/10.1016/j.fct.2009.11.004] [PMID: 19913068]

[20] Iwai K. Antidiabetic and antioxidant effects of polyphenols in brown alga *Ecklonia stolonifera* in genetically diabetic KK-A(y) mice. Plant Foods Hum Nutr 2008; 63(4): 163-9.
[http://dx.doi.org/10.1007/s11130-008-0098-4] [PMID: 18958624]

[21] Yang HW, Fernando KHN, Oh JY, Li X, Jeon YJ, Ryu B. Anti-obesity and anti-diabetic effects of *Ishige okamurae*. Mar Drugs 2019; 17(4): 202.
[http://dx.doi.org/10.3390/md17040202] [PMID: 30934943]

[22] Choi JS, Haulader S, Karki S, Jung HJ, Kim HR, Jung HA. Acetyl- and butyryl-cholinesterase inhibitory activities of the edible brown alga *Eisenia bicyclis*. Arch Pharm Res 2015; 38(8): 1477-87.
[http://dx.doi.org/10.1007/s12272-014-0515-1] [PMID: 25370610]

[23] Cho CH, Lu YA, Kim MY, Jeon YJ, Lee SH. Therapeutic potential of seaweed-derived bioactive compounds for cardiovascular disease treatment. Appl Sci 2022; 12(3): 1025.
[http://dx.doi.org/10.3390/app12031025]

[24] García Delgado N, Frías Vázquez AI, Cabrera Sánchez H, Soto del Valle RM, Sierra Gómez Y, Suárez Alfonso AM. Anti-inflammatory and antinociceptive activities of methanolic extract from red seaweed *Dichotomaria obtusata*. Braz J Pharm Sci 2013; 49(1): 65-74.
[http://dx.doi.org/10.1590/S1984-82502013000100008]

[25] Hannan MA, Dash R, Haque MN, *et al.* Neuroprotective potentials of marine algae and their bioactive metabolites: pharmacological insights and therapeutic advances. Mar Drugs 2020; 18(7): 347.
[http://dx.doi.org/10.3390/md18070347] [PMID: 32630301]

[26] Senthil KA, Murugan A. Antiulcer, wound healing and hepatoprotective activities of the seaweeds *Gracilaria crassa, Turbinaria ornata* and *Laurencia papillosa* from the southeast coast of India. Braz J Pharm Sci 2013; 49(4): 669-78.
[http://dx.doi.org/10.1590/S1984-82502013000400006]

[27] Apostolova E, Lukova P, Baldzhieva A, *et al.* Immunomodulatory and anti-inflammatory effects of fucoidan: A review. Polymers 2020; 12(10): 2338.
[http://dx.doi.org/10.3390/polym12102338] [PMID: 33066186]

[28] Khongthong S, Theapparat Y, Roekngam N, Tantisuwanno C, Otto M, Piewngam P. Characterization and immunomodulatory activity of sulfated galactan from the red seaweed *Gracilaria fisheri*. Int J Biol Macromol 2021; 189: 705-14.
[http://dx.doi.org/10.1016/j.ijbiomac.2021.08.182] [PMID: 34474051]

[29] Gono CMP, Ahmadi P, Hertiani T, Septiana E, Putra MY, Chianese G. A comprehensive update on the bioactive compounds from seagrasses. Mar Drugs 2022; 20(7): 406.
[http://dx.doi.org/10.3390/md20070406] [PMID: 35877699]

[30] Wang L, Mu M, Li X, Lin P, Wang W. Differentiation between true mangroves and mangrove associates based on leaf traits and salt contents. J Plant Ecol 2011; 4(4): 292-301.
[http://dx.doi.org/10.1093/jpe/rtq008]

[31] Mitra S, Naskar N, Chaudhuri P. A review on potential bioactive phytochemicals for novel therapeutic applications with special emphasis on mangrove species. Phytomedicine Plus 2021; 1(4): 100107.
[http://dx.doi.org/10.1016/j.phyplu.2021.100107]

[32] Dahibhate NL, Saddhe AA, Kumar K. Mangrove plants as a source of bioactive compounds. Nat Prod J 2018; 9(2): 86-97.

[http://dx.doi.org/10.2174/22103155086661809101253328]

[33]   Costa CSB, Chaves FC, Rombaldi CV, Souza CR. Bioactive compounds and antioxidant activity of three biotypes of the sea asparagus *Sarcocornia ambigua* (Michx.) M.A.Alonso & M.B.Crespo: a halophytic crop for cultivation with shrimp farm effluent. S Afr J Bot 2018; 117: 95-100. [http://dx.doi.org/10.1016/j.sajb.2018.05.011]

[34]   Gouda MS, Elsebaie EM, Alex J. Glasswort (*Salicornia* spp.) As a source of bioactive compounds and its health benefits: A review. J Food Sci Technol 2016; 13(1): 1-7.

[35]   Sung JH, Park SH, Seo DH, Lee JH, Hong SW, Hong SS. Antioxidative and skin-whitening effect of an aqueous extract of *Salicornia herbacea*. Biosci Biotechnol Biochem 2009; 73(3): 552-6. [http://dx.doi.org/10.1271/bbb.80601] [PMID: 19270393]

[36]   Kim S, Lee EY, Hillman PF, Ko J, Yang I, Nam SJ. Chemical structure and biological activities of secondary metabolites from *Salicornia europaea* L. Molecules 2021; 26(8): 2252. [http://dx.doi.org/10.3390/molecules26082252] [PMID: 33924656]

[37]   Karan S, Turan C, Sanguni K, Eliuz EAE. Bioactive compounds and antimicrobial activity of glasswort *Salicornia europaea.* Indian J Pharm Sci 2021; 83: 229-37.

[38]   Altay A, Celep GS, Yaprak AE, Baskose I, Bozoglu F. Glassworts as possible anticancer agents against human colorectal adenocarcinoma cells with their nutritive, antioxidant and phytochemical profiles. Chem Biodivers 2017; 14(3): e1600290. [http://dx.doi.org/10.1002/cbdv.201600290] [PMID: 27701810]

[39]   Sánchez-Gavilán I, Ramírez E, de la Fuente V, Baskose I, Bozoglu F. Bioactive compounds in *Salicornia patula* duval-jouve: A mediterranean edible euhalophyte. Foods 2021; 10(2): 410. [http://dx.doi.org/10.3390/foods10020410] [PMID: 33673201]

[40]   Santhanam R, Ramesh S, Sunilson AJ. Biology and Ecology of Pharmaceutical Marine Sponges CRC Press. USA: Taylor & Francis 2018; p. 342.

[41]   LaBarbera DV, Modzelewska K, Glazar AI, *et al.* The marine alkaloid naamidine A promotes caspase-dependent apoptosis in tumor cells. Anticancer Drugs 2009; 20(6): 425-36. [http://dx.doi.org/10.1097/CAD.0b013e32832ae55f] [PMID: 19369860]

[42]   Anjum K, Abbas SQ, Shah SAA, Akhter N, Batool S, Hassan SS. Marine sponges as a drug treasure. Biomol Ther 2016; 24(4): 347-62. [http://dx.doi.org/10.4062/biomolther.2016.067] [PMID: 27350338]

[43]   Karthikeyan A, Joseph A, Nair BG. Promising bioactive compounds from the marine environment and their potential effects on various diseases. J Genet Eng Biotechnol 2022; 20(1): 14. [http://dx.doi.org/10.1186/s43141-021-00290-4] [PMID: 35080679]

[44]   Dayanidhi DL, Thomas BC, Osterberg JS. Exploring the diversity of the marine environment for new anti-cancer compounds. Front Mar Sci 2021; 7: 614766. [http://dx.doi.org/10.3389/fmars.2020.614766]

[45]   Calcabrini C, Catanzaro E, Bishayee A, Turrini E, Fimognari C. Marine sponge natural products with anticancer potential: An updated review. Mar Drugs 2017; 15(10): 310. [http://dx.doi.org/10.3390/ md15100310] [PMID: 29027954]

[46]   Choi K, Lim HK, Oh SR, Chung WH, Jung J. Anticancer effects of the marine sponge *Lipastrotethya* sp. Extract on Wild-Type and p53 Knockout HCT116 Cells. Evid Based Complement Alternat Med 2017; 2017: 1-6. [http://dx.doi.org/10.1155/2017/7174858] [PMID: 28127380]

[47]   Morais SR, K C, Jeyabalan S, *et al.* Anticancer potential of *Spirastrella pachyspira* (marine sponge) against SK-BR-3 human breast cancer cell line and *in silico* analysis of its bioactive molecule sphingosine. Front Mar Sci 2022; 9: 950880. [http://dx.doi.org/10.3389/fmars.2022.950880]

[48] Murniasih T, Putra MY, Bayu A, Wibowo JT. A Review on Diversity of Anticancer Compounds Derived from Indonesian Marine Sponges. 6th International Conference on Biotechnology Engineering (ICBioE 2021). IOP Publishing Ltd 2012; 1192.
[http://dx.doi.org/10.1088/1757-899X/1192/1/012012]

[49] Elhady SS, El-Halawany AM, Alahdal AM, Hassanean HA, Ahmed SA. A new bioactive metabolite isolated from the red sea marine sponge *Hyrtios erectus*. Molecules 2016; 21(1): 82.

[50] Wilke DV, Jimenez PC, Branco PC, *et al.* Anticancer potential of compounds from the brazilian blue amazon. Planta Med 2021; 87(01/02): 49-70.
[http://dx.doi.org/10.1055/a-1257-8402] [PMID: 33142347]

[51] Nguyen TND, Feizbakhsh O, Sfecci E, *et al.* Kinase-based screening of marine natural extracts leads to the identification of a cytotoxic high molecular weight metabolite from the mediterranean sponge *Crambe tailliezi*. Mar Drugs 2019; 17(10): 569.
[http://dx.doi.org/10.3390/md17100569] [PMID: 31600933]

[52] Ortega V, Cortés J. Potential clinical applications of halichondrins in breast cancer and other neoplasms. Breast Cancer (Dove Med Press) 2012; 4: 9-19.
[PMID: 24367189]

[53] Schwartsmann G, da Rocha AB, Berlinck RGS, Jimeno J. Marine organisms as a source of new anticancer agents. Lancet Oncol 2001; 2(4): 221-5.
[http://dx.doi.org/10.1016/S1470-2045(00)00292-8] [PMID: 11905767]

[54] Warabi K, Matsunaga S, van Soest RWM, Fusetani N. Dictyodendrins A-E, the first telomerase-inhibitory marine natural products from the sponge *Dictyodendrilla verongiformis*. J Org Chem 2003; 68(7): 2765-70.
[http://dx.doi.org/10.1021/jo0267910] [PMID: 12662050]

[55] del Sol Jiménez M, Garzón SP, Rodríguez AD. Plakortides M and N, bioactive polyketide endoperoxides from the Caribbean marine sponge *Plakortis halichondrioides*. J Nat Prod 2003; 66(5): 655-61.
[http://dx.doi.org/10.1021/np030021h] [PMID: 12762801]

[56] Hamoda AM, Fayed B, Ashmawy NS, El-Shorbagi ANA, Hamdy R, Soliman SSM. Marine sponge is a promising natural source of Anti-SARS-CoV-2 scaffold. Front Pharmacol 2021; 12: 666664.
[http://dx.doi.org/10.3389/fphar.2021.666664] [PMID: 34079462]

[57] Sagar S, Kaur M, Minneman KP. Antiviral lead compounds from marine sponges. Mar Drugs 2010; 8(10): 2619-38.
[http://dx.doi.org/10.3390/md8102619] [PMID: 21116410]

[58] Appenzeller J. + 12. Agelasines J, K, and L from the Solomon Islands Marine Sponge *Agelas* cf. *mauritiana*. J Nat Prod 2008; 71 (8): 1451–54. Arch Toxicol 2017; 91(3): 1485-95.
[PMID: 27473261]

[59] Lauritano C, Ianora A. Marine organisms with anti-diabetes properties. Mar Drugs 2016; 14(12): 220.
[http://dx.doi.org/10.3390/md14120220] [PMID: 27916864]

[60] Deliorman Orhan D, Orhan N, Konuklugil B. Phenolic content, antioxidant and *in vitro* antidiabetic effects of thirteen marine organisms from mediterranean sea. Farmacia 2021; 69(1): 68-74.
[http://dx.doi.org/10.31925/farmacia.2021.1.9]

[61] Kaur KK, Allahbadia G, Singh M. Development of protein tyrosine phosphatase 1B (PTPIB) Inhibitors from marine sources and other natural products-Future of Antidiabetic Therapy: A Systematic Review. Korean J Food Health Conv 2019; 5(3): 21-33.

[62] Barde SR, Sakhare RS, Kanthale SB, Chandak PG, Jamkhande PG. Marine bioactive agents: A short review on new marine antidiabetic compounds. Asian Pac J Trop Dis 2015; 5 (1): S209-13.
[http://dx.doi.org/10.1016/S2222-1808(15)60891-X]

[63]   Arai M, Han C, Yamano Y, Setiawan A, Kobayashi M. Aaptamines, marine spongean alkaloids, as anti-dormant mycobacterial substances. J Nat Med 2014; 68(2): 372-6.
[http://dx.doi.org/10.1007 / s11418-013-0811-y] [PMID: 24414399]

[64]   Abdjul DB, Yamazaki H, Kanno S, *et al.* Haliclonadiamine derivatives and 6- *epi*-monanchorin from the marine sponge *Halichondria panicea* collected at iriomote island. J Nat Prod 2016; 79(4): 1149-54.
[http://dx.doi.org/10.1021/acs.jnatprod.6b00095] [PMID: 27035556]

[65]   Acquah KS, Beukes DR, Seldon R, *et al.* Identification of antimycobacterial natural products from a library of marine invertebrate extracts. Medicines 2022; 9(2): 9.
[http://dx.doi.org/10.3390 / medicines9020009] [PMID: 35200753]

[66]   Mostafa O, Al-Shehri M, Moustafa M. Promising antiparasitic agents from marine sponges. Saudi J Biol Sci 2022; 29(1): 217-27.
[http://dx.doi.org/10.1016/j.sjbs.2021.08.068] [PMID: 35002412]

[67]   Han B, Hong L, Gu B, *et al.* Natural Products from sponges In: Li Z (Eds) Symbiotic Microbiomes of Coral Reefs Sponges and Corals Springer, Dordrecht 2019; 329-463.

[68]   Rocha J, Peixe L, Gomes NCM, Calado R. Cnidarians as a source of new marine bioactive compounds--an overview of the last decade and future steps for bioprospecting. Mar Drugs 2011; 9(10): 1860-86.
[http://dx.doi.org/10.3390/md9101860] [PMID: 22073000]

[69]   Santhanam R, Ramesh S, Shivakumar G. Biology and Ecology of Pharmaceutical Marine Cnidarians (Series: Biology and Ecology of Pharmaceutical Marine Life) CRC Press. USA: Taylor & Francis 2019; p. 598.
[http://dx.doi.org/10.1201/9780429200038]

[70]   Hunt ME, Modi CK, Aglyamova GV, Ravikant DVS, Meyer E, Matz MV. Multi-domain GFP-like proteins from two species of marine hydrozoans. Photochem Photobiol Sci 2012; 11(4): 637-44.
[http://dx.doi.org/10.1039/c1pp05238a] [PMID: 22251928]

[71]   Kawabata T, Lindsay DJ, Kitamura M, *et al.* Evaluation of the bioactivities of water-soluble extracts from twelve deep-sea jellyfish species. Fish Sci 2013; 79(3): 487-94.
[http://dx.doi.org/10.1007/s12562-013-0612-y]

[72]   Rastogi A, Biswas S, Sarkar A, Chakrabarty D. Anticoagulant activity of Moon jellyfish *(Aurelia aurita)* tentacle extract. Toxicon 2012; 60(5): 719-23.
[http://dx.doi.org/10.1016/j.toxicon.2012.05.008] [PMID: 22652129]

[73]   Stabili L, Rizzo L, Caprioli R, Leone A, Piraino S. Jellyfish bioprospecting in the mediterranean sea: antioxidant and lysozyme-like activities from *Aurelia coerulea* (cnidaria, scyphozoa) extracts. Mar Drugs 2021; 19(11): 619.
[http://dx.doi.org/10.3390/md19110619] [PMID: 34822490]

[74]   Kim E, Lee S, Kim JS, *et al.* Cardiovascular effects of *Nemopilema nomurai* (Scyphozoa: Rhizostomeae) jellyfish venom in rats. Toxicol Lett 2006; 167(3): 205-11.
[http://dx.doi.org/10.1016/j.toxlet.2006.09.009] [PMID: 17069996]

[75]   Kang C, Munawir A, Cha M, *et al.* Cytotoxicity and hemolytic activity of jellyfish *Nemopilema nomurai* (Scyphozoa: Rhizostomeae) venom. Comp Biochem Physiol C Toxicol Pharmacol 2009; 150(1): 85-90.
[http://dx.doi.org/10.1016/j.cbpc.2009.03.003] [PMID: 19303056]

[76]   Avila C, Angulo-Preckler C. A minireview on biodiscovery in antarctic marine benthic invertebrates. Front Mar Sci 2021; 8.
[http://dx.doi.org/10.3389/fmars.2021.686477]

[77]   Singh H, Parida A, Debbarma K, Ray DP, Banerjee P. Common marine organisms: A novel source of medicinal compounds. Inter J Bio Sci 2020; 7(2): 39-49.
[http://dx.doi.org/10.30954/2347-9655.02.2020.1]

[78]   Fattorusso E, Romano A, Taglialatela-Scafati O, Achmad MJ, Bavestrello G, Cerrano C. Xenimanadins A–D, a family of xenicane diterpenoids from the Indonesian soft coral *Xenia* sp. Tetrahedron 2008; 64(14): 3141-6.
[http://dx.doi.org/10.1016/j.tet.2008.01.120]

[79]   Figuerola B, Avila C. The phylum bryozoa as a promising source of anticancer drugs. Mar Drugs 2019; 17(8): 477.
[http://dx.doi.org/10.3390/md17080477] [PMID: 31426556]

[80]   Ciavatta ML, Lefranc F, Vieira LM, *et al.* The phylum bryozoa: From biology to biomedical potential. Mar Drugs 2020; 18(4): 200.
[http://dx.doi.org/10.3390/md18040200] [PMID: 32283669]

[81]   Tian XR, Tang HF, Tian XL, Hu JJ, Huang LL, Gustafson KR. Review of bioactive secondary metabolites from marine bryozoans in the progress of new drugs discovery. Future Med Chem 2018; 10(12): 1497-514.
[http://dx.doi.org/10.4155/fmc-2018-0012] [PMID: 29788787]

[82]   Kim S, Ravichandran YD, Kim M, Kung W. Bioactive marine natural products in drug development. J Mar Biosci Biotech 2007; 2(4): 209-23.

[83]   Göransson U, Jacobsson E, Strand M, Andersson H. The toxins of nemertean worms. Toxins 2019; 11(2): 120.
[http://dx.doi.org/10.3390/toxins11020120] [PMID: 30781381]

[84]   Qi Y, Zhou J, Shen X, *et al.* Bioactive properties of peptides and polysaccharides derived from peanut worms: A review. Mar Drugs 2021; 20(1): 10.
[http://dx.doi.org/10.3390/md20010010] [PMID: 35049866]

[85]   Righi S, Forti L, Simonini R, Ferrari V, Prevedelli D, Mucci A. Novel natural compounds and their anatomical distribution in the stinging fireworm *Hermodice carunculata* (Annelida). Mar Drugs 2022; 20(9): 585.
[http://dx.doi.org/10.3390/md20090585] [PMID: 36135774]

[86]   Harnedy PA, FitzGerald RJ. Bioactive peptides from marine processing waste and shellfish: A review. J Funct Foods 2012; 4(1): 6-24.
[http://dx.doi.org/10.1016/j.jff.2011.09.001]

[87]   Šimat V, Rathod NB, Čagalj M, Hamed I, Generalić Mekinić I. Astaxanthin from crustaceans and their byproducts: A bioactive metabolite candidate for therapeutic application. Mar Drugs 2022; 20(3): 206.
[http://dx.doi.org/10.3390/md20030206] [PMID: 35323505]

[88]   Available From: https://www.apollopharmacy.in/salt/ASTAXANTHIN

[89]   Derby C. Cephalopod ink: Production, chemistry, functions and applications. Mar Drugs 2014; 12(5): 2700-30.
[http://dx.doi.org/10.3390/md12052700] [PMID: 24824020]

[90]   Santhanam R, Gobinath M, Ramesh S. Biology and Ecology of Pharmaceutical Marine Molluscs (Series: Biology and Ecology of Pharmaceutical Marine Life) CRC Press. USA: Taylor & Francis 2019; p. 218.

[91]   Pati P, Sahu BK, Panigrahy RC. Marine molluscs as a potential drug cabinet: An overview. Indian J Geo-Mar Sci 2015; 44(7): 961-70.

[92]   Tortorella E, Giugliano R, De Troch M, Vlaeminck B, de Viçose GC, de Pascale D. The ethyl acetate extract of the marine edible gastropod *Haliotis tuberculata coccinea*: A potential source of bioactive compounds. Mar Biotechnol 2021; 23(6): 892-903.
[http://dx.doi.org/10.1007/s10126-021-10073-0] [PMID: 34714443]

[93]   Esparza-Espinoza DM, Santacruz-Ortega HC, Chan-Higuera JE, *et al.* Chemical structure and antioxidant activity of cephalopod skin ommochrome pigment extracts. Food Sci Technol 2022; 42:

e56520.
[http://dx.doi.org/10.1590/fst.56520]

[94] Chakraborty K, Krishnan S, Joy M. Antioxidative oxygenated terpenoids with bioactivities against pro-inflammatory inducible enzymes from Indian squid, *Uroteuthis (Photololigo) duvaucelii*. Nat Prod Res 2021; 35(6): 909-20.
[http://dx.doi.org/10.1080/14786419.2019.1610957] [PMID: 31135235]

[95] Jeyasanta I, Patterson J. Bioactive properties of ink gland extract from squid *Loligo duvauceli*. Ecología 2019; 10(1): 9-19.
[http://dx.doi.org/10.3923/ecologia.2020.9.19]

[96] Nadarajah S, Vijayaraj R, Mani J. Therapeutic significance of *Loligo vulgaris* (Lamarck, 1798) ink extract: A biomedical approach. Pharmacognosy Res 2017; 9(5) (1): 105.
[http://dx.doi.org/10.4103/pr.pr_81_17] [PMID: 29333051]

[97] Hernández-Zazueta MS, Luzardo-Ocampo I, García-Romo JS, *et al.* Bioactive compounds from *Octopus vulgaris* ink extracts exerted anti-proliferative and anti-inflammatory effects *in vitro*. Food Chem Toxicol 2021; 151: 112119.
[http://dx.doi.org/10.1016/j.fct.2021.112119] [PMID: 33722603]

[98] Santhanam R, Ramesh S, David SR. Biology and Ecology of Pharmaceutical Marine Life: Echinoderms (Series: Biology and Ecology of Pharmaceutical Marine Life) CRC Press. USA: Taylor & Francis 2019; p. 435.
[http://dx.doi.org/10.1201/9780429060236]

[99] Ghelani H, Khursheed M, Adrian TE, Jan RK. Anti-inflammatory effects of compounds from echinoderms. Mar Drugs 2022; 20(11): 693.
[http://dx.doi.org/10.3390/md20110693] [PMID: 36355016]

[100] Cirino P, Brunet C, Ciaravolo M, *et al.* The sea urchin *Arbacia lixula*: A novel natural source of astaxanthin. Mar Drugs 2017; 15(6): 187.
[http://dx.doi.org/10.3390/md15060187] [PMID: 28635649]

[101] Khalil EA, Swelim H, El-Tantawi H, Bakr AF, Abdellatif A. Characterization, cytotoxicity and antioxidant activity of sea urchins (*Diadema savignyi*) and jellyfish (*Aurelia aurita*) extracts. Egypt J Aquat Res 2022; 48(4): 343-8.
[http://dx.doi.org/10.1016/j.ejar.2022.05.005]

[102] Soleimani S, Pirmoradloo E, Farmani F, Moein S, Yousefzadi M. Antidiabetic and antioxidant properties of sea urchin *Echinometra mathaei* from the persian gulf. J Kerman Univ Med Sci 2021; 28(1): 104-15.

[103] Vasileva EA, Mishchenko NP. Cytotoxicity of quinonoid pigments from sea urchins. Proc 2nd International Conference and Exhibition on Marine Drugs and Natural Products 2017.

[104] Milito A, Cocurullo M, Columbro A, *et al.* Ovothiol ensures the correct developmental programme of the sea urchin *Paracentrotus lividus* embryo. Open Biol 2022; 12(1): 210262.
[http://dx.doi.org/10.1098/rsob.210262] [PMID: 35042403]

[105] Vasconcelos A, Sucupira I, Guedes A, *et al.* Anticoagulant and antithrombotic properties of three structurally correlated sea urchin sulfated glycans and their low-molecular-weight derivatives. Mar Drugs 2018; 16(9): 304.
[http://dx.doi.org/10.3390/md16090304] [PMID: 30200211]

[106] Xie X, Ma L, Zhou Y, *et al.* Polysaccharide enhanced NK cell cytotoxicity against pancreatic cancer *via* TLR4/MAPKs/NF-κB pathway *in vitro/vivo*. Carbohydr Polym 2019; 225: 115223.
[http://dx.doi.org/10.1016/j.carbpol.2019.115223] [PMID: 31521276]

[107] Wu L, Yang X, Duan X, Cui L, Li G. Exogenous expression of marine lectins DlFBL and SpRBL induces cancer cell apoptosis possibly through PRMT5-E2F-1 pathway. Sci Rep 2014; 4(1): 4505.
[http://dx.doi.org/10.1038/srep04505] [PMID: 24675921]

[108] Hou Y, Vasileva EA, Carne A, McConnell M, El-Din A Bekhit A, Mishchenko NP. Naphthoquinones of the spinochrome class: Occurrence, isolation, biosynthesis and biomedical applications. RSC Advances 2018; 8(57): 32637-50.
[http://dx.doi.org/10.1039/C8RA04777D] [PMID: 35547692]

[109] Chen YC, Hwang DF. Evaluation of antioxidant properties and biofunctions of polar, nonpolar, and water-soluble fractions extracted from gonad and body wall of the sea urchin *Tripneustes gratilla*. Fish Sci 2014; 80(6): 1311-21.
[http://dx.doi.org/10.1007/s12562-014-0808-9]

[110] Lum K, Carroll A, Ekins M, *et al.* Capillasterin A, a Novel Pyrano[2,3-f]chromene from the Australian Crinoid *Capillaster multiradiatus*. Mar Drugs 2019; 17(1): 26.
[http://dx.doi.org/10.3390/md17010026] [PMID: 30621172]

[111] Dai J, Liu Y, Jia H, Zhou YD, Nagle DG. Benzochromenones from the marine crinoid *Comantheria rotula* inhibit hypoxia-inducible factor-1 (HIF-1) in cell-based reporter assays and differentially suppress the growth of certain tumor cell lines. J Nat Prod 2007; 70(9): 1462-6.
[http://dx.doi.org/10.1021/np070224w] [PMID: 17844994]

[112] Ke ZY, Chen J-W, Wu B-Y, *et al.* A new angular naphthopyrone from feather star *Comanthus parvicirrus* (Müller, 1841). J Mol Struct 2022; 1253: 132261.
[http://dx.doi.org/10.1016/j.molstruc.2021.132261]

[113] Wätjen W, Ebada SS, Bergermann A, *et al.* Cytotoxic effects of the anthraquinone derivatives 1'-deoxyrhodoptilometrin and (S)-(−)-rhodoptilometrin isolated from the marine echinoderm *Comanthus* sp. Arch Toxicol 2017; 91(3): 1485-95.
[http://dx.doi.org/10.1007/s00204-016-1787-7] [PMID: 27473261]

[114] Lum KY. Chemical and Biological Investigations of Australian Crinoids Thesis: School of Environment and Sc . Griffith University: Lum, PhD Thesis 2020.
[http://dx.doi.org/10.25904/1912/1921]

[115] Liang Q, Ahmed F, Zhang M, *et al. In vivo* and clinical studies of sea cucumber-derived bioactives for human health and nutrition from 2012-2021. Front Mar Sci 2022.
[http://dx.doi.org/10.3389/fmars.2022.917857]

[116] Santhanam R, Ramesh S. Biology and Ecology of Pharmaceutical Marine Tunicates (Series: Biology and Ecology of Pharmaceutical Marine Life) CRC Press. USA: Taylor & Francis 2019; p. 188.
[http://dx.doi.org/10.1201/9780429321788]

[117] Ramesh C, Tulasi BR, Raju M, Thakur N, Dufossé L. Marine natural products from tunicates and their associated microbes. Mar Drugs 2021; 19(6): 308.
[http://dx.doi.org/10.3390/md19060308] [PMID: 34073515]

[118] Vervoort H, Fenical W, Epifanio RA. Tamandarins A and B: New cytotoxic depsipeptides from a Brazilian ascidian of the family Didemnidae. J Org Chem 2000; 65(3): 782-92.
[http://dx.doi.org/10.1021/jo991425a] [PMID: 10814011]

[119] Badre A, Boulanger A, Abou-Mansour E, *et al.* New alkaloids from the carribean ascidian *Lissoclinum fragile*. J Nat Prod 1994; 57(4): 528-33.
[http://dx.doi.org/10.1021/np50106a016] [PMID: 8021654]

[120] Ullah S, Ahmad T. Nutritional and medical importance of fish: A mini review. Reviews Of Progress 2014; 2: 1-5.

[121] Santhanam R, Ramesh S, Nivedhitha S, Balasundari S. Pharmaceuticals and Nutraceuticals from Fish and Fish Wastes Apple Academic Press; New York 2022; 302.
[http://dx.doi.org/10.1201/ 9781003180548]

[122] WHO. Naming the coronavirus disease (COVID-19) and the virus that causes it. Available From: https://www.who.int/emergencies/diseases/novel-coronavirus-2019/technical-guidance/naming-the-coronavirus-disease-(covid-2019)-and-the-virus-that-causes-it

[123] Meštrović T. Marine resources could be promising drug candidates against SARS-CoV-2 Omicron 2022. Available From: https://www.news-medical.net/news/20220424/Marine-resources-coul--be-promising-drug-candidates-against-SARS-CoV-2-Omicron.aspx

[124] Zaporozhets TS, Besednova NN. Biologically active compounds from marine organisms in the strategies for combating coronaviruses. AIMS Microbiol 2020; 6(4): 470-94.
[http://dx.doi.org/10.3934/microbiol.2020028] [PMID: 33364539]

[125] Available From: https://www.medchemexpress.com/gallinamide-a.html

[126] Cappello E, Nieri P. From Life in the Sea to the Clinic: The marine drugs approved and under clinical trial. Life 2021; 11(12): 1390.
[http://dx.doi.org/10.3390/life11121390] [PMID: 34947921]

[127] Wu AC, Jelielek KK, Le HQ, *et al.* The 2021 marine pharmacology and pharmaceuticals pipeline. FASEB J 2022; 36: S1.
[http://dx.doi.org/10.1096/fasebj.2022.36.S1.L7586]

[128] Murugesan S. + 12. screening and druggability analysis of marine active metabolites against SARS-CoV-2: An integrative computational approach. Int J Transl Med 2023; 3(1): 27-41.

[129] Rader RA. (Re)defining biopharmaceutical. Nat Biotechnol 2008; 26(7): 743-51.
[http://dx.doi.org/10.1038/nbt0708-743] [PMID: 18612293]

[130] Available from: https: //www. bachelorsportal .com/ studies/313297/ marine-pharmaceutical -science.html

SUBJECT INDEX

A

ACE 273, 296, 297
  enzyme inhibition 273
  inhibitory activity 296, 297
Acetylcholinesterase 11, 53
Acid(s) 21, 23, 66, 69, 85, 129, 135, 140, 168,
    172, 174, 181, 238, 239, 240, 273, 306,
    312, 326, 327
  arachidonic 172, 174
  carboxylic 238
  chlorosulfonic 240
  ferulic 66
  gastric 168
  hexadecanoic 239
  hexadecenoic 306, 312
  Homogentisic 326, 327
  hydrochloric 23
  hydroxybenzoic 85
  mucopolysaccharide 273
  nucleic 21
  palmitoleic 69
  Paraminabic 181
  polyacetylenic 135
  Rumphellaoic 181
  smenotronic 129
  tartaric 23
  steroids norselic 140
  tungtungmadic 85
Acquired immune deficiency syndrome
    (AIDS) 3, 122
Action, thermo-mechanical 27
Activity 43, 56, 58, 59, 69, 106, 107, 108,
    111, 112, 116, 117, 118, 125, 128, 137,
    200, 201, 202, 203, 240, 241, 277, 297,
    300
  anti-aging 69
  anti-coronal 300
  anti-hyperlipidemia 277
  anti-hypoxia 203
  anti-oxidant 240
  anti-plasmodial 201

anti-post-stroke 202
  immunomodulatory 58, 59, 277
  neuroprotective 56
  telomerase 107
Acute pancreatitis 221
Adenocarcinoma 112, 115
Adipogenesis 55
Adipose 56, 219
  -derived stem cells 219
  tissue 56
Adrenal phaeochromocytoma cells 113
Agent, anti-diabetic 52
Alcoholic liver fibrosis 221
Allergic rhinitis 172
Alpha-glucosidase inhibitory activity 51
Alzheimer's 2, 19, 53, 152, 170, 201, 202,
    204, 278, 290
  dementia 204
  disease 2, 19, 53, 152, 170, 201, 202, 278,
    290
Amyloidosis 322
Angiogenesis 86, 240
Angiotensin-converting enzyme (ACE) 12,
    54, 208, 209, 240
Anthelmintic activity 235
Anti-aging activity 73, 221
Anti-Alzheimer's activity 201, 204
Anti-cancer 46, 119, 240
  activity 240
  agent 46
  drugs 119
Anti-dengue activity 70
Anti-diabetic activity 51, 52, 71
Anti-HIV-1 activity 124
Anti-HSV activity 47
Anti-hyperglycemic effects 51
Anti-hypertensive activity 240
Anti-inflammatory 48, 49, 69, 74, 83, 150,
    153, 219, 240, 241, 267
  activity 48, 49, 69, 74, 83, 150, 153, 219,
    240, 267
  agents 241

www.ingramcontent.com/pod-product-compliance
Lightning Source LLC
Chambersburg PA
CBHW050803220326
41598CB00006B/106

* 9 7 8 9 8 1 5 1 9 6 4 9 8 *